# Research for Advanced Practice Nurses

# Research for Advanced Practice Nurses

## From Evidence to Practice

MAGDALENA A. MATEO, PhD, RN, FAAN
KARIN T. KIRCHHOFF, PhD, RN, FAAN
EDITORS

SPRINGER PUBLISHING COMPANY
NEW YORK

Springer Publishing Company, LLC
11 West 42nd Street
New York, NY 10036
www.springerpub.com

*Acquisitions Editor: Allan Graubard*
*Project Manager: Mark Frazier*
*Cover design: Steve Pisano*
*Composition: Apex CoVantage, LLC*

Ebook ISBN: 978-0-8261-2208-7

10 11 12 13 14/ 5 4 3 2

---

**Library of Congress Cataloging-in-Publication Data**
Research for advanced practice nurses : from evidence to practice / [edited by] Magdalena A. Mateo, Karin T. Kirchhoff.
    p. ; cm.
Includes bibliographical references and index.
ISBN 978-0-8261-2207-0 (alk. paper)
1. Nursing—Research.  I. Mateo, Magdalena A.   II. Kirchhoff, Karin T.
[DNLM: 1.  Clinical Nursing Research.   2.  Evidence-Based Practice.   3.  Research
Design. WY 20.5 R43125 2009]
  RT81.5.R448   2009
  610.73072—dc22

                                                                    2009014210

---

Printed in the United States of America by Victor Graphics.

**Magdalena A. Mateo, PhD, RN, FAAN,** is Associate Professor at Northeastern University School of Nursing in Boston, where she teaches research courses at all levels. She received her BSN and MN degrees in the Philippines and her PhD from The Ohio State University. While working in clinical and academic settings as a clinical nurse specialist, and director of nursing and faculty in the Philippines, Canada, and the United States, she conducted studies and used results of studies to improve patient care. Her recent work has focused on a multidisciplinary approach to improve care for patients with memory difficulties following mild traumatic brain injury. She has taught the conduct and use of research in clinical and academic settings.

**Karin T. Kirchhoff, PhD, RN, FAAN,** is Professor Emeritus at the University of Wisconsin-Madison School of Nursing. Prior to that appointment in 2000, Dr. Kirchhoff was a professor at the University of Utah College of Nursing and research consultant at University Hospital in Salt Lake City. She is an ICU nurse who has improved care for critically ill patients and their families by both conducting studies and using the results of completed studies. Most recently she has worked to improve care at the end of life, garnering regional and national awards. She has lectured and written about the conduct and use of research since her doctoral work on diffusion of coronary precautions. She has taught this content at all educational levels and in many clinical institutions.

# Contents

# Contributors

**Susan Adams, PhD, RN**
Associate Director
Research Translation and
    Dissemination Core
Gerontological Nursing Interventions
    Research Center
College of Nursing
University of Iowa
Iowa City, IA

**Marge Benham-Hutchins, PhD, RN**
Assistant Professor
School of Nursing
Northeastern University
Boston, MA

**Mary D. Bondmass, RN, PhD**
Assistant Professor
School of Nursing
University of Nevada Las Vegas
Las Vegas, NV

**Robert J. Caswell, PhD**
Associate Professor Emeritus
Division of Health Services
    Management and Policy
Ohio State University
Columbus, OH

**Paula C. Clutter, RN, PhD, CNS-BC**
Assistant Professor
Clinical, Acute Nursing Care
The University of Texas Health
    Science Center at San Antonio
San Antonio, TX

**Ulrike Dieterle, MA, MLS**
Head of Access Services
Health Sciences Libraries
University of Wisconsin-Madison
Madison, WI

**Marquis D. Foreman, PhD, RN, FAAN**
Professor and Chair
Adult Health and Gerontological
    Nursing
College of Nursing
Rush University
Chicago, IL

**Susan K. Frazier, RN, PhD**
Associate Professor
College of Nursing
University of Kentucky
Lexington, KY

**Carol Glod, Ph.D., CS, FAAN**
Professor
School of Nursing
Director of Research
Bouvé College of Health Sciences
Northeastern University
Boston, MA

**Christopher Hooper-Lane, MA, AHIP**
Instructional Services Coordinator
Senior Academic Librarian
Ebling Library
Madison, WI

**Mary R. Lynn, PhD**
Professor, School of Nursing
Assistant Director, Operations, Office
 of Human Research Ethics
University of North Carolina at
 Chapel Hill
Chapel Hill, NC

**Lea Ann Matura PhD, RN, NP-C, CCRN**
Assistant Professor
Northeastern University
Boston, MA

**Katherine McDuffie, RN, MSN**
Doctoral Student
The University of Texas Health
 Science Center at San Antonio
San Antonio, TX

**Vivian Nowazek, PhD, MSN, RN-BC,
CNS-CC, CCRN**
Assistant Professor
University of Houston—Victoria at
 Sugar Land
Sugar Land, TX

**Beth Rodgers, PhD, RN, FAAN**
Professor and Center Scientist
Self Management Service Center
College of Nursing
University of Wisconsin—Milwaukee
Milwaukee, WI

**Leah L. Shever, PhD, RN**
Advanced Practice Nurse
Center for Nursing Quality,
 Professional Development, and
 Research
Department of Nursing Services and
 Patient Care
The University of Iowa Hospitals and
 Clinics
Iowa City, IA

**Mary Schira PhD, RN, ACNP-BC**
Associate Dean, MSN Program
School of Nursing
The University of Texas at Arlington
Arlington, TX

**Suzanne P. Smith, EdD, RN, FAAN**
Editor-in-Chief
The Journal of Nursing Administration
 and Nurse Educator
Bradenton, FL

**Kathleen R. Stevens, RN, EdD,
FANE, FAAN**
Professor and Director
Academic Center for Evidence-Based
 Practice
The University of Texas Health
 Science Center
San Antonio, TX

**Kathleen S. Stone, RN, PhD, FAAN**
Professor Emeritus
College of Nursing
Ohio State University
Columbus, OH

**Marita G. Titler, PhD, RN, FAAN**
Associate Dean for Practice and
 Clinical Scholarship
Rhetaugh Dumas Endowed Chair
University of Michigan School of
 Nursing and UMHS
Ann Arbor, MI

**Julie Johnson Zerwic, PhD, RN, FAAN**
Associate Professor and Interim Head
Department of Biobehavioral Health
 Science
College of Nursing
University of Illinois at Chicago
Chicago, IL

# Preface

The increasing focus on evidence needed for practice decisions propels us to integrate how we teach graduate students about research. The use of research summaries and the need for evidence-based quality and safety practices and for clarifying the conduct of research are all requirements for nurses functioning professionally in practice. We hope that this book meets all those needs in a single introductory volume that includes evaluation of single research reports along with summaries and guidelines that may be of use when establishing evidence-based practice (EBP). When using results from an individual report, one must have a working knowledge of the conduct of research if one is to evaluate the scientific merit and relevance of a single study.

Evidence-based practice concepts related to patient care are integrated throughout the chapters, with important points highlighted in exhibits. Clinically relevant examples present ways students and staff nurses can apply knowledge to daily clinical practice. We have also expanded, from previous versions of this book, the information on evidence-based practice and examples of clinical protocols.

*Part I: Evidence-Based Practice.* Chapters focus on an overview of EBP: the definitions of evidence-based practice that have evolved over time, types of evidence, and models of EBP. Ways of finding evidence are presented to guide the reader to respond to the mandate for EBP. This information on EBP is vital to graduate students who are developing skills that will prepare them to assume their advanced practice role in health care.

*Part II: Building Blocks for Evidence.* The section starts with appraising a single research article, a building block for evidence. Components of the research process are presented from a reviewer's perspective of using the article as supporting evidence for practice in subsequent chapters. One of the documented barriers to research utilization is that practitioners feel inadequate to read and interpret research findings. Gaining knowledge about the research process is crucial for clinicians who must read, interpret, and determine the relevance of research findings (evidence) to practice and to consider those that may be used in developing practice guidelines. It also allows them to advocate for patients who are considering whether or not to participate in research.

*Part III: Using Available Evidence.* Meta-analyses, systematic reviews, and practice guidelines from various sources such as professional organizations and government Web sites are other types of evidence that may be used in establishing EBP. Appraising information from these sources is suggested in this section. Program evaluation provides an opportunity for use of evidence. Considerations when planning and implementing EBP activities are also included in this section: identifying the focus of EBP activities (unit or organizational) and developing an EBP protocol.

*Part IV: Evaluating the Impact of EBP and Communicating Results.* Cost, outcomes, and ethical aspects are essential aspects of EBP. Communicating ideas through oral and written avenues is valuable in making EBP a reality. Techniques for acquiring oral and written methods for presenting ideas are included; such techniques are helpful in writing protocols and reporting outcomes of EBP activities.

Although graduate students are the primary audience for this book—a textbook for a graduate course in nursing research or an interdisciplinary health care, course—nurses in clinical settings also will find the book helpful in fulfilling their research role toward achieving hospital Magnet Status. Our hope is that the information provided in this book can be used to provide optimal cost-efficient care to patients that will increase their quality of life.

*Magdalena A. Mateo, PhD, RN, FAAN*
*Karin T. Kirchhoff, PhD, RN, FAAN*

# Research for Advanced Practice Nurses

# Evidence-Based Practice

# Overview of Evidence-Based Practice

KARIN T. KIRCHHOFF

To provide the best possible patient care, health professionals must obtain a quality education. After a series of publications on quality and safety in patient care, the Institute of Medicine (IOM) recommended that five core competencies be taught to ensure quality in patient care (Institute of Medicine [IOM], 2003). These are:

- Patient-centered care
- Interdisciplinary skills
- Evidence-based practice
- Quality improvement skills
- Information technology

Although evidence-based practice (EBP) had been discussed for more than a decade by this time, some nursing publications still questioned its necessity. The IOM reasoned that "clinicians are confronted with a rapidly expanded evidence base—upon which health care decisions should ideally be made—but are not consistently schooled in how to search and evaluate this evidence base and apply it to practice" (IOM, 2003). Obviously, the IOM did not consider EBP optional.

Other pressures to promote EBP also began to appear. Granting of the Magnet Hospital designation required that staff be involved in research and use evidence in practice. The Joint Commission began requiring that health care organizations demonstrate standards for the use of evidence in order to gain or sustain accreditation. Links to evidence became prompts in electronic medical records. In some settings, documentation was required as part of treatment recommendations or assessments of patients that matched them with a certain disease. Recently, the North Carolina Board of Nursing required that all schools of nursing teach EBP for state accreditation.

## DEFINITIONS OF EVIDENCE-BASED PRACTICE

In medicine, it was Gordon Guyatt who, in the 1990s, first began using the term "evidence-based medicine" (EBM). As the lead author on a series of articles, published in the *Journal of the American Medical Association,* called the Users' Guides to the Medical Literature, he and colleagues detailed how to critique and use different types of research reports (Guyatt, Sackett, & Cook, 1993; Oxman, Sackett, & Guyatt, 1993).

Definitions for evidence-based medicine (EBM) have changed over time. In 2000, Sackett (Sackett, Straus, Richardson, Rosenberg, & Haynes), in the 2nd edition of *Evidence-Based Medicine,* defined it as the "Integration of best research evidence with clinical expertise and patient values." Some of the early criticism of EBM was that the expertise of the clinician was not valued and that everyone was treated the same—in other words, cookbook medicine. This definition in 2000 counters the notion of evidence as the sole criterion upon which to make medical decisions. The 3rd edition added the notion of circumstances (Straus, Richardson, Glaziou, & Haynes, 2005, p. 1): "Integration of best research evidence with clinical expertise and patient values and circumstances."

The use of evidence has a different history in nursing than in medicine. Early studies on whether or not research was used in practice were conducted by Ketefian (1975), who asked about the correct use of glass thermometers, and by Kirchhoff (1982), who surveyed nurses' use of coronary precautions. Because there was a desire to promote the use of research in practice, several studies were funded to provide summaries of research for use, such as the 10 medical-surgical protocols for practice developed by Joann Horsley (Horsley, Crane, Crabtree, & Wood, 1983) and the thematic conferences at the University of North Carolina scheduled by Sandra Funk (Funk, Tornquist, Champagne, Copp, & Wiese, 1989).

These efforts in nursing, called research utilization (RU), were defined as the application of research findings in patient care (Kirchhoff, 1991) or the process of using research findings as a basis for practice (Titler, Mentes, Rakel, Abbott, & Baumler, 1999). A number of nurses developed models for RU (Kirchhoff, 2004).

After physicians at McMaster began the evidence-based medicine movement, however, a number of nursing leaders in research utilization followed suit by updating their RU models as EBP models. Kirchhoff (2004) listed a number of advantages of EBP over RU. In EBP many groups produce high-quality summaries of the evidence, at times inclusive of studies in several languages, and post the summaries and their recommendations on the Internet for ease of access. These group members are frequently experts in the area and may be government sponsored, with reports made available without charge to the public. The evidence is graded, and expert opinion is used to supplement weak or missing evidence.

In contrast, RU work might be done at a clinical site by a nursing group searching for answers to a clinical problem. The nurses were required to identify and summarize the literature and to make decisions for practice with little help from topic experts. RU was seen as based on a dichotomy (was there or was there not sufficient evidence for practice), rather than as a graded, strength-of-evidence approach like EBP.

Most nursing EBP models begin with a problem to be solved through use of evidence. Titler et al. (1994) included knowledge-focused triggers, which occur when a useful guideline or summary is published, as well as problem-focused triggers.

## RESEARCH UTILIZATION AND EVIDENCE-BASED PRACTICE

The term *EBP* has been used in the nursing literature interchangeably with *RU*. EBP and RU, however, are not identical. If one accepts the definition of EBP as the integration of clinical expertise with the best scientific evidence from systematic research, then the sources for EBP are broader than those for RU. Both qualitative and quantitative studies are employed in RU; in addition, RU does not limit itself to findings from randomized controlled trials (RCT). EBP is not limited to RCTs but values those studies as offering the highest level of evidence for or against the use of an intervention. In RU, the studies found require integration, which includes accessing, appraising, and summarizing findings. Then practice decisions can be made and changes in practice implemented institutionally.

EBP includes some steps in RU but adds other sources besides research, such as scientific principles of pathophysiology, case report data, and expert opinion, when studies are lacking. In some cases, the best available evidence may be case reports or expert opinion. The steps required in RU—finding the studies, appraising them, and summarizing—also are done by clinical experts when EBP sources are used, resulting in time and quality improvements. And, while appraisal is still done in EBP research, it is done at the level of the summary (guideline or systematic review), rather than at the level of the individual study (as in RU). The application to practice and evaluation of impact are the same for both EBP and RU.

## ONE MODEL OF EVIDENCE-BASED PRACTICE

### Steven's ACE Star Model of Knowledge Transformation

Steven's ACE Star Model of Knowledge Transformation (Stevens, 2004) is graphically displayed as a 5-point star. This model follows the development of evidence from the initial study to the evaluation of the impact of summaries and translation of that evidence. Point 1 is *Discovery*—a knowledge-generating stage. Research results are generated through the conduct of a single study, which becomes a brick in the wall of evidence.

Point 2 is *Evidence Summary,* where a number of studies are synthesized into a single, meaningful statement of what we now know. The Cochrane Handbook (Cochrane Collaboration, 2008) lists the steps in this process. The Agency for Healthcare Research and Quality uses the term *evidence synthesis* in this regard. When *meta-analysis* (a statistical procedure) occurs, the authors have combined the results of several studies that address a set of related research hypotheses. Other terms such as *review of literature* and *state of the science reviews* are seen as less rigorous and, therefore, less reliable summary processes. Producing high-level research summaries is now termed the *science of research synthesis.*

Point 3 is *Translation,* where evidence summaries are transformed into clinical recommendations so that they can be brought into actual practice. These recommendations are called *practice guidelines* or *clinical practice guidelines.* Statements should appear on how care should be performed, with links to strengths of evidence and strength of recommendation.

Point 4 is *Integration,* with care recommendations disseminated to all clinicians and institutions involved. It will be necessary to find ways to implement necessary changes so that the recommended practice becomes the norm, including changes at the individual and at the organization level. How to foster the adoption and overcome the barriers that prevent the adoption of evidence is a focus of much effort (Dopson, FitzGerald, Ferlie, Gabbay, & Locock, 2002; Sinuff, Cook, Giacomini, Heyland, & Dodek, 2007).

Point 5 is *Evaluation.* The impact of the practice change should be evaluated in order to see if the desired effect was obtained. If not, one must ask whether the plan was implemented consistently. Are there differences in the setting that might have prevented the desired effect? Possible outcomes to be measured include patient health outcomes, provider and patient satisfaction, efficacy, efficiency, economic analysis, and health status impact.

## Competencies

Stevens developed competencies in EBP for the 5 points of the star arranged by educational levels (Stevens, 2005). For example, under star point 2, Evidence Summary, an undergraduate would be expected to locate a systematic review, a graduate student would be expected to do the same using multiple sources, and a doctoral student would be expected to conduct an evidence synthesis with an interdisciplinary team.

## APPLICATION OF EVIDENCE TO PRACTICE

Types of evidence that can be used in practice have become numerous over time. Initially, only single articles were available as evidence for specific topics of care. At that time, that was considered the best evidence available. Recently, summaries of single articles on the same topic have been written, and these summaries overcome the inconsistency in findings and methodological shortcomings of one single study. These summaries or systematic reviews (if done according to scientific standards) have a close cousin, *meta-analysis,* which combines statistical findings into a common metric across all studies related to the topic. Although these two types of summaries tell us what "we know," they might not make it sufficiently clear what "we do" in practice. Another form of evidence, guidelines, provides that type of guidance. Where, then, does one start in the application of evidence?

Although nurses might be involved in the entire process, as outlined in the ACE Star Model, or at a single step in that process, nurses most commonly use evidence compiled by others. When using such evidence, however, it is important to look for a summary in the form of a guideline that tells us "what to do." If no guidelines are available or relevant to our population because of recency or specificity of the practice, then the next best source of evidence is a systematic review or a meta-analysis. These summaries should detail the decisions made about which studies to include because of quality and what conclusion(s) prevail(s). Although this evidence clearly depicts "what we know," "what to do" requires additional work. When both categories are not available or helpful, searching for original research articles becomes imperative. More detail on searching for guidelines, summaries, and research articles is found in Chapter 2, "General Searching: Finding Research Reports."

The important Web site of the Agency for Healthcare Research and Quality (AHRQ), with links to the National Guideline Clearinghouse (NGC) (www.guideline.gov) and the U.S. Preventive Services Task Force (USPSTF) (http://www.ahrq.gov/clinic/uspstfix.htm), is a gold mine. These guidelines are of a more general nature. The Centers for Disease Control & Prevention (CDC) (www.cdc.gov) has guidelines about immunizations, infection control, prevention, and so on. Guidelines for specific clinical conditions may be found on professional Web sites such as those for the American Diabetes Association, the Society for Critical Care Medicine, and the Oncology Nursing Society. Another useful site is UpToDate (www.uptodate.com), which provides evidence derived from a number of resources, including but not limited to hand-searches of more than 375 peer-reviewed journals, electronic searches of databases, including those of Medline, the Cochrane Database, Clinical Evidence, and ACP Journal Club, as well as consensus guidelines, information (such as reports from the Food & Drug Administration [FDA], the CDC, and the National Institutes of Health [NIH]), and proceedings of major national meetings.

Once a guideline is found that seems relevant, appraisal is the next step. One site that offers an appraisal form for use by several raters is the AGREE collaboration (http://www.agreecollaboration.org/pdf/agree instrumentfinal.pdf). Another system of appraisal is called GRADE (Atkins et al., 2004). In both, the quality of the evidence, the importance of outcomes, and the considerations of benefits and harms are used to appraise the guideline. The issue of timeliness of the guideline is relative, since some clinical topics change rapidly in terms of their knowledge base, whereas knowledge about other topics remains more stable. Be that as it may, guidelines must be updated at least every 5 years. Guidelines on rapidly changing topics may be updated more frequently to keep them current.

When guidelines do not provide clinical answers, the next best source of evidence includes high-quality systematic reviews, such as the preferred Cochrane Collaboration, where great effort is made to secure publications of high quality in all languages. As the Cochrane Database of Systematic Reviews on clinically relevant topics, with more than 660 topics, requires a subscription, it is available at most large universities and medical centers. The Database of Abstracts of Reviews of Effects (DARE), with more than 2,700 topics, is available without a subscription but only in the form of abstracts. Other free evidence-based summaries are found at the AHRQ Evidence-Based Practice Centers (EPCs) (http://www.ahrq.gov/clinic/epcindex.htm). If a topic has been selected by a center, helpful summaries of the research will be found there. Another federally sponsored site is the Physician Data Query (PDQ) at the Web site of the National Cancer Institute (http://www.cancer.gov/cancer topics/pdq). The PDQ cancer information summaries are peer reviewed and are updated monthly by six editorial boards made up of specialists in adult treatment, pediatric treatment, supportive care, screening and prevention, genetics, and complementary and alternative medicine. The boards review current literature from more than 70 biomedical journals, evaluate its relevance, and synthesize it into clear summaries.

The bibliographic databases, such as PubMed and CINAHL, can be searched with limits to find published guidelines and systematic reviews. The limit is publication type and the terms to be selected for the PubMed database are *practice-guideline, review,* and *meta-analysis* to find summaries; *randomized controlled trial* or *clinical trial* for research; and *consensus development conference* (with or without NIH) to find expert consensus. CINAHL's terms with publication type as limit are *abstract* or *research* to pull research summarized in clinical journal; *clinical innovation* or *practice guidelines* for guidelines; and *systematic review;* if enough are not found, the search can be expanded to all *review* articles (also a publication type).

The advantage of systematic reviews is that they are frequently preformed when evidence accumulates or are *evidence driven.* Guidelines, on the other hand, tend to be *necessity driven* and developed because of a need in practice (Straus et al., 2005, p. 166). The evidence may not be rich in the guideline and some of the interventions will vary in the strength of their support.

Another interesting source of evidence is Bandolier, a monthly print and Internet journal about health care that uses evidence-based medicine techniques to provide advice about particular treatments or diseases for health care professionals and consumers (http://www.jr2.ox.ac.uk/bandolier/index.html). The content is tertiary publishing, distilling the information from (secondary) reviews of (primary) trials and making it comprehensible. PubMed and the Cochrane Library are searched for systematic reviews that can be rewritten for ease of understanding. Bandolier also writes its own systematic reviews.

The TRIP database is set up to be the Database of databases (http://www.tripdatabase.com/index.cfm). A search box takes a term and then returns articles, summaries, guidelines across Web sites, and databases. A membership allows access to additional functions on the site. The site gives direct, hyperlinked access to the largest collection of evidence-based material on the Web, as well as to articles from premier online journals such as the *British Medical Journal*.

When systematic reviews or meta-analyses are found, they also require appraisal. One helpful site is http://www.cche.net/usersguides/overview.asp, where such a review is labeled an *overview*. The topics covered include the results, the validity of those results, and whether they are helpful to the patient.

Last, when there is little evidence, reliance on expert opinion or consensus is preferable to guessing. The sources for this weaker type of evidence are professional societies' Web sites and information obtained by using a search limit, *consensus conference*, for publication type.

Although many professionals turn first to Medline or CINAHL, when one is advocating for practice changes, use of guidelines and systematic reviews is preferable to reliance on single research articles that have not been replicated or quality filtered. Medline has more than 11 million references, and finding the right ones can be difficult. It is the most up-to-date database, and, where recency is critical, it may provide the answers. Having finely honed searching skills has become ever more critical, and, as technology changes, researchers should take classes at a health science library to make sure their skills are current. Some people are deluded by the retrieval of a large number of articles, but quantity alone is not adequate and may mislead the researcher. The strength of the evidence

presented in the studies consulted should be ev
for articles and finds differing results. It is criti
the study's findings to the local setting be eva
may not be the same in the two settings. Impl
quires careful planning and the coordination
make the change; institutional support might
of documentation or policy changes. Last, aft__ __
should be done to determine whether the guideline was impi__
correctly and whether the desired outcomes were seen. This last stage can
be performed through the usual quality and safety monitoring.

## SUMMARY

In summary, EBP is an excellent way to communicate about practice
across disciplines where the focus is on the evidence, rather than on
the discipline of the practitioner. Using available evidence is easier than
reinventing summaries of research and is more likely to be comprehensive, especially when the information has been found on high-quality
Web sites, but, in order to find all these sources, nurses will need to
develop new search skills.

## SUGGESTED ACTIVITIES

1    Select a topic or clinical problem. Go to several of the recom-
     mended Web sites to find any information available in summaries
     or guidelines. Is the information on these sites as up-to-date as
     the results of a Medline or CINAHL search on the same topic?
     How do you explain any discrepancies in your findings?
2    Use the same topic and find a professional organization that
     might have a guideline for it. Was this the same guideline that
     you found with your bibliographic database?

## REFERENCES

Atkins, D., Best, D., Briss, P. A., Eccles, M., Falck-Ytter, Y., Flottorp, S., et al. (2004).
     Grading quality of evidence and strength of recommendations. *British Medical Jour-
     nal, 328*(7454), 1490.
Cochrane Collaboration. (2008). Cochrane handbook for systematic reviews of interven-
     tions. Retrieved April 27, 2008, from http://www.cochrane-handbook.org/

itzGerald, L., Ferlie, E., Gabbay, J., & Locock, L. (2002). No magic tar-
anging clinical practice to become more evidence based. *Health Care Man-
ev, 27*(3), 35–47.

S. G., Tornquist, E. M., Champagne, M. T., Copp, L. A., & Wiese, R. A. (1989).
*Key aspects of comfort: Management of pain, fatigue, and nausea.* New York: Springer
Publishing.

Guyatt, G. H., Sackett, D. L., & Cook, D. J. (1993). Users' guides to the medical literature II: How to use an article about therapy or prevention. A. Are the results of the
study valid? Evidence-based medicine working group. *Journal of the American Medical Association, 270*(21), 2598–2601.

Horsley, J. A., Crane, J., Crabtree, M. K., & Wood, D.J. (1983). *Using research to improve nursing practice: A guide.* Orlando, FL: Grune & Stratton.

Institute of Medicine (IOM). (2003). *Health professions education: A bridge to quality.*
Washington, DC: National Academies Press.

Ketefian, S. (1975). Application of selected nursing research findings into nursing practice. *Nursing Research, 24,* 89–92.

Kirchhoff, K. T. (1982). A diffusion survey of coronary precautions. *Nursing Research,
31*(4), 196–201.

Kirchhoff, K. T. (1991). Who is responsible for research utilization? *Heart and Lung,
20*(3), 308–309.

Kirchhoff, K. T. (2004). State of the science of translational research: From demonstration projects to intervention testing. *Worldviews Evidence-Based Nursing, 1*(Suppl. 1),
S6–S12.

Oxman, A.D., Sackett, D. L., & Guyatt, G. H. (1993). Users' guides to the medical literature. I. How to get started. The evidence-based medicine working group. *Journal of
the American Medical Association, 270*(17), 2093–2095.

Sackett, D. L., Straus, S. E., Richardson, W. S., Rosenberg, W., & Haynes, R. B. (Eds.).
(2000). *Evidence-based medicine* (2nd ed.). Edinburgh: Churchill Livingstone.

Sinuff, T. M. D. P., Cook, D. M. D. M., Giacomini, M. P., Heyland, D. M. D. M., &
Dodek, P.M. D. M. (2007). Facilitating clinician adherence to guidelines in the intensive care unit: A multicenter, qualitative study. *Critical Care Medicine, 35*(9), 2083–
2089.

Stevens, K. R. (2004). *ACE Star Model of EBP: Knowledge transformation.* Academic
Center for Evidence-Based Practice. Retrieved March 1, 2005, from www.acestar.
uthscsa.edu

Stevens, K. R. (2005). *Essential competencies for evidence-based practice in nursing.* San
Antonio: Academic Center of Evidence-Based Practice, University of Texas Health
Science Center at San Antonio.

Straus, S., Richardson, S. W., Glaziou, P., & Haynes, R. B. (2005). *Evidence-based medicine: How to practice and teach EBM* (3rd ed.). Edinburgh: Elsevier Churchill Livingstone.

Titler, M. G., Kleiber, C., Steelman, V., Goode, C., Rakel, B., Barry-Walker, J., et al.
(1994). Infusing research into practice to promote quality care. *Nursing Research,
43*(5), 307–313.

Titler, M. G., Mentes, J. C., Rakel, B. A., Abbott, L., & Baumler, S. (1999). From book to
bedside: Putting evidence to use in the care of the elderly. *Joint Commission Journal
on Quality Improvement, 25*(10), 545–556.

# 2

# General Searching: Finding Research Reports

ULRIKE DIETERLE AND CHRISTOPHER HOOPER-LANE

Conducting a literature review in the 21st century poses challenges for the researcher. The emphasis on evidence-based decision making in health care, the exponential increase in the volume of scientific literature, and the growing dependence on ever-changing computer technologies result in a more complicated research environment. The changing shape of information, how it is retrieved and evaluated, has profound effects at every level of the research process. While the core concepts of research have remained relatively consistent, new tools, new technologies, and new information destinations continue to evolve and multiply. This chapter discusses the search for evidence as a systematic process consisting of four distinct phases, including activities to promote literature reviews that yield helpful information.

A brief review of significant information trends related to the health sciences will illustrate the impact on the advanced practice nurse's (APN) search for evidence to support practice. One of the most dramatic changes in the past 10 years affecting all types of information gathering has been the shift from print to electronic resources. It is estimated that original information is increasing at a rate of approximately 30% a year, and most of this new information appears for the first time in digital formats (Lyman & Varian, 2003). Action verbs used 15 years ago for information-gathering activities—scanning, browsing, retrieving—conjure very different mental pictures today. As research tools continue to develop, APNs find it difficult to refresh computer skills and to keep up-to-date in their fields. Staying current, as information resources evolve, takes time, appropriate skill sets, and attention (Skiba, 2005). Researchers now find themselves spending the bulk of their research hours with computers and virtual research partners, often performing searches alone and developing their final papers in digital spaces. And, while the information explosion continues, the skills to navigate through denser, more crowded information landscapes seldom keep pace (Tanner, Pierce, & Pravikoff, 2004).

Another recent trend is the appearance of new information destinations. One variant of this is the open-access movement, which was spurred on by the library community and influential research-granting institutions such as National Institutes of Health. This movement promises to dramatically increase public access to full-text scientific articles. A significant milestone was reached on December 26, 2007, when the FY 2008 appropriations process (Consolidated Appropriations Act of 2007 [H.R. 2764]) included wording to make articles reporting publicly funded research freely available to the world. As vendor-providers find their inventories disappearing from behind their proprietary firewalls, even more information destinations will arise, adding to the existing "information diasporas." With additional places to look, it will become increasingly important to chart the research course in more detail in advance, identify resources more precisely, and evaluate the right skill sets early in the process.

The heightened focus, in recent years, on improving clinical outcomes through support of scientific knowledge has resulted in a greater emphasis on the integration of evidence-based practices (EBP) at all levels of health care (Brancato, 2006). As nursing students and health care professionals learn to incorporate EBP into their clinical work flow, they must learn to identify evidence-based information resources and construct related information-seeking strategies. Practitioners now have mandates to adopt effective EBP recommendations to their practices. Effective EBP practices will be increasingly important in saving clinicians' time and energy and, ultimately, in achieving improved clinical outcomes (Polit & Beck, 2008).

## PHASES IN THE SEARCH FOR EVIDENCE

### Phase I: Preparation and Planning

While much attention is traditionally paid to the process of formulating search statements and selecting appropriate search terminology, databases and strategies, a literature review consists of more than this. It is, in a very real sense, a project waiting to be managed. Thinking of and identifying its many parts before embarking on the active searching will benefit the searcher and instill order in what can seem to be string of chaotic activities. The preliminary literature review preparation phase, that is, Phase I., will be discussed first.

A real-world, kitchen-table analogy may work here. Everyone has been challenged by the prospect of preparing a new recipe. It is a known fact that it is best to first read the entire recipe from beginning to end before assembling the ingredients for the dish. One then gathers appropriate ingredients and needed utensils. After preparing the same recipe a number of times, one finds that the preparation is much easier. It becomes second nature. As the cook gains more assurance, more certainty in the procedure, a pattern begins to develop. As patterns develop, variations are incorporated with ease and confidence increases over time.

Research is much the same. If searching a database is a rare occurrence, it will continue to be a slow and laborious process. Once evidence-based research is fully integrated into clinical cultures and professional work flow, it will become second nature.

## Ask Questions

Before diving head-first into database searching, it is important to ask a few questions to guide subsequent actions. Pre-search preparation will tease out existing strengths and weaknesses. It will define the skills needed and pinpoint knowledge gaps. Asking the right questions *before* beginning a project is a valuable exercise in charting the most effective and efficient research course. Questioning the purpose of the literature review will determine the intent and the appropriate intensity, depth, and scope of the search(es).

A literature review may be undertaken for a variety of reasons:

1  To answer a clinical question
2  To prepare for a thesis, conduct a topical survey, or ready a scholarly research for a publication
3  To conduct a systematic review, respond to a professional curiosity, or some variation on these

An inclusive search for all relevant literature, such as demanded by systematic reviews and meta-analyses, requires more time and involves more databases than a selective review of limited scope. Which resources are best for the research question? It is advisable to identify the best information resources for the topic before constructing search strategies. Good preparation prevents distracting detours and lost time, resolves confusion, and serves to sequence the order in which databases are searched. In Phase I, exploratory searches are important for discovery and to determine the viability of the research topic.

Medline (PubMed), for example, is an ideal choice for initial exploratory searches because it is the largest biomedical database available. It provides article citations in all levels of the evidence hierarchy, from the "gold standard" of systematic reviews to the most casual, subjective opinions.

What are the best search strategies? Because databases have their own "personalities," it is best to understand not only the basic features common to all but also the unique characteristics of each selected database before initiating the search process. Researchers who make repetitive use of a database will develop degrees of comfort and form patterns of recognition useful in attaining precision. Expert searching is an acquired skill developed over time with practice. Even seasoned researchers can benefit from added search acuity. Exhibit 2.1 lists factors to consider when searching relevant literature.

Most online databases provide tutorials or help manuals that give at least rudimentary point-of-need assistance. Medline (PubMed) has an extensive series of tutorials accessible from the PubMed home page, presented in well-defined learning increments. Medical librarians at academic health sciences libraries, hospitals, and clinics are also available to provide database suggestions, search guidance, and training opportunities.

Exhibit 2.1

### QUESTIONS TO ASK DURING PHASE I

- What is the purpose of the literature review?
- Which resources are best for the research question?
- How are the resources best searched?
- Where can help be obtained?
- What resources are available?
- Is time a limiting factor?
- Which bibliographic management tools will be used?
- How is the information evaluated?

What other resources are available? Is time a limiting factor in this project? Which bibliographic management tools will be used, if any? How does the researcher evaluate the information? Self-assessment questions similar to these will help to make necessary components transparent to the researcher and allow time to prepare. Conducting the literature review involves many intersecting, nonlinear processes, including planning, discovery, preparation, contemplation, search skills, and evaluation.

These phases do not always progress in a strict linear fashion from point A to point B. In fact, research is much like lining up the colors on a Rubik's cube, more a process of moving forward, pushing back, sliding sideways, re-evaluating, and refining. It is more a series of overlapping loops that propel momentum forward (Mellon, 1984). Through repeated checks, evaluations, confirmations, and reflections along the way, the APN avoids unplanned detours down a foggy path. Finding oneself in a research fog of uncertainty is not unusual but can be minimized by planning and preparation. The uncertainties faced by novice researchers are often inadvertently magnified, setting up needless hoops and hurdles. The aid of a multipart schematic for research success is a helpful tool.

## Define Search Goal

Defining the scope of the planned research is an important element in moving forward. Assessing the intended outcome of the search provides clarity of purpose and direction. Is the impending literature review a class assignment with specific guidelines, requirements, and deadlines? Is it generated by unanswered health care questions that need immediate attention? Is it part of a team project leading to the creation of evidence-based guidelines in the clinical setting? Is the literature review part of a long-term research project to publish? Answers to these questions may drive the momentum of the literature review down slightly varying search paths. Decisions made at this juncture will also impact the choice of databases and resources consulted. One size does not fit all. A small-size research goal does not warrant an extensive research approach. Each literature review is a sum of its smaller parts.

## Gather Background Information

One important preliminary step is to understand how the research topic fits into its related field of knowledge. The APN must attain some degree of comfort with the nomenclature and the topic-at-large before moving into serious search phases. Background builds an information foundation that will support increased awareness of vocabulary (important when searching) and related issues. Background information can be found in many places, including textbooks, trusted Web sites, reference resources, and review articles. If the topic is interdisciplinary, as many nursing topics are, the information destinations will be broader in scope, more numerous, and, often, less familiar. Reaching across disciplines can be a stretch, especially for the less experienced searcher. During the background gathering, it is advisable to clearly list and expand related terminology to aid in search strategy construction later.

## Construct Searchable Question

First, formulating a searchable or answerable question is a technique that focuses on the most basic elements of the research topic. By focusing on only the core elements of a complex health care scenario, the researcher clarifies the central question and achieves a more precise definition of the subject. Precision and focus are also enhanced by the use of the PICO method. The PICO mnemonic (P = patient, population, problem, I = intervention, C = comparison, O = outcome) provides a useful instrument in peeling away the outer layers of the research question and directs the focus to only the most essential components. This concentrated effort removes other "noisy" narrative that may prove distracting when constructing search strategies. Not every query fits neatly into the PICO format, but the approach of deconstructing the parts to their meaningful essence, clarifies the purpose and helps develop more effective search strategies.

## Eliminate Search Barriers

Nursing literature is replete with documentation of potential barriers to the integration of evidence-based methods into practice. The most commonly identified barriers include the perceived lack of value of EBP to practice, time constraints, lack of access to computers and databases at the point of need, limited database searching skills, and continued underutilization of evidence-based information in health care environments. Even trusted online resources are not as accessible or viewed as useful as consultation with a colleague (Dee & Stanley, 2005; Pravikoff, Tanner, & Pierce, 2005).

An overestimation of difficulties related to the research process can cause uncertainty, which, in turn, may lead the APN to avoid research or even bring about the onset of research rigor mortis (Downs, 1969). Uncertainties surrounding the research process can inhibit forward momentum. It is important to identify and manage research uncertainties early and throughout the process. According to Klein (2003), there are five basic sources of uncertainty, which are displayed in Exhibit 2.2. These sources are: missing or inaccessible information; unreliable or untrustworthy information; information that is inconsistent or conflicting; information that is confusing and that clouds decision making; and "noisy" or distracting information, which can result in time wasted sifting through unrelated resources.

Researchers are advised to follow a basic prescription when contemplating literature reviews: (1) spend pre-search time on discovery, planning, reflection, then (2) choose the appropriate information destinations and execute well-formulated searches, (3) critically evaluate and expand search parameters and (4) sort, store, and organize information gathered throughout the process. Keeping in mind the topic and essential information listed in Exhibit 2.3 could promote effective search strategies.

Above all, remember that one size does not fit all research situations. Allow for slippage, expect some detours, and reach out for help before spinning those research wheels needlessly. Timely consultations with subject experts, faculty, and medical librarians can decrease frustration. The process of conducting a literature review will, with time, actually become an interesting and rewarding journey.

Exhibit 2.2

### FIVE SOURCES OF UNCERTAINTY

- Missing information
- Unreliable information
- Conflicting information
- "Noisy" information
- Confusing information (Klein, 2003)

Exhibit 2.3

**CHECKLIST—PHASE I**

| | |
|---|---|
| Research Topic | ☐ |
| Due Date | ☐ |
| Background Info | ☐ |
| Citation Manager | ☐ |
| PICO or Searchable Question | ☐ |
| Major Databases | ☐ |
| Knowledge Gaps | ☐ |

## Phase II: Mining the Literature Databases

### Choose the Best Resources

Once a well-formulated question is created, researchers and practitioners must look for the best evidence to answer the question. Succeeding in this venture will require an understanding of the EBM hierarchy, adequate searching skills, and access and to appropriate resources. There is a remarkable amount of health research now published. Mulrow (1994) estimated that more than 2 million research papers on biomedical topics were published annually. Therefore, it is essential that a researcher know the kind (or level) of evidence needed to answer the question and a good grasp of the resources.

### Start With Reviews

From an evidence-based perspective, the best bet is to start by using resources containing the secondary literature, that is, articles that summarize or review peer-reviewed research on a topic. The term *review* has many meanings. A *literature review* tends to be a body of text that states the current knowledge on a topic from a wide variety of sources. A *systematic review,* on the other hand, is a type of literature review that focuses on a specific clinical topic and uses explicit methods to perform a thorough literature search and to appraise individual studies on that topic. Some also place *practice guidelines* into the review category. This is true only if their statements are based on rigorous scientific evidence (i.e., systematic reviews and randomized controlled trials) found in the literature. In addition, a true evidence-based guideline includes a section that documents the process used to develop the statements and grades the strength of the evidence used in making clinical recommendations.

## Search the Primary Literature

The value and body of secondary literature have grown phenomenally in the past few years; however, much of the evidence, particularly in nursing and allied health fields, still lies within the *primary literature,* that is, individual reports of findings. These single studies are the building blocks from which the systematic reviews and evidence-based guidelines are built. As one might guess, studies are not created equal, and there is a broad spectrum of publication types found in the journal literature. All levels of the evidence hierarchy, from double-blinded randomized controlled trials to cohort studies to case studies to qualitative and descriptive studies, are found in journals. So, researchers and clinicians should initiate a search in the review literature and turn to primary literature to fill in the gaps (both in content and in currency).

## Select Resources to Search

There are literally thousands of electronic and print resources that cover the scholarly output of the health sciences. Some are freely available on the Internet through government agencies, health organizations, and even commercial enterprises; others are restricted to individuals and/or institutions with subscription that are at times costly. Nonetheless, the highest quality health research is found in the published peer-reviewed primary and review literature among the journals and literature databases that cover them. Literature databases are indices (now almost exclusively Web-based) of journal or magazine articles, containing citations, abstracts, and often either the full text of the articles indexed or links to the full text. So it is in the best interest of the researcher or clinician to commence with searches in core databases. The two most familiar literature databases are Medline (PubMed) and CINAHL. Certainly, these databases are the best starting point for both clinical and research topics in the health sciences. For a list of core database descriptions and features, see Table 2.1.

There are other large databases, however, with specific content that might be useful, if not integral, to the searcher depending on the topic.

Table 2.1

## SELECTED CORE LITERATURE DATABASES

| | COVERAGE | PUBLICATION TYPES | FEATURES | FINDING REVIEWS |
|---|---|---|---|---|
| **CINAHL** (http://www.cinahl.com) | Comprehensive source for nursing & allied health journals, providing coverage of 1,000 journals along with 80 other publication types | Systematic Reviews Guidelines Primary Literature Dissertations Book and Book Chapters Audiovisual Pamphlet Etc. | Controlled Vocabulary (CINAHL Headings) Explode Major Concept Allows Boolean Limits | Use the Systematic Review publication-type limit or the Evidence-Based Practice special-interest filter |
| **Cochrane Central Register of Controlled Trials (CENTRAL)** (http://www.cochrane.org) | Includes citations and summaries culled from literature databases and other published and unpublished sources used to create Cochrane Reviews | Primary Literature | Controlled Vocabulary (MeSH) Allows Boolean | NA |
| **Cochrane Database of Systematic Reviews** (http://www.cochrane.org) | Includes ~5,000 reviews and protocols involving therapy and prevention in all areas of health care | Systematic Reviews Protocols (detailed plan to create a systematic review) | Controlled Vocabulary (MeSH) Allows Boolean Limits (Systematic Review or Protocol) | If available, use the Restrict to Reviews limit |

| Database | Description | Content | Features | Tips |
| --- | --- | --- | --- | --- |
| **Database of Abstracts of Reviews of Effects (DARE)** (http://www.crd.york.ac.uk/crdweb/) | Covers health related interventions and fields as diverse as diagnostic tests, public health, health promotion, pharmacology, surgery, psychology, and the organization and delivery of health care. Complements the Cochrane Database by including reviews not yet completed by the Cochrane Collaboration | Abstracts of Systematic Reviews | Controlled Vocabulary (MeSH) Allows Boolean Can Restrict Searches by: author, title, record type, language, publisher name, country | All contents are reviews |
| **Medline (PubMed)** (http://www.pubmed.gov) | Largest health database, covering more than 5,000 journals in all areas of the health sciences | Systematic Reviews Guidelines Primary Literature | Controlled Vocabulary (MeSH) Explode Focus Allows Boolean Limits Filters (Clinical Queries) | Use Clinical Queries: Systematic Review filter or the Systematic Reviews subset limit |

For instance, EMBASE, a large international health database, contains unique global literature, particularly in the drug-related fields; ERIC (Education Resources Information Center) should be tapped to find evidence to answer education questions; and PsycINFO, as its name implies, has strong coverage in the psychology literature. Table 2.2 lists secondary databases that may include worthwhile content to complement the core databases.

## Speak the Database Language

Nurses have identified a lack of searching skills as a barrier to evidence-based practice (Melnyk et al., 2004; Pravikoff et al., 2005). Therefore, it is essential that database users develop a skill set to gain confidence and search efficiently. This chapter will proceed with a discussion of some of the basic search concepts and tools that all searchers should exploit. However, a session at a health library or institution, a consultation with a librarian, or even a few moments spent reviewing resource-specific help and tutorials might pay great dividends if the resource is central to the topic.

The terms chosen for a topic often have a significant bearing on the quality of the results. Terminology in the health science literature is replete with synonyms (different words, same definition) and homonyms (same word, different definition). When a searcher enters terms into a search box of a literature database, challenging decisions need to be made regarding the selection of appropriate terms for the concepts to be searched. For example, the concept *cancer* can be entered in a database as *cancer, tumor, malignancy, neoplasm, mass,* and so on.

In some cases, using common or everyday language is effective and appropriate. This is called *free-text* or *keyword* searching. However, searching with terms offered from database-specific thesauri, often referred to as *controlled vocabularies,* often proves the best way to improve the breadth and accuracy of the retrieval set.

## Search Using Keywords

Keyword (free-text, natural language, common language) searches are the most common form of text search on the Internet (e.g., Google), and all literature databases also allow searchers to place basic terms into search boxes. Keyword searches are by nature fairly restrictive, as records retrieved by the database must have the exact term(s) entered in the search box. For example, if an author of an article uses the term *ascorbic*

Table 2.2

## SELECTED PERIPHERAL LITERATURE DATABASES

| DATABASES | COVERAGE |
|---|---|
| **Allied & Complementary Medicine Database** (http://www.bl.uk/collections/health/amed.html) | AMED covers references to articles from around 596 journals, in three separate subject areas: professions allied to medicine, complementary medicine, and palliative care. The scope of coverage is mainly European. |
| **British Nursing Index** (http://www.bniplus.co.uk/) | From the partnership of Bournemouth University, Poole Hospital NHS Trust, Salisbury Hospital NHS Trust, and the Royal College of Nursing, BNI covers 200 journal titles from all the major British nursing and midwifery titles and other English-language titles. |
| **EMBASE** (http://www.embase.com) | EMBASE is a large international biomedical and pharmacological database containing more than 11 million records from 5,000 biomedical journals from 70 countries. EMBASE features good coverage of Drug Research, Pharmacology, Pharmacy, Pharmacoeconomics, Pharmaceutics and Toxicology, Human Medicine (Clinical and Experimental), Basic Biological Research, Health Policy and Management, Public, Occupational and Environmental Health, Substance Dependence and Abuse, Psychiatry, Forensic Science, and Biomedical Engineering and Instrumentation. |
| **ERIC** (http://www.eric.ed.gov/) | Sponsored by the U.S. Department of Education, ERIC provides free access to more than 1.2 million records of journal articles from 600 + journals and other education-related materials and, if available, includes links to full text. |
| **Maternity and Infant Care Database** (http://www.midirs.org/) | MIC contains more than 120,000 references with abstracts to journal articles from more than 550 international English-language journals, books, and grey literature relating to the midwifery profession, pregnancy, labor, birth, postnatal care, and neonatal care and the first year of an infant's life. Journals indexed in the database are international from the United States and Canada, Europe, Australia/New Zealand, the United Kingdom, Africa, and the Middle East. In addition, grey literature is covered, such as pamphlets, reports, Web journals, press releases, newspaper articles, and chapters in books. |
| **PsycINFO** (http://www.apa.org/psycinfo/) | Produced by the American Psychological Association, PsycINFO provides abstracts and citations of the literature in the behavioral sciences and mental health. All levels of the evidential literature are included, so use the methodology limit: Systematic Review and/or Meta-Analysis. |

*acid* and the searcher enters *Vitamin C*, the searcher will retrieve only the articles with the term *Vitamin C*, not those with *ascorbic acid.*

Keyword searches can be used to find good information on a topic and are appropriate in certain circumstances. Experts often begin the process of searching a database by entering a few important keywords to obtain a quick and dirty initial retrieval set. This set is then perused to better focus a more formal search strategy, as well as to uncover any appropriate terms needed to refine the query.

Although the use of keywords may not be the best way to search a given resource (see the next section, Search Using a Controlled Vocabulary), there are techniques that will help you improve the results of your search. *Truncation,* also called stemming, allows searching for various word endings and spellings of a keyword term simultaneously. Databases that allow truncation designate database-specific characters, or wildcards, to initiate the truncation feature. The asterisk (*) and question mark (?) are commonly used wildcards. For example, a search in PubMed using the keyword *communit** will retrieve records with the terms *community, communities, communitarian, communitarians,* and much more. Some resources also allow for internal (wom?n) or beginning truncation ($natal). *Phrase searching* is a good way to search for specific phrases or words that are unusually formed. Many resources allow a searcher to place brackets, parentheses, or quotes (depending on the resource) around a phrase; only the results with a phrase matching all of the words enclosed in brackets are considered a match. This modification can reduce irrelevant results by requiring that the component words appear consecutively and in the order specified. For example, a search for *community acquired pneumonia* will find only results containing that exact string of words.

## Search Using a Controlled Vocabulary

A *controlled vocabulary* is a carefully selected, standardized list of terms, or thesaurus, that indexers (librarians who review individual articles before including them in a database) use to determine the major and minor topics discussed in the article. These terms may or may not be the same words the author uses to describe his or her writings, but they are placed within the database record. Therefore, a searcher using a controlled term will retrieve an article if the concept is covered by an author regardless of the ambiguity of terms. Many studies have shown that utilizing a controlled term improves searches in both size and accuracy. Be aware that not all health databases use a controlled vocabulary system, and, even in databases that do, it takes time to incorporate a new concept or term into its thesaurus. For example, the term *AIDS* was coined in 1981, but it took two years before it was introduced into Medline's Medical Subject Heading (MeSH) thesaurus. In these cases, a searcher must resort to a keyword search.

There are many examples of a controlled vocabulary in the health literature, and many are database specific:

- MeSH (*Medical Subject Headings*) is the National Library of Medicine's thesaurus for Medline's (PubMed) controlled vocabulary. MeSH is a hierarchy of more than 25,000 descriptive terms covering virtually all medical concepts.
- The CINAHL database uses a different set of controlled vocabulary, named CINAHL Subject Headings. Although CINAHL Subject Headings follow the structure of MeSH, they were developed to reflect the terminology used by nursing and the allied health professionals. This controlled-vocabulary thesaurus should be used when searching the CINAHL database.

Some databases have addressed the ease, as well as the problems, associated with keyword searches by developing a built-in term mapping system where free-text terms are matched against a controlled-vocabulary translation table. For example, although Medline's MeSH list includes 45,000 terms, another 200,000 synonyms are included in the translation table. So a search with term *Vitamin C* will be matched (and searched) with the proper MeSH term, *ascorbic acid*. Although this can be reliable for many common health terms, not all have such straightforward and successful mapping.

## Explode and Focus Terms

The subject headings of a controlled vocabulary are often presented in a hierarchical structure. For example, in Medline's MeSH thesaurus, the term *Depressive Disorder* is presented alongside broader and narrower terms:

Mood Disorders

Affective Disorders, Psychotic

**Depressive Disorder**

Depression, Postpartum

Depressive Disorder, Major

Dysthymic Disorder

Seasonal Affective Disorder

Many databases allow searchers to *explode* subject headings. This tells the database to search for the requested subject heading, as well as any more specific or narrower terms that are related to the topic. In Medline, a search query with the exploded MeSH term *Depressive Disorder* will search not only the MeSH term *Depressive Disorder* but also the terms *Depression, Postpartum Depressive Disorder, Major Dysthymic Disorder,* and *Seasonal Affective Disorder.*

The *focus* (e.g., major concepts) command instructs the database to retrieve only those articles in which the subject term selected is considered to be a primary focus of the article. This command narrows your search by eliminating articles that discuss the topic of the subject heading only peripherally.

## Combine Concepts (Boolean Operators)

Boolean logic defines the relationship between terms in a search. There are three Boolean operators: AND, OR, NOT. Database searchers can use these operators to create broader or narrower searches:

- *AND* combines search terms so that each search result contains all of the terms. The *AND* operator is generally placed between different concepts. For example, the search *St Johns Wort AND Depression* will retrieve articles that contain both terms *St Johns Wort* and *Depression.*
- *OR* combines search terms so that each search result contains at least one of the terms. The *OR* operator is generally placed between synonyms of the same concept. For example, *St Johns Wort OR Hypericum* retrieves results that contain either term, *St Johns Wort* or *Hypericum.*
- *NOT* excludes terms so that each search result does not contain any of the terms that follow it. For example, *St Johns Wort NOT*

*Adolescent* will retrieve results that contain the term *St Johns Wort* but not the term *Adolescent.* Searches should use the *NOT* operator with caution, since it may exclude relevant results with only a passing mention of the term *NOTed* out.

For more efficient searching using Boolean operators, parentheses can be used to nest search terms within other search terms. By nesting terms, searchers can specify the order in which the database interprets the search. It is generally recommended that synonyms (that is, terms *ORed* together) should be nested; an example is *(St Johns Wort OR hypericum) AND (depression OR depressive disorder).*

## Advanced Versus Basic Search Modes

Several resources offer the searcher an option of using a *basic* search interface with limited and rudimentary options for conducting and refining a search or a more *advanced* mode that provides more sophisticated search features and allows searchers to employ many of the techniques discussed in this section. The advanced search mode is the only choice for earnest researchers.

## Utilize Filters and Limits

To aid in retrieval relevancy and precision, databases may offer options to filter or to limit searches by certain parameters. Several databases have devised valuable and effective filters for researchers and clinicians specifically to help them find the evidence to answer clinical questions. One example is PubMed's *Clinical Queries,* which offers two essential built-in evidence-based medicine search filters: *Find Systematic Reviews,* which restricts the retrieval set to systematic reviews, meta analyses, reviews of clinical trials, guidelines, and consensus development conferences, and *Search by Clinical Study Category,* which restricts the retrieval set to top-level evidence for single trials and studies on a topic (e.g., randomized controlled trials for therapy scenarios). Other examples include the *Evidence-Based Practice* special-interest limit or the *Systematic Review* publication-type limit within CINAHL. Both can be particularly helpful in finding the best evidence on a topic.

There are also many limits available in most literature databases. However, searchers must be careful in applying limits, especially if a comprehensive or exhaustive search of the literature is warranted. Common limits include:

- Date—Allows searchers to restrict the publication dates of the articles retrieved. Keep in mind that newer literature is not always better.
- Language—Articles from many countries and languages are included in databases, so it may be helpful to limit the results of a search to a specific language.
- Publication type—Journal articles are not created equal. Case reports, cohort studies, controlled trials, editorials, systematic reviews, comments, practice guidelines, audiovisuals, book chapters, dissertations, and so on are found in the journal literature.
- Age—Some databases offer limits by specific age groups. For example, by selecting the *All Infant* limit in CINAHL or Medline, you can retrieve articles concerning this age range.
- Full-text—Most databases include a small selection of free full-text (entire) articles. Use of the full-text limit will restrict the results to only items that include, or provide links to, the full text. This limit tends to greatly reduce the search results and gives no guarantee of the quality of the items retrieved. In addition, many health organizations, centers, and academic institutions, have the ability to embed a much larger set of full-text content into a database that will not be picked up by the generic full-text limit. If the purpose of your search is to produce a systematic review, you should not use this limit. If the purpose is only to obtain a quick grasp of a clinical problem, this route might be useful.

## Phase III: Beyond the Literature Databases: Mining the Internet

*Target Health Web Sites for Guidelines, Reviews, and Reports*

There are plenty of quality health-related Web sites that provide information that both researchers and clinicians should target. It is essential to venture beyond the literature databases to find guidelines, reports, consensus statements, and other documents not necessarily published in the commercial literature. Table 2.3 presents a selective list of valuable sites for evidence-based practice.

Table 2.3

## SELECT EXAMPLES OF WEB SITES

| WEB SITE | NOTES |
|---|---|
| **ACP Clinical Practice Guidelines** (http://www.acponline. org/clinical_information/ guidelines/) | ACP Clinical Practice Guidelines cover many areas of internal medicine, including screening for cancer or other major diseases, diagnosis, treatment, and medical technology. Guidelines are created following a rigorous development process and are based on the highest quality scientific evidence. |
| **Agency for Healthcare Research and Quality Evidence Based Practice Centers** (http://www.ahrq.gov/clinic/ epcix.htm) | A collection of high-quality reports, reviews, and technology assessments based on rigorous, comprehensive syntheses and analyses of the scientific literature on topics relevant to clinical, social science/behavioral, economic, and other health care organization and delivery issues. |
| **Agency for Healthcare Research and Quality U.S. Preventive Services Task Force** (http://www.ahrq.gov/clinic/ uspstfix.htm) | The U.S. Preventive Services Task Force is an independent panel of experts in primary care and prevention that systematically reviews the evidence of effectiveness and develops recommendations for clinical preventive services. |
| **American Heart Association Scientific Statements and Guidelines** (http://www.americanheart. org/presenter.jhtml? identifier=9181) | A collection of AHA's scientific statements and practice guidelines that are published in *Circulation; Stroke; Arteriosclerosis, Thrombosis, and Vascular Biology; Hypertension; Circulation Research,* and other journals. |
| **Bandolier** (http://www.ebandolier.com) | A quirky, independent online electronic journal and database written by Oxford University scientists. Each month PubMed and the Cochrane Library are searched for systematic reviews and meta-analyses, and the reviews that look interesting are read and discussed in bullet points in Bandolier, first in the paper version and, after six months, on the Web site. |
| **CMA Infobase** (http://mdm.ca/cpgsnew/ cpgs/index.asp) | Guidelines produced or endorsed in Canada by a national, provincial/territorial, or regional medical or health organization, professional society, government agency, or expert panel. |
| **The Community Guide** (http://www.thecommunity guide.org/) | Developed by the nonfederal Task Force on Community Preventive Services, whose members are appointed by the Director of the Centers for Disease Control and Prevention (CDC), the Community Guide summarizes what is known about the effectiveness, economic efficiency, and feasibility of interventions |

*(Continued)*

Table 2.3

## SELECT EXAMPLES OF WEB SITES (CONTINUED)

| WEB SITE | NOTES |
|---|---|
| **Infectious Diseases Society of America Practice Guidelines** (http://www.idsociety.org/ Content.aspx?id=9088) | Includes standards, practice guidelines, and statements developed and/or endorsed by IDSA. |
| **Institute for Clinical Systems Improvement** (http://www.icsi.org/ guidelines_and_more/) | ICSI is a collaboration by medical groups, hospitals, and health plans that provide health care services to people who live and work in the state of Minnesota and in adjacent areas of surrounding states. Included on the Web site are guidelines, order sets, protocols, guideline impact studies, patient education resources, and technology assessment reports. |
| **The Joanna Briggs Institute** (http://www.joannabriggs. edu.au/about/home.php) | JBI is an initiative of Royal Adelaide Hospital and the University of Adelaide. The Institute provides "a collaborative approach to the evaluation of evidence derived from a diverse range of sources, including experience, expertise and all forms of rigorous research and the translation, transfer and utilization of the 'best available' evidence into health care practice." Many resources are available only to member institutions, although selected systematic reviews and best practices information sheets are available to nonmembers. |
| **National Cancer Institute Clinical Trials** (http://www.cancer.gov/ clinicaltrials) | Allows users to search browse recent clinical trial results by type of cancer or topic or to search NCI's list of thousands of clinical trials now accepting participants. Also included are educational materials about clinical trials, a list of noteworthy clinical trials, and more information for research teams interested in conducting clinical trials. |
| **National Guidelines Clearinghouse** (http://www.guidelines. gov/) | Developed by the Department of Health and Human Services, the National Guideline Clearinghouse collects best-practice guidelines produced by medical facilities, agencies, and organizations around the world. The site is searchable by disease, and there is a guideline comparison tool that allows different guidelines for the same disease to be compared. Guidelines can be downloaded to a PDA. |

*(Continued)*

Table 2.3

## SELECT EXAMPLES OF WEB SITES (CONTINUED)

| WEB SITE | NOTES |
| --- | --- |
| **National Kidney Foundation** (http://www.kidney.org/ professionals/KDOQI/ guidelines.cfm) | The National Kidney Foundation Web site includes 20+ clinical practice guidelines published under NKF's KDOQI brand. All guidelines follow the rigorous KDOQI process, are developed by independent volunteer work groups, and are funded by more than a dozen companies within the kidney disease field. |
| **Netting the Evidence** (http://www.shef.ac.uk/ scharr/ir/netting/) | A multipurpose Web site that provides support and access to evidence-based medicine organizations and learning resources, such as an evidence-based virtual library, software, and journals. |
| **SUMSearch** (http://sumsearch.uthscsa. edu/) | A free meta-search engine for evidence-based medical information, scanning databases (Medline, DARE, and National Guidelines Clearinghouse), as well as various high-impact medical journals. To automate searching, SUMSearch combines meta- and contingency searching. Meta-searching is designed to scan multiple databases and sites simultaneously and returns one single retrieval document to the user. If a high number of results are obtained, more restrictive searches (called contingency searches) are conducted by activating additional filters. Conversely, if the result is small, more databases are added to the search. |
| **TRIP** (http://tripdatabase.com) | A free meta-search engine that aims to provide quick access to a collection of evidence-based and other high-quality medical information resources via a single interface. TRIP identifies and searches numerous high-quality Internet resources that allow access to their content, such as Medline, Cochrane, National Guidelines Clearinghouse, ACP Journal Club, and top peer-reviewed journals. These resources are then categorized by type: Evidence-Based Synopses, Clinical Questions, Systematic Reviews, Guidelines, Core Primary Research, E-textbooks, and Calculators. |

Some sites look and act much like commercial literature databases and provide access to information created by others (called meta-sites). *TRIP Database*, for example, is a sophisticated tool, that searches 150 evidence-based resources (in addition to the millions of articles in Medline) and more than 80,000 other documents, including, reviews and guidelines. *SUMSearch* also searches the Internet for evidence-based medical information by scanning literature databases and high-impact medical journals and employs a unique method of searching and filtering for the best results.

Whereas large meta-sites include citations from a wide variety of documents, others are designated as repositories for specific publication types. Practice guidelines are valuable components in the delivery of evidence-based health care practice. Therefore, clinicians and researchers should have some familiarly with sites focusing on guidelines, such as *National Guidelines Clearinghouse* (NGC).

Government agencies and professional associations that have developed clinical guidelines may include them on their Web sites. For example, the *National Kidney Foundation* Web site offers a collection of its published K/DOQI guidelines.

Web sites of health agencies and associations organized around specific diseases or conditions also frequently post valuable reviews, reports, and studies that may or may not be included in the pages of journals. For example, the Web site for the *Agency for Healthcare Research and Quality* delivers agency-funded evidence-based research reports on health care outcomes, quality, and cost, use, and access. The *National Cancer Institute* and the *National Kidney Foundation* Web sites list summaries of recently released results from clinical trials.

## Search the Whole Internet

There is never one perfect location to find information on a health topic. Some people quickly turn to the ease of the Internet as a starting place, which can be quite useful if you know where to look or how to search for pertinent and reliable information, as we have seen. There are benefits to exploring a topic on the Internet as a complement to a formal search within relevant literature databases; Web sites are often very current. The capability for "publishers," whether they are health care institutions, corporate entities, government agencies, or even individuals, to quickly and inexpensively publish permits immediate information transfer to the Internet user. This also allows groups to distribute potentially important relevant information that may go unpublished through commercial channels. This type of literature is often referred to as the *grey literature.* Examples include scientific and technical reports, guidelines, care plans, patent documents, conference papers, internal reports, government documents, newsletters, fact sheets and theses.

The information available via the Internet is neither trustworthy nor well organized. There are numerous popular search engines that scour the Web to retrieve materials that match keywords entered in the search box. These search engines use specific algorithms to sort retrieved results. In many cases, order depends on a mixture of keyword matches, currency, and other factors (not necessarily quality of content). To eliminate some of the vagaries of Internet searching, there are techniques to improve the quality and reliability of the retrieval. First is to try a selective search engine. A good example of a selective multidisciplinary search engine is *Google Scholar* (http://scholar.google.org), which restricts an Internet search to "scholarly" publications such as journal articles, technical reports, preprints, theses, books, and vetted Web pages from academic publishers, professional societies, preprint repositories, universities, and other scholarly organizations. Another good technique is to look for and use an *advanced search* option, which may offer numerous options for making searches more precise and getting more reliable results. Additional approaches that promote the retrieval of pertinent information are presented in Exhibit 2.4.

Exhibit 2.4

### STRATEGIES TO DETERMINE WEB SITE QUALITY

1. Read through the web pages associated with the site, looking for the credentials of the author and identification of the site sponsor.
2. Look for the date when the page was produced or revised.
3. View the HTML or page source of Web pages to look for author identification and/or publication date.
4. If you are not already knowledgeable about the topic, ask someone who is to review the information.
5. Find reviews of Internet resources by reviewers in reputable print and online sources, or use selective subject directory/electronic library collections you trust to identify resources.
6. Go to related sites you trust to see whether there is a link to the site you are questioning.
7. Email the person or organization identified as responsible and ask them about their credentials (Kovacs & Carlson, 2000).

## Be Aware of Emerging Resources

Searching for, perusing, and validating either the review or the primary literature found in these databases takes skill and precious time. New practical resources to support evidence-based decisions are becoming readily available to practitioners. *Clinical Summary Databases* (CSDs) are designed to act as a quick, single-stop, point-of-care tool that connects the health practitioner to the current knowledge of a condition or treatment. The best CSDs summarize current high-quality research for answers to specific clinical questions, often adding practice implications specifically supported by a rationale and pertinent, current evidence. The centerpiece of these products includes hundreds of entries on the treatment and prevention of medical conditions, which are developed from synthesized information obtained by searching quality evidence-based medicine resources and health-related literature databases. Creation of these entries is generally overseen by recognized experts and clinical specialists. Most CSDs tend to be updated monthly, although some are updated quarterly and insert news items and urgent updates as needed. Although there is great variation in searchability, most interfaces offer browsable tables of contents and rudimentary search boxes; some include means to target or narrow search results. Examples of CSDs are listed in Table 2.4.

Most researchers and clinicians commonly scan a fairly narrow set of journals to find articles of interest. To broaden their radar, readers should consider utilizing specialty resources that survey large sets of journals in selected disciplines. These *surveillance tools* summarize important

Table 2.4

### CLINICAL SUMMARY DATABASE EXAMPLES

- **NursingConsult (Evidence-Based Practice Section)**
  (http://www.nursingconsult.com/)
- **UptoDate**
  (http://uptodate.com)
- **BMJ's Clinical Evidence**
  (http://clinicalevidence.bmj.com/)
- **DynaMed**
  (http://www.ebscohost.com/dynamed/)
- **ACP PIER**
  (http://pier.acponline.org/index.html)

articles that warrant the attention of their readership. In general, editors associated with these resources scan the health literature (often hundreds of journals) and highlight published topic reviews and individual studies from prominent journals. With few exceptions, reviews or studies that appear in these sources are sound and have met established quality criteria. Much like the clinical databases, these resources boil down lengthy systematic reviews and detailed studies to a consumable package of value added information. Selected examples of sources that provide this service are listed in Table 2.5.

## Phase IV: Pulling It All Together

The search for evidence does not end with successful retrieval from a database or Web site. The relevant information needs to be retained and organized for further analysis and full-text copies of articles, reports, and guidelines, and similar documents need to be tracked down and stored. In addition, any search queries used should be retained and available for future searches on the topic.

### Save Your Search Query

Experienced searchers are well aware of the benefits of saving database search queries at the conclusion of a search. One good motivation to do so is to prevent that sting of frustration when a search gets interrupted or misplaced and the entire search progression needs to be retraced. Another reason is simply to be in a position to quickly rerun a search at designated intervals to keep atop of the literature on the particular topic.

Table 2.5

**CLINICAL SUMMARY DATABASE EXAMPLES**

- **Evidence-Based Nursing**
  (http://ebn.bmj.com/)
- **ACP Journal Club**
  (http://www.acpjc.org/)
- **bmjupdates+**
  (http://www.bmjupdates.com/)
- **Essential Evidence Plus: Daily POEMs**
  (http://essentialevidenceplus.com)

As a valuable convenience, databases now allow users to create individual accounts that retain user information, search queries, and search results. MyNCBI (PubMed) and My EBSCOhost are examples of user-created personal accounts within databases.

## Invest in a Citation Manager

Databases allow searchers to output their retrieval sets in a variety of displays and a range of output formats. The most common display options are normally citation only, citation with abstract, or full record, which includes descriptors, accession numbers, and other useful data. Databases also offer different output options so that material can be saved as a text file or a Microsoft Word file, preserved in an e-mail, or sent to a printer. Web sites, on the other hand, give virtually no output choice other than the browser-supported PRINT and SAVE AS options.

The most efficient researcher, however, will enlist the help of commercial software called a *citation manager* to transfer, store, and manage the bibliographic references and citations retrieved from databases or Web sites. Commonly used citation managers in the health sciences include:

- EndNote (http://www.endnote.com)
- Reference Manager (http://wwwrefman.com/)
- Pro-Cite (http:///www.procite.com/)
- RefWorks (http:.refworks.com)
- Zotero (http;//www.zotero.org/)
- CiteULike (http://citeulike.org/)

These products consist of a database in which full bibliographic citations (e.g., abstracts, subject headings) can be entered or imported, as well as a system for generating selective lists or articles in the different formats required by publishers. Citation managers can be integrated with word processors so that a list of citations in the appropriate format (e.g., MLA, APA) is produced automatically as an article is written. There are many citation managers available on the market and the best of them allow:

- Direct export from online databases such as Medline, CINAHL, PsycINFO, and ERIC into the citation manager.
- Folders and subfolder organization of citations

- Output to formatted bibliographies in all major styles (e.g., MLA, APA)
- Automatic integration with word processor formats (e.g., Microsoft Word, RTF, HTML)
- Items (e.g., image files, Adobe PDFs, Microsoft Word docs) to be attached to a citation within the database for opening at a later time

## Find the Full Article (Full-Text)

One of the barriers to completing a successful review is simply getting one's hands on the full-text article or report. Access to full-text articles has improved dramatically with the growth of electronic publishing; yet, this usually remains a multistep process. The majority of databases and Web sites tend to provide only citations to (and often abstracts of) items of interest, but the entire articles are not always immediately available online. Certain databases are making an effort to assist the user by allowing publishers and academic institutions to insert buttons within item records to lead users to the full article. Keep in mind that commercial and academic publishers charge fees, some exorbitant, to grant access to a single article. A searcher may want to first contact a local clinic, hospital, academic, or even public library. Very often, libraries have established access to journal collections or offer interlibrary loan services. If none are available in your area, an inexpensive alternative is the National Library of Medicine's *Loansome Doc* service for ordering documents through PubMed.

*Keep up with the topic.* Keeping abreast of the published information on any given topic is no longer difficult. Several databases now offer *alert* or *current awareness* services that allow users automatically to receive new results (via e-mail) from saved search queries at prescribed intervals. Search queries can involve topics of interest or can pertain to specific authors or a set of relevant journals.

*RSS* (Really Simple Syndication) is an emerging technology that many predict will revolutionize the way researchers and clinicians retrieve information from favorite sources. RSS is more or less an electronic table-of-contents service where one can quickly scan the contents (called feeds) of any number of the latest journals, headlines from favorite news sources, news from relevant organizations, entries from blogs and Web sites, and even updates from literature searches at one location (called a feed reader) with no nagging e-mail clutter. There are many free feed readers available. Here are some selected examples:

- Google Reader (http://reader.google.com)
- Bloglines (http://bloglines.com)
- Sage (for Firefox Internet browser) (http://sage.mozdev.org)
- Thunderbird RSS (e-mail based) (http://www.mozilla.com/thunder bird/)

Most RSSs are Web-based, such as *Google Reader* or *Bloglines*. Others are browser-based. such as Mozilla Firefox's *Sage* or email-based, such as Mozilla's *Thunderbird RSS*. Getting started with RSS is relatively easy and is likely to become an indispensable tool for keeping a researcher or clinician current and for saving time.

## SUMMARY

In summary, literature reviews are not mysterious manifestations of scholarly pursuits. Nor should they be merely academic exercises. They are, and are increasingly being required, as a vital component of quality health care.

Literature reviews are the sum of many definable parts and the application of systematic procedures, as illustrated in this chapter, in four phases: (1) pre-search preparations and planning, (2) mining of major literature databases for evidence-based information, (3) mining of additional resources across the Internet, and (4) using new technologies to organize, store, and update found information. The process is unfolded to reveal a researcher's toolkit, which can be adapted to meet individual needs and the information demands of the current evidence-based research topic.

## SUGGESTED ACTIVITIES

You are planning to conduct a study to find out adherence of diabetic people to their diet. Do a literature search of articles published in the last 3 to 5 years to find out ways diabetics conform to their prescribed diets. Use two types of databases (e.g., CINAHL and Medline) to find articles that can be used for the background and significance of the topic.

Compare and contrast the types of articles you retrieve from CINAHL and from Medline.

## REFERENCES

Brancato, V. C. (2006). An innovative clinical practicum to teach evidence-based practice. *Nurse Educator, 31*(5), 195–199.

Dee, C., & Stanley, E. E. (2005). Information-seeking behavior of nursing students and clinical nurses: Implications for health sciences librarians. *Journal of the Medical Library Association, 93*(2), 213–222.

Downs, F. S. (1969). Some critical issues in nursing research. *Nursing Forum, 8*(4), 393–404.

Klein, G. A. (2003). *Intuition at work: Why developing your gut instincts will make you better at what you do* (1st ed.). New York: Currency/Doubleday.

Kovacs, D. K., & Carlson, A. L. (2000). *How to find medical information on the Internet: A print and online tutorial for the healthcare professional and consumer.* Berkeley, CA: Library Solutions Press.

Lyman, P., & Varian, H. R. (2003). *How much information? 2003* University of California-Berkeley. Retrieved February 21, 2008, from http://www.sims.berkeley.edu/how-much-info-2003

Mellon, C. A. (1984). Process not product in course-integrated instruction: A generic model of library research. *College & Research Libraries, 45*(6), 471.

Melnyk, B. M., Fineout-Overholt, E., Feinstein, N., Li, H., Small, L., Wilcox, L., et al. (2004). Nurses' perceived knowledge, belief, skills, and needs regarding evidence-based practice: Implications for accelerating the paradigm shift. *Worldviews on Evidence-Based Nursing, 1*(3), 185.

Mulrow, C. D. (1994). Rationale for systematic reviews. *BMJ (Clinical Research Ed.), 309*(6954), 597–599.

Polit, D. F., & Beck, C. T. (2008). *Nursing research: Generating and assessing evidence for nursing practice* (8th ed.). Philadelphia: Wolters Kluwer Health/Lippincott Williams & Wilkins.

Pravikoff, D. S., Tanner, A. B., & Pierce, S. T. (2005). Readiness of U.S. nurses for evidence-based practice. *The American Journal of Nursing, 105*(9), 40–51; quiz 52.

Skiba, D. J. (2005). Preparing for evidence-based practice: Revisiting information literacy. *Nursing Education Perspectives, 26*(5), 310–311.

Tanner, A., Pierce, S., & Pravikoff, D. (2004). Readiness for evidence-based practice: Information literacy needs of nurses in the United States. *Medinfo, 11*(Pt. 2), 936–940.

# 3

# Research and the Mandate for Evidence-Based Practice, Quality, and Patient Safety

KATHLEEN R. STEVENS, KATHERINE McDUFFIE, AND PAULA C. CLUTTER

The development of science for nursing and health care is a response to needs for knowledge to address the health of the public. The applied science of nursing has the ultimate aim of discovering effective interventions to resolve actual and potential health problems and to provide knowledge about effectiveness of interventions in producing desired health-related outcomes. Although nursing research has been well institutionalized since 1984, with the establishment of the NIH National Institute for Nursing Research (originally, National Center for Nursing Research), only in the recent past has health care's research interests swung dramatically to examine how to move research findings into practice. Not only is there public demand for moving new knowledge into practice, but also there is also demand for doing this in ways that increase quality and safety of care and increase the likelihood of realizing the intended health outcomes. In the past 5 years, research to build the science of quality and safety has grown.

This chapter presents events and findings that have influence on this new scientific interest in health care quality and safety. Included are descriptions of the underlying reasons for the new emphasis on quality and safety, frameworks for conceptualizing and studying quality and safety, methods used for such investigations, and new resources and future trends in quality and safety research.

**43**

chapter explores how evidence-based practice
ety in health care are reflected in nursing theory,
ce in meeting the mandate for quality and safety. To
ad context, our discussion first presents an overview of
ionship among research, EBP, quality, and safety, providing a
nework through which to view these facets of health care. Sections
of the chapter are devoted specifically to quality and to safety, highlighting the dominant thinking and research advances in each area. The
chapter concludes with a look to the future of quality and safety, examining recent advances and suggesting directions in theory, research, and
science.

## OVERVIEW: RESEARCH, EBP, QUALITY, AND SAFETY

Quality and safety are top priorities in contemporary health care. The
responsibility and accountability for ensuring effective and safe care are
inescapable for all health professionals and are a social obligation to every
health care agency. Delivering the right care at the right time in the right
setting is the goal of efforts to advance safety and quality. This challenge
requires that well-prepared nurses play key roles in moving research
into action to overhaul today's health care system.

For nurses to effectively guide the movement for quality and safety,
skills are required that reflect improvement science and principles of
high-reliability industries.

The morbidity and mortality toll of both ineffective care and unsafe
care requires that all health professionals take a serious look at what
must be done to address lapses in quality and to avoid the cost of hundreds of thousands of lives. To meet this challenge, it is vital to ensure
that health care is error free, that all existing best (research-based) practices are used, and that everyone implements the highest quality and
most reliable processes for every patient. The narrow notion of safety as
the absence of medication errors or falls has been broadened. This is the
challenge of quality and patient safety in health care. The foundation
of success is translation of research results into clinical care; the infrastructure of success is conducting research to elucidate change interventions that improve clinical care processes at the individual clinician,
organization, system, environment, and policy levels. Thus, research is
key to determining clinical effectiveness of care and translation is key to
redesigning health care systems that are safe and effective.

## SEVERE PROBLEMS IN HEALTH CARE QUALITY

Research has built a large body of science about "what works" in health care, yet actual care lags behind what has been reported be effective (Institute of Medicine [IOM], 2001). The end result is health care that is ineffective in producing intended patient health outcomes and care that is unsafe. These circumstances are prevalent in nursing and across all health professions. even though massive numbers of research reports provide "best evidence" for care. Health care processes and outcomes could be greatly improved if research results were put into practice.

## QUALITY AND EBP

The quality of health care is based on the degree to which decisions about patient care should are guided by "conscientious, explicit, and judicious use of current best evidence" (IOM, 2008, p. 3). The definition of health care quality emphasizes this point:

**Definition: Quality of Health Care**

Degree to which health services for individuals and populations increase the likelihood of desired health outcomes and are consistent with current professional knowledge. (IOM, 1990)

This definition makes clear that evidence is a core element in producing intended health outcomes. Unless patient care is based on the most current and best evidence, it falls short of quality.

The aim of EBP is to standardize health care practices to science and best evidence and to reduce illogical variation in care, which leads to unpredictable health outcomes. Development of evidence-based practice is fueled by public and professional demand for accountability in safety and quality improvement in health care. It is imperative that health care be based on current professional knowledge in order to produce the quality necessary for intended patient outcomes.

Leaders in the field have defined EBP as the "Integration of best research evidence with clinical expertise and patient values" (Sackett, Straus, Richardson, Rosenberg, & Haynes, 2000, p. ii). Therefore, EBP melds research evidence with clinical expertise and encourages individ-ualization of care through incorporation of patient preferences and the circumstances of the setting.

Just as evidence and quality are linked, so are safety and quality. The ties among safety, errors, quality, and caring are explained as concentric circles or subsets of a common flaw (Woolf, 2004). The innermost con-centric circle is safety, followed by errors, then quality, and, finally, caring as the outermost circle. The model suggests that safety is a subcategory of health care errors. Such errors include mistakes in health promotion and chronic disease management that cost lives but do not affect safety—these are errors of omission. Following this model, errors are a subset of quality lapses, which result from both errors and systemic problems. Sys-temic problems that reduce quality in health care may stem from lack of access, inequity, and flawed system designs. Finally, this model suggests that lapses in quality are a subset of deficient caring; such deficiencies can be seen in lack of access, inequity, and faulty system designs (Woolf, 2004). In nursing research, such a model can serve to frame investiga-tions of health care safety and quality.

Health care quality and safety emerged as a principal concern only recently. In 1990, interprofessional opinion leaders began an intensive initiative to improve the quality of health care (IOM, 1990). These lead-ers proclaimed that there is a chasm between what we *know* (through research) to be best health care and what we *do*. In a series of influen-tial reports, these national advisers called for one of our nation's most far-reaching health reforms, called the IOM Quality Initiative. A series of reports known as the *Quality Chasm Series* dissected health care problems and recommended fundamental and sweeping changes in health care (IOM, 2001). The directions set by the *Quality Chasm Series* continue to have marked impact on every aspect of health care. Each of the trend-setting IOM reports (2001, 2003a, 2003b, 2008) identifies evidence-based practice (EBP) as *crucial* in closing the quality chasm. This movement is likely to continue beyond the next decade. The follow-ing discussion summarizes the IOM reports.

In 2000, the Institute of Medicine (IOM) reviewed studies and trends and concluded that 48,000 to 98,000 Americans die annually in hospitals due to medical errors caused by defective systems rather than caregivers themselves. *To Err Is Human* (IOM, 2000) offered impres-sive documentation regarding the severity and pervasive nature of the nation's overall quality problem. In fact, using statistical approaches, the report documented that more people die from medical mistakes each year than from highway accidents, breast cancer, or AIDS. In addition to deaths, it was noted that medical errors cause permanent disabilities and unnecessary suffering. This report raised the issue of patient safety to high priority for every health care provider, scientist, agency leader, and policymaker.

The next report in this series further unfolded the story of quality in American health care. In *Crossing the Quality Chasm: A New Health System for the 21st Century* (IOM, 2001), health care leaders reviewed research that highlighted other widespread defects in our health care system. Defects included overuse, misuse, and underuse of health care services and described a wide gulf between ideal care (as supported by research) and the reality of the care that many Americans experience. The *Quality Chasm* report presented research evidence documenting a lack of quality in health care, cost concerns, poor use of information technology, absence of progress in restructuring the health care system, and underutilization of resources. Throughout these analyses of health care safety and quality, a deep-rooted problem was highlighted: While health science and technology were advancing at a rapid pace, the health care delivery system were failing to deliver high-quality health care services (IOM, 2001). The reports emphasized that a major part of the problem is that research results are not translated into practice and that practice lags behind research-generated knowledge.

The profession of nursing is central to many of the interprofessional and discipline-specific changes that must be accomplished to provide safe and effective care. The Interdisciplinary Nursing Quality Research Initiative (INQRI) supported by Robert Wood Johnson Foundation funded studies to discover how nurses contribute to and can improve the quality of patient care (RWJF, 2008).

Since the purpose of research ultimately is to uncover causal relationships, the primary goal is to determine which interventions are most effective in assisting patients and clients to resolve actual and potential health problems. In other words, research shows us "what works" best to produce the intended health outcome for a given health problem. Knowledge discovered through research is then translated into practice guidelines and ultimately affects health policy through commonly accepted health care practices.

## NURSING, RESEARCH UTILIZATION, AND EBP

In health professions, research is conducted to build a case for specific practices and interventions. Since the very reason for conducting research is to illuminate effective (best) practices, then it follows that research must be translated into clinical decision making at the point of care. Although this goal is clear, nurses have struggled to achieve research utilization since the 1970s.

Nursing has struggled with ways to move research results into practice; however, early attempts were not fully successful. Barriers to knowledge translation became a crucial topic of investigation in nursing in the early 1990s. A number of research utilization models were developed to explain the barriers and challenges in applying research results in practice. One program of study established a dissemination model (Funk, Tornquist, & Champagne, 1989) and developed a scale with which to quantify nurses' perception of barriers to applying research in practice (Funk, Champagne, Wiese, & Tornquist, 1990). Still widely used today, the BARRIERS scale is framed in the old paradigm of research utilization, in which results of a single study were examined for direct application, and clinical nurses were expected to read, critique, and translate primary research reports into point of care practice, and to devote time to these activities.

This early work in research utilization resulted in a clearer focus on clinical investigations. Nurse scientists who conducted research, largely in academic settings, were criticized for their shortcomings in making research results clinically meaningful. Such criticism included claims that research did not address pressing clinical problems, results were not expressed in terms understood by clinicians, and clinicians were not in positions to apply the results in care. In tandem, nurse scientists gathered momentum to establish what is today the National Institute for Nursing Research, dedicated to funding clinical research.

Initial research utilization models were developed prior to the emergence of EBP. The Stetler model (Stetler, 1994) mapped a step-by-step approach that could be used by individual clinicians to critique research, restate findings, and consider the findings in their own decision making. The model focuses on a bottom-up approach to change in clinical practice. The Iowa Model outlined a process to guide implementation of research results into clinical practice in context of provider, patient, and infrastructure (Titler et al., 2001). The Iowa Model gives heavy emphasis to nurse managers as key instruments of change. Both models have moved from their original roots in research utilization to reflect a broader approach used in EBP. These early efforts underscored the importance of moving research into direct patient care.

## SHIFT FROM RESEARCH UTILIZATION TO EBP

Frequently, research results are either inadequately translated into clinical practice recommendations or applied inconsistently in the delivery of health care. Additionally, poor health care system design contributes to the chasm; health care design inadequacies include a lack of interprofessional teams to provide comprehensive and coordinated care and a complex system that is a maze to patients and that fails to provide to patients the services from which they would likely benefit (IOM, 2001).

As growth in the EBP movement grew, it became apparent that the hurdles to translating research to practice required complex answers not yet discovered. The EBP movement has provided new scientific means with which to overcome these hurdles.

Until recently, much importance in the use of research was placed on what it was we *did not know,* and this became the basis for the clinician's action: designing and conducting research studies. In the EBP approach to the use of research, the knowledge itself has become the basis for action: improving care processes and outcomes with knowledge about clinical effectiveness. In EBP, the importance is placed on what we *do know* and on increasing the clinical utility and usefulness of the knowledge. It became clear that knowledge transformation must occur as research results are translated into practice (Stevens, 2004).

As the health care quality paradigm shifted to evidence-based practice, additional hurdles in transforming research results into common practice became apparent. Evidence-based practice approaches, derived from clinical epidemiology, provided new insights and changed the paradigm for thinking about translating research. With the paradigm shift, hurdles became apparent. Two primary hurdles include (a) the large volume and complexity of health research literature and (b) the low clinical utility of the form of knowledge that is available to the clinician (Stevens, 2004). The EBP movement offers techniques to overcome these two hurdles, including the transformation of knowledge reflected in the ACE Star Model: evidence summary, translation into clinical guidelines, integration into practice, and evaluation of outcomes and impact (Stevens, 2004).

### Evidence Summary

To overcome the hurdle posed by the large volume of research, a new approach was developed in the mid-1990s. The most rigorous scientific method for synthesizing all research into a single summary is called a *systematic review*. A systematic review is defined as a scientific investigation that focuses on a specific question and uses explicitly, preplanned scientific methods to identify, select, assess, and summarize similar but separate studies.

These EBP approaches produce a concise and comprehensible statement about the state of the science regarding clinical effectiveness. The new research method, systematic review, is the keystone to understanding whether a clinical intervention works (IOM, 2008). Indeed, it is now known that an evidence summary is requisite to "getting the evidence [about intervention effectiveness] straight" (Glasziou & Haynes, 2005). The sobering flip-side of this logic is that *not* conducting an evidence summary (*not* getting the evidence straight) leads to a misinformed clinical decision. Nursing care must be driven by research evidence—not knowing the state of the science about clinical effectiveness results in ineffective, unnecessary, or harmful care. From EBP, we now realize that basing care on results of a single primary research study can lead to the selection of a wrong intervention. With this new realization, we have moved away from using single research studies to change practice to a much more rigorous knowledge form—the evidence summary.

Systematic reviews (SRs) serve two important knowledge functions in health care. First, a systematic review provides evidence about the clinical effectiveness of a particular intervention in relation to specified outcomes. Second, a systematic review provides a view of gaps in the scientific field and points to further research needed to fill these voids. A prime advantage of an evidence summary, such as a systematic review, is that all research results on a given topic are transformed into a single, harmonious statement (Mulrow, 1994). In this way, the state of the science on a given topic is placed at the fingertips of the clinician in terms of what is known and what remains to be discovered. With regard to providing evidence-based direction for clinical care, a systematic review offers other advantages (Mulrow 1994) as outlined in Exhibit 3.1.

## Guidelines

The next stage of knowledge transformation is in the form of the evidence-based clinical practice guidelines (CPGs). To overcome low point-of-care use of research, evidence-based clinical practice guidelines are used to translate the evidence summary into recommendations for clinical practice. Clinical practice guidelines are defined as "systematically defined

Exhibit 3.1

## ADVANTAGES OF A SYSTEMATIC REVIEW

1. Reduces information into a manageable form
2. Increases power in cause and effect
3. Assesses consistencies across studies
4. Integrates information for decisions
5. Establishes generalizability—participants, settings, treatment variations, study designs
6. Reduces bias and improves true reflection of reality
7. Reduces time between research and implementation
8. Offers basis for continuous update as new knowledge is discovered
9. Points to further research to address gaps

Adapted from "Rationale for Systematic Reviews," by C. Mulrow, 1994, *British Medical Journal, 309,* pp. 597–599.

statements that are designed to help clinicians and patients make decisions about appropriate health care for specific clinical circumstances" (IOM, 1990, p. 38). The utility of CPGs is enhanced by inclusion of specification and rating of supporting evidence. Evidence-based CPGs have the potential to reduce illogical variations in practice by encouraging use of clinically effective practices.

## Integration

Once the evidence is straight-through summaries and guidelines, it becomes necessary to introduce the evidence-based practice into ongoing care. The challenges of changing the provider's practices are many and complex. New approaches to studying organizational change, complex adaptive systems, and culture shifts are adding to our understanding of the challenge of integration. Research will fill the gap in what we know about "getting the straight evidence used" (Glasziou & Haynes, 2005) in practice.

## Evaluation

Once integrated, the practice change is evaluated for its impact on the care process, the patient health outcome, or both. The quality of the care process is equal to the degree to which the care reflects best (evidence-based) practice. A number of important quality indicator research initiatives are discussed in the section on the future of quality.

## MANDATE

In view of the size and pervasiveness of the problem of quality in America's health care system, leaders issued an urgent call for fundamental change to close the "quality gap." This call and accompanying actions were detailed in the *Quality Chasm* report (IOM, 2001). Sweeping systemic changes were recommended. A blueprint for change outlined immediate action to improve all aspects of care over the next decade.

The plan offered strategies to implement change and specified six aims to improve quality while redesigning the health care delivery system so that patients will experience safer, more reliable, more responsive, more integrated, and more available care. These six aims include making sure that health care is safe, effective, patient-centered, timely, efficient, and equitable (IOM, 2001). In the changes in health care, these six principles have been identified as the following:

Health care must be redesigned to be:

**S**afe

**T**imely

**E**ffective

**E**fficient

**E**quitable

**P**atient-centered

The "STEEEP" redesign principles are now woven throughout quality and safety initiatives at many levels of our health care institutions. For example, the Institute for Healthcare Improvement (IHI) identifies the STEEEP principles as foundational to their corporate philosophy (IHI, 2008), and the new Health Care Innovations Exchange of the Agency for Healthcare Review and Quality (AHRQ) identifies the STEEEP principles in its criteria for inclusion of improvement projects (AHRQ, 2008a).

In these reports, EBP was identified as foundational to quality of care and safety. Recommendations included creating an environment that supports evidence-based practice (IOM, 2001); emphasizing the need for evidence-based practice to reduce unwarranted variations in care where knowledge for improvement was available (IOM, 2003a); and establishing EBP as a basic competence in all health professions (IOM, 2003b). The most recent report sets a blueprint for the nation to assess clinical effectiveness and provide credible information about what really works in health care (IOM, 2008). The recommendations are to set priorities and manage systematic reviews of clinical effectiveness and to generate credible clinical practice guidelines.

Health care facilities are reacting to the new quality and safety agenda health care with unprecedented speed. Few other movements in health care have gained such widespread and rapid momentum. Nurses have risen to the occasion to join and lead evidence-based quality efforts through improvement efforts, development of explanatory models and science of EBP, educational program revision, and development of oversight and regulatory programs.

## SHIFTS IN NURSING RESEARCH COMPETENCIES

Because of these forces and shifts in emphasis, the relationship between research and clinical care has changed. In the past, primary research was conducted to test the effectiveness of interventions; now, researchers investigate ways to render health care systems and processes effective and safe. In addition, clinicians are expected to integrate research into practice—to transform knowledge into clinical practice. Clients demand that health care be based on best scientific evidence in combination with client preferences and the clinician's expertise (the definition of EBP).

This new paradigm of EBP requires a shift in thinking about research competencies that are needed in clinical care. Prior to the new knowledge forms offered by EBP, education programs prepared nurses to "conduct" investigations that would discover new knowledge. While an important function, conducting research is insufficient to achieve evidence-based quality improvement. Increasingly, advance practice nurses assume roles that emphasize evidence-based quality improvement—competencies not widely included in basic and professional development education. These competencies include both knowledge and the skill to translate research into practice (Stevens, 2005). Systematic identification of these new competencies makes clear the distinction between conducting research and translating research into practice. National consensus on 83 EBP competencies (Stevens, 2005) has galvanized changes in nursing education programs as EBP is integrated through undergraduate, graduate, and professional development education. Additional work is under way in identifying learning outcomes for quality and safety education (Cronenwett et al., 2007), which also will contribute to this growing effort toward a workforce that is prepared to translate research into practice.

## CHANGES IN NURSING RESEARCH

The focus of nursing research has recently expanded to include health care quality and patient safety. In the past, nursing research produced knowledge about individual clients through primary research studies, largely based on research designs used to investigate individual client treatment and experiences (such as experimental psychology and anthropology). These research reports were found to be difficult to translate into practice.

Today's health care redesign and evidence-based quality initiatives call on nurse scientists and clinicians also to embrace what is known about best (effective) practices and system change to support quality health care. New research methods and models, such as systematic reviews and complex adaptive systems, are being added to prior methods and models, such as true experiment and King's theory of mutual goal setting. New competencies to translate research into practice are being added to prior investigative competencies to conduct primary research studies. Nurse researchers are realigning previous research approaches and adopting new research designs as part of translational science teams that produce knowledge about effective health care and systems.

## PATIENT SAFETY

Safety research is rapidly emerging as the nation's top priority in health care research. While the epidemiology of errors receives much attention, investigating prevalence of adverse events is hindered by the prevalent culture of blame. This culture squelches adequate reporting of adverse events and prevents health care providers from making adverse events visible for further analysis and correction of causes of unsafe care.

Enhancing patient safety in health care includes three complementary actions: (1) preventing adverse events, (2) making adverse events visible, and (3) mitigating the effects of adverse events when they occur (World Health Organization [WHO], 2005). These three actions have stimulated development of theories to guide safety and the testing of those theories to produce safety science.

Safety science in health care is relatively new. *To Err Is Human* (IOM, 2000) raised awareness of the hazards associated with health care, identifying errors as the eighth leading cause of death in the United States. Safety science was well established in other industries, such as the airlines and the gas industries. Such high-risk industries are inherently dangerous and have developed safety management systems that nurture a culture of safety, thereby reducing errors and risks for errors. Safety practices established in these high-risk industries are now being adapted and tested in health care.

As in any new field of science, key concepts must be defined, theories generated to guide investigations, and new methods employed to study the topic. Likewise, theories and models with which to frame the investigation must be developed and tested.

An *adverse event* is defined as an untoward and usually unanticipated outcome that occurs in association with health care. *Patient safety* has been defined by AHRQ as the freedom from accidental injuries during the course of medical care and encompasses actions taken to avoid, prevent, or correct adverse outcomes that may result from the delivery of health care.

Reason (2000) advanced one of the most widely used theories on human error, one that has been used extensively in high-risk industries and cited in IOM reports. In Reason's model, human error is recognized as being inevitable. Reason identified two ways to view human error: the person approach and the system approach. The person approach has been the longstanding tradition in health care that focuses on individual providers, blaming providers for forgetfulness, inattention, or moral weakness. The systems approach holds as its basic premise that humans are fallible and errors are to be expected. The theory suggests that, to avert or mitigate errors, interventions must focus on conditions under which individuals work and must build defenses against error (Reason, 2000).

It is the management of errors and risks that becomes everyone's priority in a safety organization. Organizations that have fewer accidents than normal as a result of a change in organizational culture are high-reliability organizations.

## Safety Cultures

A culture of safety has emerged as a crucial element in providing safe patient care. A culture shares norms, values, and practices associated with a nation, organization, or profession. The model of cultural maturity (Westrum, 2004) explains stages in the evolution of a safety culture. These stages progress from a pathological stage where safety is a problem of the worker; the business is the main driver and the goal is to avoid being caught by regulators. Reactive cultures take action only after an error occurs. In a calculative culture, safety is driven by management, which collects much data and imposes safety on the worker. In a proactive culture, workforce involvement begins to move away from the top-down approach, focusing instead on improving performance where the unexpected is a challenge. The final evolutionary stage of an organizational culture is the generative stage, where everyone participates in safety because all workers understand that safety is an inherent part of the business.

## Safety Models in Nursing

There are four safety models that are seen as an integral part of the culture of safety. These models are Reason's Swiss Cheese Model of Systems Accidents; Helmreich's Threat and Error Management (TEM) Model for Medicine, which was developed from aviation's Crew Resource Management (CRM); Marx's Just Culture; and Complex Adaptive Systems.

The Swiss Cheese Model of System Accidents describes high-technology systems that have many defensive layers; when holes in these defenses momentarily line up, the opportunity for accidents occurs. The hole in any one defensive layer does not normally cause a bad outcome. There are two reasons that holes occur in the defensive layers: active failures and latent conditions. An active failure is an unsafe act committed by people who are in direct contact with the system. Latent conditions arise from decisions made by designers, builders, procedure writers, and management. Latent conditions may lie dormant in a system for years until they combine with active failures and local triggers create an accident opportunity (Reason, 2000). Human-error research in nursing has been valuable in examining barriers to safety in a neonatal intensive care unit (Jirapaet, Jirapaet, & Sopajaree, 2006).

Threat and error management (TEM) was developed to analyze adverse events, define training needs for medical personnel, and define organizational strategies to recognize and manage threat and error (Helmreich, 2000). Threats are factors that can increase the likelihood of an error being committed. In this model, threats are either latent or overt and serve as settings or overarching variables that increase the potential for error to occur. Latent threats are aspects of the hospital or medical organization that are not always easily identifiable but that predispose it to the commission of errors or the emergence of overt threats; examples are failure to maintain equipment and high nurse-patient staffing ratios. Overt threats include environmental factors such as poor lighting and excessive noise, individual factors such as fatigue, team- and staff-related factors such as poor communication, and patient-related factors such as low acuity level. For example, Pape (2003) significantly reduced nursing distractions during medication administration by having staff use protocols from high-risk industries (Pape, 2003).

Marx's Just Culture describes four behavioral concepts (evils) that are necessary to the comprehension of the interrelationship between discipline and patient safety: human error, negligent conduct, knowing violation of rules, and reckless conduct (Marx, 2001). Human errors are the mistakes, slips, and lapses that occur in our everyday behaviors. Negligence is a legal term used when a person has been harmed by a failure to provide reasonable and safe care in a manner consistent with that of other prudent health care workers. Intentional rule violations occur when an individual knowingly works around policy and procedures while performing a task or skill. Reckless conduct is the conscious disregard of obvious and significant risk; it differs from negligence in that negligence involves a failure to recognize the risk. The purpose of a Just Culture is to promote nonpunitive reporting of errors, either anonymously or confidentially, without eliminating individual or organizational responsibility.

The most prominent theory in complexity science is the complex adaptive systems (CAS) theory. CASs are collections of different agents, individuals, or groups that interact with other groups and with their environment in a way that allows them to learn and act in ways that are not always predictable. These systems are dynamic and evolve over time. CASs encompass individual, interdisciplinary, and systems facets of quality and safety. Characteristics of CASs are their ability to self-organize, the emergence of new patterns from nonlinear interactions, and their co-evolution as the agent and the environment mutually transform in response to the interactions (Stroebel, McDaniel, Crabtree, Miller, Nutting, & Stange, 2005). The complexity of the health care system has been a challenge to those trying to adapt safety models of other high-risk industries. Usually, in other high-risk industries, the individuals involved in the fatal error die themselves, unlike in health care, where the health care worker is not directly harmed by the actions or the error. CAS helps researchers understand the complexity of the work of the clinician (Ebright, Patterson, Chalko, & Render, 2003; Ebright, Urden, Patterson, & Chalko, 2004).

## Risk Management Models

Incident reports are the primary method for data collection on errors. Other high-risk industries have criticized health care for not having a standardized method of investigation, documentation, and dissemination of information on medication errors. Studies have been conducted on failures within the incident reporting system. The current incident reporting system is voluntary. The present rate of medical errors underestimates the full scope of the problem because of the incomplete reporting in the medical field. Studies have shown that nurses use the incident report system more frequently than physicians and other health care workers, which results nurses appearing to commit a disproportionate number of medication errors.

Root Cause Analysis (RCA) is a retrospective approach to error analysis that has been widely used in high-risk industries. The Joint Commission mandated the use of the multidisciplinary RCA in 1997 to investigate sentinel events in hospitals. RCA are uncontrolled case studies (qualitative approach) that predominantly use Reason's taxonomy of error to uncover the latent errors that underlie a sentinel event. The majority of RCAs reported were on serious adverse events that resulted in patient death. Limitations of the RCA are the hindsight bias of the investigators and the voluntary nature of reporting. The Joint Commission suggests that hospitals underreport incidents because they fear being put on probationary status and because of the legal implications of the disclosure of a sentinel event. Nursing researchers have used RCA to change current nursing practice in the transport of sick newborns in an effort to improve patient outcomes (Mordue, 2005).

Most errors that affect patient safety occur at the microsystem level within a hospital macrosystem. For example, as part of an effort to increase error reporting and to capture Reason's active failures, *near miss* or *close call* (errors that do not reach the patient) incident reporting has improved with The Good Catch Pilot Program at M. D. Anderson Cancer Center (AHRQ, 2008a). Three strategies were employed to improve reporting of close-call errors. First, the terminology for a potential error was changed to *good catch.* Second, an end-of-shift safety report was implemented that gave nurses an opportunity to identify and discuss patient safety concerns that had come up during the shift. Third, awards and other patient safety incentives were sponsored by executive leadership to recognize the efforts of individual nurses to improve patient safety. For example, in one hospital, scores based on the anonymous reporting by individual nurses on the various units were kept at the unit level. Buy-in by the upper level of nursing management was instrumental in promoting open discussions about patient safety and the distribution of Good Catch pins to unit team members. At nine weeks, more than 800 potential errors were reported, and at 6 months that number had increased to 2,744, which represents an increase of 1,468% in the reporting of potential errors. Changes that occurred as a result of the Good Catch program were highlighted in a weekly nursing newsletter as a source of feedback to employees (Mick, Wood, & Massey, 2007).

The IHI Failure Modes and Effects Analysis (FMEA) tool has been adapted from high-risk industries outside health care. Its purpose is to assess risks of failures and harm within a system and to identify the most important areas for improvement. This process is conducted with a multidisciplinary team approach that identifies any and all possible failure modes and causes, assigns Risk Priority Numbers to these failures, and then plans, implements, and evaluates interventions to reduce potential failures. The FMEA tool is available online (http://www.ihi.org/IHI/Topics/PatientSafety/SafetyGeneral/Tools/Failure+Modes+and+Effects+Analysis+%28FMEA%29+Tool+%28IHI+Tool%29.htm) through IHI, which also offers online monitoring and tracking of the FMEA tool (http://www.ihi.org/ihi/workspace/tools/fmea/).

## Instruments, Tools, and Resources for Measuring Patient Safety

There are various approaches to quantifying variables important in patient safety research. Through methodological research designs, scientists have developed and estimated psychometric qualities (reliability and validity) of a number of such instruments. The following describes several important instruments used in quality and safety research, including Hospital Survey on Patient Safety Culture (AHRQ, 2004). Some of the surveys have been adapted from other high-risk industries, as was the Safety Attitudes Questionnaire (SAQ). The SAQ was developed in partnership with AHRQ. The Practice Environment Scale of the Nursing Work Index (PES-NWI) was developed specifically to address issues relevant to nursing in Magnet Hospitals (Lake, 2002).

A valuable instrument is the Hospital Survey on Patient Safety Culture (AHRQ, 2004). The survey gathers data about staff opinions regarding patient safety issues, medical error, and event reporting. It provides hospitals with basic knowledge necessary to assess safety culture and to help them evaluate how well they have established a culture of safety in their institution. In addition, benchmarking based on data voluntarily provided by other, similar hospitals can be accomplished (AHRQ, 2008b). The highly reliable 42-item questionnaire measures 12 domains: openness of communication, feedback and communication of errors, frequency of events, handoffs and transitions, management support, nonpunitive response to error, organizational learning, overall perceptions of patient safety, staffing, manager expectations, actions that promote patient safety, teamwork across units, and teamwork within units.

The Safety Attitudes Questionnaire (SAQ) was adapted from the Flight Management Attitudes Questionnaire (FMAQ), which has been used in aviation worldwide. Six attitudinal domains that have been identified as necessary components of a safety culture are measured in the SAQ: teamwork climate, job satisfaction, perceptions of management, safety climate, working conditions, and stress recognition (Sexton et al., 2006).

The Practice Environment Scale of the Nurse Work Index was developed to measure five subscale domains of the hospital nursing practice environment. Two of the subscales measure the hospital wide environment: Nurse Participation Hospital Affairs and Nursing Foundations for Quality of Care. The other three subscales are more unit-specific: Nurse Manager Ability, Leadership, and Support; Staffing and Resource Adequacy; and Collegial Nurse-Physician Relations.

## THE FUTURE OF QUALITY AND SAFETY RESEARCH

Research in health care quality and safety is evolving at an unprecedented speed. As health care is redesigned, providers, administrators, and policymakers look to scientists to develop and evaluate sound approaches. In response, scientists are developing and evolving new research designs, theories, and measurement approaches. Top priorities for health care organizations include providing high-quality and safe patient care. The quality and patient safety movement is accelerating in health care organizations, and progress is evident (Buerhaus, 2007).

Key national quality reports have been a major impetus for health care improvements in quality and safety. The Institute of Medicine (IOM) report *Crossing the Quality Chasm: A New Health System for the 21st century* (IOM, 2001) identified the need for fundamental change in the U.S. health care system. The redesign of the health care system involves providing health care that is safe, timely, effective, efficient, equitable, and patient centered. In addition, the IOM's *Health Professions Education: A Bridge to Quality* (2003b) was another key report that identified five core competencies needed by health care professions to provide quality care in the 21st century. The essential five core competencies identified were (1) providing patient-centered care, (2) working in multidisciplinary teams, (3) using evidence-based practice, (4) applying quality improvement, and (5) using informatics.

National agencies such as the Agency for Healthcare Research and Quality (AHRQ), the Joint Commission, and the Institute of Healthcare Improvement (IHI) have been instrumental in setting initiatives designed to advance quality and safety in the health care arena. The AHRQ's 14 Evidence-Based Practice Centers (EPCs) and the AHRQ's Translating Research Into Practice (TRIP) initiatives are important resources that assist in translating evidence-based research into clinical practice promoting quality and patient safety in health care. In addition, the AHRQ Health Care Innovations Exchange project is an exciting new program created to support health care professionals in sharing and adopting innovations that improve the quality of health care. The AHRQ Health Care Innovations Exchange Web site provides resources and guidance to assist health care organizations in stimulating innovations and promoting quality and safety (AHRQ, 2008a). Summary snapshots of innovations provide vital information such as the description of the innovation, the results, the evidence rating, factors regarding the planning and development process, resources used and skills needed, and adoption considerations related to getting started with the innovation and, more important, sustaining the innovation (AHRQ, 2008a).

The Institute for Healthcare Improvement's 100,000 Lives and 5 Million Lives campaigns are outstanding examples of how national initiatives can improve quality and safety and incorporate evidence-based knowledge into clinical practice. The 100,000 Lives campaign focused on six interventions to reduce morbidity and mortality. The six interventions were (1) deployment of rapid response teams, (2) improvement of care of patients with acute myocardial infarction by delivering reliable evidence-based care, (3) prevention of adverse drug events through medication reconciliation, (4) prevention of central line infections, (5) prevention of surgical site infections, and (6) prevention of ventilator-associated pneumonias. This initiative involved the participation of 3,100 hospitals and saved an estimated 122,000 lives in 18 months (IHI, 2008).

IHI expanded the quality and safety focus with the 5 Million Lives campaign to address the issue of protecting patients from 5 million incidents of medical harms between December 2006 and December 2008. The 5 Million Lives campaign continues with the six interventions in the 100,000 Lives campaign, in addition to six new interventions targeted on harm: (1) preventing harm from high-alert medications (i.e., anticoagulants, sedatives, narcotics, and insulin), (2) reducing surgical complications, (3) preventing pressure ulcers, (4) reducing Methicillin-Resistant Staphylococcus Aureus (MRSA) infection, (5) delivering reliable, evidence-based care for congestive heart failure, and (6) defining the roles of hospital Boards of Directors in promoting and sustaining a culture of safety. Frequent new initiatives introduced by IHI are adding greatly to the nation's quality movement.

The Joint Commission is another national agency that focuses on improving quality and safety of health care. The Joint Commission's annual National Patient Safety Goals are reviewed by health care organizations to ensure that their clinical practices are addressing these quality and safety areas. In addition, the Joint Commission's Patient Safety Practices is an online resource providing more than 800 links that health care professionals can use to address patient safety issues (Joint Commission, 2008). These goals have stimulated many innovative interventions the impact of which is evaluated using research approaches.

## QUALITY INDICATORS, MEASURES, AND REPORTING

Performance measures are necessary to determine the impact of ongoing quality improvement efforts. Such efforts require that specific quality indicators be identified and measurement approaches validated through research. In the recent past, a number of health care entities responded to the need for such indicators by developing consensus on indicators that should be tracked and by launching annual quality reports from national surveys. These efforts are reflected in the work of the Agency for Health care Research and Quality (AHRQ) and the National Quality Forum. Other groups have undertaken efforts to create nursing-sensitive quality indicators reflected in the following sources: National Database of Nursing Quality Indicators, Veterans Affairs Nursing Sensitive Outcomes Database, Military Nursing Outcomes Database, and California Nursing Outcomes Coalition Database.

These groups note that many barriers to the widespread adoption of consensus standards exist and that overcoming them will require significant resources. Despite progress in quality improvement, challenges remain. These include inadequately developed measures, lack of standardization of performance measures and quality indicators, the need to refine measures, misalignment of measures of outcomes and baseline measures, and the burdens of data collection.

## AHRQ NATIONAL HEALTHCARE QUALITY REPORTS

Since 2003, AHRQ has reported on progress and opportunities for improving health care quality. One of the key functions of the AHRQ National Healthcare Quality Report (NHQR) is to track the nation's progress in providing safe health care. For 5 years, the reports have presented a snapshot of the safety of health care provided to the American people. NHQR surveys the health care system through quality indicators, such as the percentage of heart attack patients who receive recommended care when they reach the hospital or the percentage of children who receive recommended vaccinations. In all, 218 measures are used, categorized across four dimensions of quality—effectiveness, patient safety, timeliness, and patient centeredness (AHRQ, 2007).

As a result of such research efforts in improvement science, a clearer picture of health care safety is beginning to emerge. The 2007 report assessed the state of health care quality using 41 core report measures that represent the most important and scientifically credible measures of quality for the nation (AHRQ, 2007). The report shows that, 5 years after the first NHQR and 7 years after the IOM's landmark publication *To Err Is Human* (2000), it is still difficult to document progress, although more information on patient safety is now available. The report reflects slow progress in improvements in quality and safety. Between

2000 and 2007, patient safety improved at an annual rate of only 1%. The report identifies three themes:

- "Health care quality continues to improve, but the rate of improvement has slowed."
- "Variation in quality of health care across the Nation is decreasing, but not for all measures."
- "The safety of health care has improved since 2000, but more needs to be done." (AHRQ, 2007)

## QUALITY INDICATORS: THE NATIONAL QUALITY FORUM

The National Quality Forum (NQF) is a nonprofit organization with diverse stakeholder membership from the public and private health sectors, including consumers, health care professionals, providers, health plans, public and private purchasers, researchers, and quality improvement organizations. Established in 1999, NQF seeks to implement a national strategy for health care quality measurement and reporting. The NQF mission includes improving health care by "setting national goals for performance improvement, endorsing national consensus standards for measuring and publicly reporting on performance, and promoting the attainment of national goals through education and outreach programs" (NQF, 2008).

Since the formation of NQF, health care quality has become a major public policy issue. The diverse NQF stakeholders agreed on standards by which the health care industry would be measured, and data on these measures are publicly reported. Together with the other forces in effect, NQF has fostered public reporting of performance. Such reporting, once a rare event, is becoming the norm. NQF-endorsed™ voluntary consensus standards are widely viewed as the "gold standard" for the measurement of health care quality.

## SELECTED NURSING PERFORMANCE QUALITY INDICATORS

Because of the sheer number of nurses and the frequency of contact with patients, nurses have a major impact on patient safety and health care outcomes (NQF, 2007a). Research points to the influence of nursing on patient outcomes (e.g., IOM, 2004); however, only recently have advances in building a platform for public reporting reflecting nursing sensitive performance measures been made.

## National Quality Forum 15

NQF recently endorsed a set of 15 consensus-based nursing sensitive standards. These uniform metrics will increase understanding of nurses' influence on inpatient hospital care and advance internal quality improvement. The measures are recommended to evaluate the impact that nurses in acute care settings have on patient safety, health care quality, and professional work environment (NQF, 2007a).

### Definition: Nursing-Sensitive Performance Measures

"Nursing-sensitive performance measures are processes and outcomes—and structural proxies for these processes and outcomes (e.g., skill mix, nurse staffing hours)—that are affected, provided, and/or influenced by nursing personnel—but for which nursing is not exclusively responsible. Nursing-sensitive measures must be quantifiably influenced by nursing personnel, but the relationship is not necessarily causal." (NQF, 2007a)

The "NQF-15" includes measures from three perspectives: patient-centered outcome measures, nursing-centered intervention measures, and system-centered measures. The NQF-15 is expected to grow as nursing research continues to advance other measurement and reporting initiatives (NQF, 2007a).

NQF undertook a 15-month study to better understand the adoption of NQF-15 and to identify the successes, challenges, and technical barriers experienced by those implementing the measure. In 2006 and 2007, interviews were conducted with critical leaders, hospital representatives, quality organization leaders, and representatives of implementation initiatives. Interview data were augmented with a Web-based survey. Content and descriptive analyses led to recommendations to accelerate adoption of the NQF-15. The 10 recommendations focus on aligning the NQF-15 with priorities, advancing science, improving regulatory and reporting requirements, fostering adoption of the standard through education, holding nurses accountable for public reporting, and creating a business case for nursing quality measurement (NQF, 2007b). The NQF-15 measures were drawn largely from existing nursing performance measurement databases, including National Database of Nursing Quality Indicators, and from several other initiatives.

## National Database of Nursing Quality Indicators

Another major quality and safety measurement effort is reflected in the National Database of Nursing Quality Indicators (NDNQI). The American Nurses Association developed the NDNQI in 1998. The NDNQI is designed to assist health care organizations in patient safety and quality improvement initiatives by supplying research-based national comparative data on nursing care and its impact on patient outcomes. The NDNQI reflects nursing-sensitive indicators related to the structure, process, and outcomes of nursing care. Structure of nursing care is reflected by the supply, skill level, and education and certification of nursing staff. Process indicators reflect nursing care aspects such as assessment, intervention, and RN job satisfaction. Outcome indicators reflect patient outcomes that are nursing sensitive; these improve with both greater quantity and greater quality of nursing care (e.g., pressure ulcers, falls, and IV infiltrations) (NDNQI, 2008).

## KEY INITIATIVES IN FUTURE QUALITY AND SAFETY

A number of initiatives are proving to be key in the forefront of quality and safety. These include additional IOM reports, the Magnet Recognition Program, and the Interdisciplinary Nursing Quality Research Initiative, each of which is described here.

The IOM report *Keeping Patients Safe: Transforming the Work Environment of Nurses* (2004) identified mandates for quality and safety. The report emphasized a call for change for health care organizations, federal government, state boards of nursing, educational institutions, professional organizations, labor organizations, and professional nurses and urged them to take an active role in improving quality and safety in health care. This report identified essential patient safeguards in the work environment of nurses, calling for (1) governing boards that focus on safety, (2) leadership and evidence-based management structures and processes, (3) effective nursing leadership, (4) adequate staffing, (5) organizational support for ongoing learning and decision support, (6) mechanisms promoting multidisciplinary collaboration, (7) work designs promoting safety, and (8) organizational culture the enhances patient safety. Additional research addressing patient safety is necessary in the following areas: information on nurse's work, including on how nurses divide their time among various activities, information on nursing-related errors, safer nursing work processes and workspace design, standardized measurements of patient acuity, and safe nursing staff levels on various nursing units (IOM, 2004).

## Magnet Recognition Program

The Magnet Recognition Program developed by the American Nurses Credentialing Center has been a driving factor urging nursing to develop a research agenda focused on evidence-based practice, quality, and safety. The Magnet Recognition Program was developed to recognize health care organizations that provide nursing excellence and to provide a channel for spreading successful nursing practices. Providing high-quality and safe patient care and integrating evidence-based knowledge into clinical practice are important components in achieving the esteemed magnet recognition certification (AACN, 2008). The program has had a significant impact on quality and safety in nursing and in increasing the amount of attention paid to employing evidence-based practice and conducting research.

## Interdisciplinary Nursing Quality Research Initiative (INQRI)

Robert Wood Johnson Foundation (RWJF) is a leading funder of research on nursing quality care. The primary goal of the Interdisciplinary Nursing Quality Research Initiative (INQRI) is to "generate, disseminate and translate research to understand how nurses contribute to and can improve the quality of patient care" (RWJF, 2008). The program of research seeks to fill the gaps in what is known about nurses' effect on quality and on keeping patients safer and healthier. The ultimate goal is to support research to reduce health care errors and improve patient care. To date, 29 studies have been funded to discover how nursing is causally related to quality outcomes (RWJF, 2008).

## SUMMARY

Patient safety and the national effort to ensure that health care systems provide quality and safe care will continue to be top priorities for health care professionals. Nurses are essential in creating and sustaining a culture of safety, translating evidence-based research into clinical practice in health care, and creating the science of safety and quality to improve the quality of health care and maximize positive health outcomes.

## SUGGESTED ACTIVITIES

1   Explore the AHRQ Health Care Innovations Exchange. Search and locate the profile of an innovation of interest. Review the section "Did It Work," and analyze the approach to evaluating the impact of the innovation. How was the resulting evidence rated? What does the rating mean?

2   Search a bibliographic database such as CINAHL. Locate a research study using "complex adaptive systems" or chaos theory as a framework. List the primary variables in the investigation. Relate the results to quality and/or safety in health care.

## REFERENCES

Agency for Healthcare Research and Quality. (2004, November 10). *New AHRQ survey helps hospitals measure and improve patient safety culture.* Press Release. Retrieved from http://www.ahrq.gov/news/press/pr2004/hospcult2pr.htm

Agency for Healthcare Research and Quality. (2007). *National Healthcare Quality Report.* AHRQ Pub. No. 08–0040.

Agency for Healthcare Research and Quality. (2008a). *AHRQ health care innovations exchange.* Retrieved June 2008 from http://www.innovations.ahrq.gov

Agency for Healthcare Research and Quality. (2008b). *Patient Safety Culture Surveys.* Retrieved April 26, 2009, from http://www.ahrq.gov/qual/patientsafetyculture/

American Nurses Credentialing Center. *Magnet Recognition Program.* Retrieved June 2, 2008, from http://www.nursecredentialing.org/Magnet.aspx

Berwick, D. M. (2008). The science of improvement. *Journal of the American Medical Association 299*(10), 1182–1184.

Buerhaus, P. (2007). Is hospital patient care becoming safer? A conversation with Lucian Leape. *Health Affairs, 26*(6), w687–w696.

Cronenwett, L., Sherwood, G., Barnsteiner, J., Disch, J., Johnson, J., Mitchell, P., Sullivan., D. T., et al. (2007). Quality and safety education for nurses. *Nursing Outlook, 55*(3), 122–131.

Ebright, P. R., Patterson, E. S., Chalko, B. A., & Render, M. L. (2003). Understanding the complexity of registered nurse work in acute care settings. *Journal of Nursing Administration, 33*(12), 630–638.

Ebright, P. R., Urden, L., Patterson, E., & Chalko, B. (2004). Themes surrounding novice nurse near-miss and adverse-event situations. *Journal of Nursing Administration, 34*(1), 531–538.

Funk, S. G., Champagne, M. T., Wiese, R. A. & Tornquist, E. M. (1990). BARRIERS: The barriers research utilization scale. *Applied Nursing Research, 4*(1), 39–45.

Funk, S. G., Tornquist, E. M., & Champagne, M. T. (1989). Application and evaluation of the dissemination model. *Western Journal of Nursing Research, 11*(4), 486–491.

Glasziou, P., & Haynes, B. (2005). The paths from research to improved health outcomes. *ACP Journal Club, 142*(2)(Suppl.), A-8–A-10.

Helmreich, R. L. (2000). On error management: Lessons from aviation. *British Medical Journal, 320*(7237), 781–785.

Institute of Medicine (IOM). (1990). *Clinical Practice Guidelines: Directions for a new program.* Edited by M. J. Field & K. N. Lohr Washington, DC: National Academies Press.

Institute of Medicine (IOM). (2000). *To err is human: Building a safer health system.* Edited by L. T. Kohn, J. M. Corrigan, & M. S. Donaldson. Washington, DC: National Academies Press.

Institute of Medicine (IOM). (2001). *Crossing the quality chasm: A new health system for the 21st century.* Washington, DC: National Academies Press.

Institute of Medicine (IOM). (2003a). *Priority areas for national action: Transforming health care quality.* Washington D.C: National Academies Press.

Institute of Medicine (IOM). (2003b). *Health professions education: A bridge to quality.* Edited by A. Greiner & E. Knebel. Washington, DC: National Academies Press.

Institute of Medicine (IOM). (2004). *Keeping patients safe: Transforming the work environment of nurses.* Edited by A. Page. Washington, DC: National Academies Press. Retrieved from http://www.iom.edu/?id=19376

Institute of Medicine (IOM). (2008). *Knowing what works: A Roadmap for the nation.* J. Eden, B. Wheatley, B. L. McNeil, & H. Sox (Ed.). Washington, DC: National Academies Press.

Institute for Healthcare Improvement (IHI). (2008). *About us.* Retrieved April 2, 2008, from http://www.ihi.org/ihi/about

Jirapaet, V., Jirapaet, K., & Sopajaree, C. (2006). The nurses' experience of barriers to safe practice in the neonatal intensive care unit in Thailand. *JOGNN: Journal of Obstetric, Gynecologic, & Neonatal Nursing, 35*(6), 746.

Joint Commission (2008). *National patient safety goals.* Retrieved June 7, 2008, from http://www.jointcommission.org/patientsafety/nationalpatientsafetygoals/

Lake, E. T. (2002, June). Development of the practice environment of the Nursing Work Index. *Research in Nursing & Health, 25*(3), 176–188.

Marx, D. (Ed.). (2001). *Patient safety and the "Just Culture": A primer for health care executives.* New York: Trustees of Columbia University.

Mick, J. M., Wood, G. L., & Massey, R. L. (2007). The Good Catch pilot program. *Journal of Nursing Administration, 37*(11), 499–503.

Morduo, B. C. (2005). A case report of the transport of an infant with a tension pneumopericardium. *Advances in Neonatal Care, 5*(4), 190–200.

Mulrow, C. D. (1994). Systematic reviews: Rationale for systematic reviews. *British Medical Journal, 30* (6954), 597–599.

National Dataset of Nursing Quality Indicators. (2008). Retrieved March 20, 2008, from www.nursingquality.org

National Quality Forum (NQF). (2006). *Compendium 2000–2005.* Washington DC: NQF. Retrieved July 24, 2008, from http://qualityforum.org/pdf/reports/compen dium.pdf

National Quality Forum. (2007a). *Nursing performance measurement and reporting: A status report.* Washington DC: National Quality Forum. Retrieved July 24, 2008, from http://216.122.138.39/pdf/news/IB_july2007.pdf

National Quality Forum. (2007b). *Tracking NQF-endorsed consensus standards for nursing sensitive care: A 15-month study.* Washington DC: National Quality Forum. Retrieved July 12, 2008, from http://www.qualityforum.org/pdf/reports/Nursing70907.pdf

National Quality Forum. (2008). *National Quality Forum endorses National Consensus Standards promoting accountability and public reporting.* Retrieved August 15, 2008, from http://www.qualityforum.org/news/releases/080508-endorsed-measures.asp

Pape, T. M. (2003). Applying airline safety practices to medication administration. *Medsurg Nursing, 12*(2), 77–94.

Reason, J. (2000). Human error: models and management. *British Medical Journal, 320,* 768–770.

Robert Wood Johnson Foundation (RWJF). (2008). *Program overview of the Interdisciplinary Nursing Quality Research Initiative.* Retrieved August 16, 2008, from http://www.inqri.org

Sackett, D. L., Straus, S. E., Richardson, W. S., Rosenberg, W., & Haynes, R. B. (2000). *Evidence-based medicine: How to practice and teach EBM* (2nd ed.). Edinburgh: Churchill Livingstone.

Sexton, J. B., Helmreich, R. L., Neilands, T. B., Rowan, K., Vella, K., Boyden, J., et al. (2006). The Safety Attitudes Questionnaire: Psychometric properties, benchmarking data, and emerging research. *BMC Health Services Research, 3,* 6.

Stetler, C. B. (1994). Refinement of the Stetler/Marrram model for application of research findings to practice. *Nursing Outlook, 42*(1), 15–25.

Stevens, K. R. (2004, October). *ACE Star Model of Knowledge Transformation: Utility in practice and education.* Proceedings of the NIH State of the Science Conference.

Stevens, K. R. (2005). *Essential competencies for evidence-based practice in nursing.* San Antonio: Academic Center for Evidence-Based Practice (ACE) of The University of Texas Health Science Center.

Stroebel, C. K., McDaniel, R. R., Crabtree, B. F., Miller, W. L., Nutting, P. A., & Stange, K. C. (2005). How complexity science can inform a reflective process for improvement in primary care practices. *Journal on Quality and Patient Safety, 31*(8), 438–446.

Titler, M. G., Kleiber, C., Steelman, V. J., Rakel, B. A., Budreau, G., Everett, L.Q., et al. (2001). The Iowa Model of evidence-based practice to promote quality care. *Critical Care Nursing Clinics of North America, 13,* 497–509.

Westrum, R. (2004). A typology of organizational cultures. *Quality and Safety in Health Care, 13*(2), ii22–ii27.

Woolf, S. H. (2004). Patient safety is not enough: Targeting quality improvements to optimize the health of the population. *Annals of Internal Medicine, 140,* 33–36.

World Health Organization (WHO). (2005). WHO draft guidelines for adverse event reporting and learning systems. Geneva: WHO Document Production Services.

# Building Blocks for Evidence

PART
II

# 4

# Appraising a Single Research Article

MARY SCHIRA

Whether one is reading a research article for translation of findings into evidence-based practice or as a building block for a proposed study, the process begins with a single research article. One of the most frequent barriers noted by individuals to incorporating research findings (and therefore providing evidence-based care) into practice is a lack of confidence in their ability to read and interpret research findings. Nurses use critical thinking skills in practice every day. These same skills can be expanded to incorporate the new skill of reading and interpreting research.

Reading and evaluating research is a critical skill in the research process. Previous chapters have addressed how to locate the research literature and ensure that once the literature is located, it can be retrieved; chapters that follow provide additional detail regarding elements of a research study and the article where the results are published. The purpose of this chapter is to introduce the reader to sections of a single research article and to provide an organized approach to reading and interpreting the strength and relevance of the research. Components of a research article to consider include the abstract, background, and significance of the study, methods, data analysis, findings and results, discussion, and implications for practice.

The purpose of reading a research article is to evaluate the adequacy of each section and determine the strengths, weaknesses, and usefulness of the research findings (Schira, 1999). Research articles are written with a similar organization; the logic of the researcher's thinking should be clear enough so the reader has few questions about how and why the study was conducted. By the end of the article, the reader should be able to determine how the research results fit into current knowledge and whether the findings are appropriate for implementation into practice. As the reader progresses through the report, each section builds on the previous information. Exhibit 4.1 provides a summary of key elements to consider as the reader appraises a research article; the exhibit may be used as a guide or checklist.

## ABSTRACT

The first part of a research article is the abstract. The abstract is a brief, targeted summary of the full article that follows. The summary gives the reader enough basic information about the study to evaluate whether the study is of interest or applies to the reader's practice setting or population (DiCecco, 2007). Most readers use the abstract as a screen to determine whether or not to read the entire research article.

## BACKGROUND AND SIGNIFICANCE

The first section of a research report provides an overview of and a context for the research. The aim of the first few paragraphs is to provide the reader with a thorough understanding of the background of the study, why the study was conducted, and why the study was important (significance). Gaps in current knowledge should be noted and how the study proposed to fill the gaps addressed. Near the end of the section (or set apart), the purpose or problem statement of the study is presented. Both or only one may be included in a published report, as they are closely related. The purpose or problem statement should be clearly stated and provide the variables (independent and dependent) studied. The author may also include research questions, hypotheses tested in the study, or both. In any case, the reader will know the population (who) and phenomenon (what) that was studied. The reader can use the information to assess the rest of the report.

Exhibit 4.1

## KEY QUESTIONS IN EVALUATING A SINGLE RESEARCH ARTICLE

PROBLEM STATEMENT/PURPOSE
  What was studied? What variables were measured (independent and
    dependent)?
  Does the purpose (or research question) relate to the problem?
  Does the purpose clearly address the problem?

LITERATURE REVIEW
  Are all variables included in the literature review?
  Is the literature current? Relevant?
  Is the research literature summarized and evaluated?
  Are gaps in the literature noted?
  How likely is it that the current study will provide additional information to
    close the gap?

DESIGN
  What is the overall design of the study? Quantitative or qualitative?
  Is the design a good match with the problem statement or purpose of
    the study?

METHOD
  Ethics—How was the protection of human subjects ensured?
  Sample—How was the sample identified? Do the subjects have the
    characteristics needed to answer the research question?
  Instruments—What instruments were used? Were they reliable? Valid?

STUDY PROCEDURE
  Was the procedure realistic?
  If an independent variable was manipulated, was it done consistently?
  How were instruments or tools administered? In what environment?

DATA ANALYSIS
  How were data analyzed?
  Were statistical tests used appropriately?
  If the research is a qualitative study, how were themes and meaning elicited?

FINDINGS AND RESULTS
  What were the outcomes of the study?
  Were all aspects of the problem statement addressed?
  How do the findings fit with previous research?

DISCUSSION
  What conclusions did the researcher draw from the findings?
  Do the findings make sense and relate to the problem?
  How do the findings compare with other research findings in the literature?
  What limitations are noted?
  Can the results be generalized to other populations?
  How will limitations affect generalizability of the findings?

IMPLICATIONS
  Are implications for practice and research noted?
  Do the implications flow from the results?

## LITERATURE REVIEW

In some cases, the background section includes a review of the literature. In other articles, the literature review is specifically set apart as a separate section in the article. The review of the literature should be appraised for both content and relevance. The literature presented should be relevant to the study, relate to the variables that were studied, and be current. The literature review often includes both theoretical and research (data-based) sources. The previous research studies included in the discussion should at minimum address the purpose, sample, design, and findings and a brief critique of the study's strengths and weaknesses (Burns & Grove, 2008). Another approach in reporting the research literature is to present a synthesis of numerous studies and an overall evaluation of the body of knowledge. Whichever approach is used, the reader should have an understanding of the current knowledge and how the study plans fill or address gaps in knowledge. The existing research literature included in the review may be directly or indirectly related to the purpose of the study. Indirectly related studies should be linked for relevance.

The reader should specifically check the dates of the literature cited in the article's literature review and reference list and judge whether or not it is (at least reasonably) current. While some studies are considered classics, much of the cited literature should be recent and reflect up-to-date thinking and understanding of the study's focus. This is especially important in practice areas undergoing rapid change (e.g., genomics) and in areas that are time sensitive (e.g., attitudes, opinions). The reader's personal knowledge and level of expertise in the content area are valuable in determining the currency and strength of the literature review included in the research report.

## METHOD

A large section of the research report is the method section, which describes how the study was conducted. The method section includes design, sample, instruments, and specific procedures for data collection (Russell, 2005). The method section is a critical part of a research article and deserves careful attention. While reading the method section, the reader should be alert for any problems in the way the study protocol was implemented, such as sample bias, inconsistencies in data collection among subjects, and weaknesses of the instruments or tools used to collect the data. The strength of the method section helps the reader determine the generalizability of the results that will follow.

## Design

The study design is identified early in the method section if it has not already been implied in the purpose or problem statement. The author should identify whether the study used a quantitative, qualitative, or *mixed-method* design. Quantitative studies use designs that result in numerical data that can be used in statistical (mathematical) analysis and assess the size of relationships among variables (DiCecco, 2007). Variables of interest in quantitative designs may be measured using physiologic instruments (e.g., blood pressure, weight), questionnaires with fixed responses (e.g., scale of 1 to 5), or variables that can be assigned a number (e.g., gender). In addition, quantitative research designs may be further identified as experimental, quasi-experimental, or nonexperimental, depending on how subjects were chosen, whether and how study variables were manipulated, and how the data to measure the variables were collected.

Qualitative studies also identify a specific study approach but do not result in numbers for statistical analysis. The most common qualitative designs are ethnographic, phenomenological, historical, and grounded theory approaches. Just as in quantitative designs, there are specific and distinguishing elements among the qualitative designs. The goal of studies that use qualitative designs is to explore the phenomenon of interest from the perspective of individuals experiencing the phenomenon. As a result, qualitative designs yield descriptions that can then be analyzed for themes, common elements, and shared meaning among subjects (Vishnevsky & Beanlands, 2004). The end result of a qualitative design may be new knowledge or the beginning of a theory, whereas the end result of a quantitative study is often acceptance or rejection of current knowledge or theory.

In some instances, study design may include both qualitative and quantitative elements, resulting in a mixed-method design. In such a design, the reader should evaluate whether the design was appropriately used and followed in gathering the specific data. The specific qualitative and quantitative design aspects must be compatible. For example, sample size in a mixed-method study may be a challenge. Quantitative and qualitative design approaches can differ greatly, with quantitative designs often seeking large sample sizes and random selection whereas some qualitative designs have small samples obtained from a narrowly recruited group of individuals. Regardless of the overall research design, the key question for the reader to consider is how well the design used is likely to fulfill the purpose of the study and answer the research question.

## Sample

The number of subjects who participated in the study (sample size) should be clearly stated in the article. Additional information in the article should describe how the sample size was determined and specific inclusion and exclusion criteria for participants. In a quantitative study, sample size is determined by completing a power analysis, a mathematical determination based on the researcher's desired level of statistical significance, estimates of variability, and effect size. In a pilot study, this detail is not included because a primary purpose of a pilot study is to obtain beginning information to justify and guide larger studies (Oliver & Mahon, 2006). In many qualitative studies, the researcher describes how it was determined that the (often small) sample size was sufficient to answer the research question.

The demographic characteristics of study participants (e.g., age, gender) are usually described and help the reader evaluate how closely the study sample matches the reader's population of interest. Sample characteristics are also important in determining whether or not the study findings might be applicable for practice. The more closely the sample matches the reader's population, the more likely the reader is to implement the findings into practice if all other criteria are met (no contradictory study results, other studies with similar results). In addition, the number of subjects and a brief description of subjects that did not complete the study or study procedures should be included so that the reader can make a judgment whether individuals who completed the study were different from those who did not complete the study, a potential source of bias called *attrition*.

In quantitative studies, random selection of subjects and random assignment of subjects to treatment groups is ideal but often difficult to accomplish because of the constraints that accompany research on human subjects in a clinical environment. As a result, a convenience sampling method that does not contain apparent selection bias is often appropriate and is strengthened when the design incorporates random assignment to treatment groups. The reader needs to make a judgment regarding bias in the sample and the appropriateness of the sampling plan in answering the problem.

## Research Instruments and Data Collection Tools

Each research tool or instrument used in the study should be described in detail. The instruments should measure the variables of interest. If an existing tool or instrument was used (e.g., Depression Scale), the number of items and a brief description of what the tool measures should be described. Measures of reliability, the consistency of the tool or instrument, and validity, whether the tool actually measures the phenomenon under study, are important considerations and should be reported in the article. An advantage of using research instruments that have already been used is that reliability and validity data may already be established (Oliver & Mahon, 2006). If the researcher developed a tool for the study, a full description of the instrument and a discussion of how reliability and validity were established should be included. Whether an existing research instrument was used or a tool was created for the study, a lack of information regarding reliability and validity leads to questions regarding whether or how well the variables in the study were actually measured.

## Study Procedures

The procedure section provides a detailed description of how the study was conducted, including exactly how and when data were collected and under what conditions. The information should be clearly presented so that the reader could replicate the study by following the description. The reader should see a logical flow in the data collection process and consider any extraneous variables in the setting that may affect the data.

## Ethics

The methods section should also include a short description of how ethical considerations in conducting the study were addressed. Alternatively, the protection of human subjects may be addressed as the first part of the description of the study procedure. In either case, a statement regarding review of the study by an institutional review or research ethics board prior to the beginning of the study is generally included. In addition, procedures for obtaining subjects' consent to participate in the study and how consent was obtained should be detailed. If the subjects were minors or were incompetent to provide informed consent personally, the author should fully describe consent procedures and mention whether any difficulties were encountered.

## DATA ANALYSIS

By the time the reader comes to the data analysis section of the research article, he or she will know a great deal about the study. The reader has formed beginning opinions about the strength and potential usefulness of the study and is, in most cases, looking forward to reading the findings and results. The data analysis section begins with a description of how the data obtained from the research instruments were summarized and analyzed to bring meaning to the data. In a qualitative study, the data analysis approach is described, including how themes or patterns were elicited from the data. In a quantitative report, the data are analyzed using statistical methods and tests. There are numerous statistical procedures and tests available. The key issue in evaluating the statistical analysis is to determine that the method used is appropriate for the research question and how the data were measured (Burns & Grove, 2008; DiCecco, 2007). For the novice reader, the data analysis section may be the most difficult and potentially intimidating part of the research article. This discomfort is often due to limited exposure to and understanding of the statistical tests used and uncertainty about whether the appropriate test has been applied to the data. Resources that will aid the reader as skills develop include a basic statistics book and colleagues with an understanding of data analysis techniques. As with any skill, the more the reader gains in understanding, the easier reading the analysis section becomes.

## FINDINGS AND RESULTS

Perhaps the most enjoyable section of a research article to read is the findings of the study. Each previous section has been building to this part of the article, and it essentially solves the puzzle or problem that was introduced in the very beginning of the article. Simply put, the findings tell the reader what the researcher discovered as a result of the data that were collected, collated, and analyzed. As the findings of a study are presented, whether a qualitative or quantitative design was used, the reader learns whether the research question was answered and how completely the question or problem statement was addressed. All results and data that address the research question or problem statement are included in a discussion of the findings (Schira, 1999). If the study was analyzed using statistical methods, the statistical significance of the results is noted. In the results section, the data and outcomes of statistical analysis are presented but generally not explained or discussed. The intent of the findings section is to present the factual outcome of data analysis, rather than explain the meaning of the data. While this section may seem dry or unimaginative, the advantage of this approach is to allow the reader to make beginning judgments regarding the study outcomes in the absence of the opinion or interpretation of meaning from others. In addition to a narrative summary of the results, most articles present findings in a table for easier review.

Qualitative study findings, depending on the specific qualitative design used in the study, are presented quite differently from quantitative results. In a qualitative study, direct quotes or summaries of participant responses are often included in the results section or may be presented in a combined Results/Discussion section. The author may group the findings according to themes or patterns that became apparent during the data analysis. As a result, many qualitative studies provide data using a narrative approach and describe results in terms of richness and depth of the data.

Some readers prefer to read the results section immediately after reading the problem or purpose of the study. This may be due to curiosity about the outcome or to a wish to decide whether or not to read the entire article. The dedicated reader will then go back to the beginning of the article and read it entirely. There is nothing inherently wrong with reading the results out of sequence as long as the reader recalls that, in order to use the findings in practice or to build additional research studies, the previous sections of the article are critical in evaluating the strength of the findings. In addition, this approach may encourage a reader to fully read only those articles that report significance or that reinforce current ways of thinking. Studies that do not demonstrate statistical significance are often as revealing as those that do and encourage us to challenge existing perceptions. Finally, because the results section presents but does not discuss the findings, the reader may overlook studies with clinical (but no statistical) significance.

## DISCUSSION

In the discussion section of an article, the authors present the conclusions they drew from the findings, acknowledge any limitations of the study, and suggest how findings may be generalized to individuals or groups beyond the study sample. In the discussion, a description of how the results fit into the current body of knowledge in general and previous research in specific should be presented. The author should compare and contrast the study findings with those of the previous research that was cited in the review of the literature earlier in the article. A critical comparison by the author demonstrates to the reader that the researcher evaluated the findings with an open mind.

## CONCLUSIONS

The author's conclusions provide the researcher's interpretation of the study findings. In contrast to the factual presentation of the study outcomes in the findings section, the conclusions present the meaning of the results from the author's perspective. The conclusions drawn by the researcher should flow from the scope of the study and directly relate to the purpose of the study; they should be confined to the variables that were studied.

## LIMITATIONS

The author's identification of the study's limitations recognizes that, while no study is perfect, results can provide valuable information for future researchers (Oliver & Mahon, 2006). At the same time, limitations cannot be used as an excuse for a poor design or flawed study procedures. Among the limitations often cited in research reports are problems with data collection (e.g., unexpected intervening variable that occurred during data collection), small sample size, problems with how the sample was obtained (e.g., convenience sample), and limitations inherent in the study's research design (e.g., nonrandom assignment of subjects to groups). In most cases, the reader has already identified limitations and is not surprised by those noted by the author.

## GENERALIZABILITY

The generalizability of study findings is an essential evaluation of a study's outcome. Studies are conducted with subjects that have specific characteristics and in settings with unique environments. In addition, manipulation of the independent variable and measurement of the dependent variable may be done in more than one way, and researchers may use comparable research instruments or tools or very different ones. As a result, the meaning of the findings and how the findings may be implemented with other populations and in other settings must be addressed in the article. An understanding of the limitations of the study also affects generalizability. A study with numerous or key limitations results in findings that have minimal or narrow generalizability beyond the population or setting in the study. This is especially likely when bias is present in the sample. Bias may be a design flaw or may be unintentional and discovered during data analysis.

## IMPLICATIONS

The final major aspect of a research article is implications for practice and research. An important goal of research is to provide evidence to further explain phenomena, validate current thinking and practice, or change current practice and approaches. Depending on the purpose of the study, the strength of the study's design, and the statistical and clinical significance of findings, it is important for the author to suggest to the reader how the findings may actually be used. Implications may be noted for direct patient care practice, education, or the delivery of health care services. The implications should have direct links to the findings, be realistic, and be suggested within the limitations of the study as previously noted by the author. Again, the reader will critically evaluate the information presented and determine the extent to which the reader agrees or disagrees with the author's perspective.

Implications for future research are similarly important. Authors commonly cite a need for replication of the study, recognizing that changes in clinical practice are rarely made on the basis of a single study. In addition, the author should make suggestions for further studies that might expand scientists' understanding of the phenomenon or problem studied. In the case of an article based on a pilot study, the author should make specific recommendations for a larger study that may incorporate additional variables, change the study design, or revise or change the research tools.

## SUMMARY

Reading a single research article is the first step in progressing down the path of implementing evidence-based care, planning a research study, or both. Like most skills in nursing, comfort and proficiency in reading research studies increase with diligent practice. The critical thinking skills that nurses use in clinical practice provide useful building blocks for critically evaluating each section of a research article.

## SUGGESTED ACTIVITIES

Read two research articles—one quantitative and one qualitative—in your area of expertise or interest. Compare and contrast the two studies in the following areas:

1 Evaluate the methods section of the articles and note the following:
   - What specific type of design did the research use?
   - Does the design "match" the purpose of the study? Will the design provide the information to achieve the purpose or answer the problem stated?
   - How was the sample obtained? Based on the specific quantitative/qualitative design of the study, was the sampling plan appropriate?
   - In the quantitative study, were the reliability and the validity of the research instrument(s) described? In the qualitative study, how did the researcher record and organize the data?
   - Were data obtained in the same manner from all subjects?
2 Evaluate how the data were analyzed.
   - In the quantitative study, were the statistical tests appropriate to the type of data collected?
   - In the qualitative study, were the data analyzed in a way consistent with the type of qualitative design?

**3**   In both studies, are conclusions consistent with the data? Are limitations identified?
**4**   How could the study's findings be used—in practice, to plan further research?

## REFERENCES

Burns, N., & Grove, S. (2008). *The practice of nursing research. Appraisal, synthesis, and generation of evidence* (6th ed). Philadelphia: Elsevier.

DiCecco, K. (2007). Medical literature. Part II: A primer on understanding scientific design. *Journal of Legal Nurse Consulting, 18*(2), 3–11.

Oliver, D., & Mahon, S. (2006). Reading a research article. Part III: The data collection instrument. *Clinical Journal of Oncology Nursing, 10*, 423–426.

Russell, C. (2005). Evaluating quantitative research reports. *Nephrology Nursing Journal, 32*, 61–64.

Schira, M. (1999). Looking in the literature. In M. Mateo & K. Kirchhoff (Eds.), *Using and conducting nursing research in the clinical setting* (2nd ed., pp. 201–214). Philadelphia: Elsevier.

Vishnevsky, T., & Beanlands, H. (2004). Qualitative research. *Nephrology Nursing Journal, 31*, 234–238.

# 5 Identifying a Focus of Study

## LEA ANN MATURA AND VIVIAN NOWAZEK

There are numerous sources of ideas for identifying the focus of an inquiry. The literature review presents what is currently known about the topic of interest and the gaps in the literature. Once a thorough search and evaluation of the available evidence have been conducted, the focus of the study can be defined in the form of a purpose, objectives, and specific aims, along with well-developed research questions. This chapter delineates the components needed to define a research topic. Examples are included to illustrate the concepts and to facilitate practice in critically evaluating material from an evidence-based perspective.

## SOURCES OF TOPICS AND PROBLEMS

When a researcher is identifying a topic of inquiry, several sources can provide guidance in determining the question or problem to investigate. Some areas previously identified as starting points include clinical practice, continuous quality improvement, the research literature, professional organizations, and conferences (Mateo & Newton, 1999). Likewise, there are multiple examples from varying clinical settings or domains of health care where ideas may be generated; Clinical problems or questions; the literature; regulatory agencies; new diagnoses; media coverage; sentinel events; and legislative issues are briefly discussed and are only a few possibilities, but, these examples may stimulate thoughtful reflection on practice as we look forward to future studies. Once an idea is generated, a search of the literature is the next step in discovering what is already known and not known about the topic.

## Clinical Problems or Questions

The clinical setting is an excellent place to generate research questions. For example, a nursing unit may have protocols that define "routine vital signs," or perhaps a health care provider's order reads "Vital signs every 4 hours." Where is the evidence to support how often vital signs should be recorded? Are there studies that have explored the relationship between how often or when vital signs are performed and patient outcomes?

Another pervasive problem in health care is the prevention of pressure ulcers. Standard practices recommend turning patients every 2 hours, although there continues to be little support for this practice. A recent review of the literature searched for evidence on how best to prevent pressure ulcers (Reddy, Gill, & Rochon, 2006). The authors reviewed 59 randomized controlled trials (RCTs). Of the 59, only 2 trials were found to specifically address repositioning. One study found that turning every 4 hours on a specialty mattress reduced the number of pressure ulcers (Defloor, Bacquerb, & Grypdoncka, 2005). A study compared lateral and supine positioning to positioning at a 30-degree and a 90-degree angle (Young, 2004). The investigators did not find any difference between the two groups. These studies demonstrate no support for the common practice of repositioning patients every 2 hours and suggest the need for more research.

## Literature

Reading and critiquing the literature are other mechanisms for identifying gaps in what is known and not known in clinical practice. For example, researchers conducted a RCT to investigate whether telephone-only motivational interviewing increased physical activity among rural adults (Bennett, Heather, Nail, Winters-Stone, & Hanson, 2008). They found that the intervention did not increase physical activity, but they suggested that more investigation is needed to determine whether winter weather influenced the sample or whether a longer intervention period would have provided a positive result. Because a telephone intervention is a relatively inexpensive tool to improve care, especially in rural areas, more investigation is needed, and this area offers an ideal opportunity for more nursing research.

## Regulatory Agencies

Regulatory agencies such as The Joint Commission (http://www.joint commission.org) and the Centers for Medicare and Medicaid Services (CMS) (http://www.cms.hhs.gov/) are rich sources for research. The Joint Commission collaborated with the American Heart Association and the American College of Cardiology to develop performance measures, or core measure sets, for acute myocardial infarction (AMI). These measures specify evidence-based interventions necessary to provide patients with quality care. These measures include such interventions as smoking-cessation education. Nursing is in an excellent position to test interventions that assist patients in their smoking-cessation efforts.

## Technology

Advances in technology, such as electronic medical records (EMRs) and telemedicine, afford opportunities for nurses to use technology in caring for patients. One of the largest challenges in health care is implementing EMR for patients. Researchers described how primary care practices within the Practice Partner Research Network implemented EMRs in a national quality improvement project, Accelerating Translation of Research into Practice. They evaluated performance on 36 process and outcome indicators across eight domains common to primary practice, such as cardiovascular disease, diabetes, and cancer. They found that nursing plays an important role in facilitating quality improvement within primary care practices (Nemeth, Wessell, Jenkins, Nietert, Liszka, & Ornstein, 2007). More research will be necessary to determine whether the use of EMRs improves health care delivery.

Telemedicine is another area that is expanding to provide improved health care, especially for chronic conditions such as heart failure. A randomized controlled trial was conducted to determine whether telehomecare, a telephone-based data transfer, could affect outcomes such as hospitalization and mortality (Dansky, Vasey, & Bowles, 2008). They found patients in the telehomecare group had lower rates of both hospitalization and emergency department visits at 1- and 2-month follow-up periods and fewer symptoms than the control group. A limitation to this study is that the power analysis suggests that a larger sample was needed; therefore, this study should be replicated with a larger sample size. There are many more patient populations with chronic illnesses that need to be studied to determine whether telemedicine can help deliver and improve health care.

## New Diagnoses

Health care continues to make new discoveries, including new diagnoses, especially because of research in genetics. As new syndromes are defined and new diseases and diagnoses are discovered, there will be an increasing need for research in these areas. Infectious diseases are continuing to emerge. For example, the World Health Organization (WHO) in October 2008 investigated an unknown disease in South Africa and Zambia (WHO, 2008). An employee of a safari tour company in Zambia died from an unknown case. The paramedic and the nurse caring for the patient also became ill and died. The reported signs and symptoms were fever, headache, diarrhea, myalgia, a rash, and liver dysfunction. To date, the infection does not seem to be a type of hemorrhagic fever. Nursing can play a key role in assisting in the care of and infection control practices for these patients, which are all sources for investigation.

An example of a new genetic syndrome is a microdeletion of 15q13.3, which causes mental retardation, epilepsy, and facial and digital dysmorphisms (Sharp et al., 2008). Although this disorder is thought to affect about 3 out of 1,000 individuals with mental retardation, there is a need for further investigation to determine the impact of this syndrome on patients and their caregivers. This again gives nursing an excellent opportunity to investigate the impact of this syndrome and possible interventions to improve patient care.

Similarly, a new genetic syndrome discovered by researchers in 2003 revealed a microduplication of chromosome 22q11.2 in patients previously diagnosed with DiGeorge/velocardiofacial (DG/VCFS) syndrome (Ensenauer et al., 2003). The phenotypic features of this new syndrome are widely spaced eyes and superior placement of the eyebrows with increased distance from the eyebrow to upper eyelid crease, downslanting palpebral fissures, and a long narrow face. These features are different from the DB/VCRS syndrome, which led researchers to conclude that this is a new syndrome. To date, there is only one other publication referencing this new syndrome (Yobb et al., 2005). This gives researchers opportunities to conduct studies from a nursing perspective to potentially improve the care and lives of these patients and patients' families.

## Media

The media represent another avenue for generating ideas for investigation. Media include television, radio, newspapers, and the Internet. The media report issues that are important to patients. A good example has been the recent media attention to the GARDASIL® [Human Papillomavirus Quadrivalent (Types 6, 11, 16, 18) vaccine, recombinant] vaccine, including discussion of adverse events reported by recipients of the vaccine. GARDASIL® was approved by the U.S. Food and Drug Administration (FDA) (http://www.fda.gov) on June 8, 2006, for females between 9 and 26 years of age to prevent cervical cancer, precancerous genital lesions, and genital warts due to human papillomavirus (HPV) types 6, 11, 16, and 18 (U.S. Food & Drug Administration, 2006). There have been reports of adverse reactions to the vaccine, to which the media have called attention. When the search engine Google™ is used, for example, a search for *GARDASIL® adverse events or media reports* returns between 24,900 and 34,000 results. In July 2008, the FDA reported that the manufacturer had distributed more than 16 million doses of GARDASIL® and that there had been 9,749 Vaccine Adverse Event Reporting System (VAERS) reports following GARDASIL® vaccination. Ninety-four percent were classified as nonserious, while 6% were categorized as serious, including 20 deaths. Other serious VAERS reports included Guillian-Barre Syndrome and thromboembolic disorders. The FDA and the Centers for Disease Control and Prevention (http://www.cdc.gov) have investigated and reviewed these VAERS reports and have found that GARDASIL® continues to be safe and effective. To date, there has been no change in any recommendations for the use of GARDASIL®. As researchers involved in monitoring the safety and efficacy of GARDASIL® continue to follow reactions to the vaccine, this will offer a prime opportunity for nurses to investigate those who file a VAERS report to determine how their health has been affected and to identify possible interventions to help them improve or regain their health. Other research possibilities include how reports influence the decision making of parents, girls, and women as they choose whether to receive the GARDASIL® vaccine or other vaccines (U.S. Food & Drug Administration, 2008).

## Sentinel Events

Unfortunately, untoward, or sentinel, events sometimes occur. The Joint Commission defines a sentinel event as "an unexpected occurrence involving death or serious physical or psychological injury, or the risk thereof. Serious injury specifically includes loss of limb or function" (Joint Commission, 2007).These events may be related to system problems, knowledge deficits, equipment malfunction, or a variety of other related problems. Some examples of Sentinel Event alerts issued in 2008 concerned the prevention of errors relating to commonly used anticoagulants; behaviors that undermine a culture of safety; the prevention of pediatric medication errors; and the prevention of accidents and injuries in the magnetic resonance imaging (MRI) suite. Nurses are well poised to study how these important occurrences happen and to develop effective interventions for prevention.

Several studies have described disruptive behavior or workplace bullying and how it potentially affects patient safety and nurse retention (Martin, 2008; Rosenstein, 2002; Rosenstein & O'Daniel, 2005). Next steps, as outlined by the Joint Commission, can be skills-based training for management on relationship building, collaborative practice, and conflict resolution. Cultural assessment instruments can be used to determine whether attitudes are changing over time as a result of the training. Another potential study might focus on the development of a system for assessing staff perceptions of the seriousness of unprofessional behavior and the risk of harm to patients. All of these are areas that need further investigation to keep patients and the health care team safe and to improve the delivery of quality care.

## Legislative Events

Other opportunities for nursing research are related to legislative issues. Nursing is in a unique position for studying health policy and legislation. In an earlier section, we discussed the vaccine GARDASIL®. Some states have considered making the vaccine mandatory for young girls, with Texas leading the way (Napoli, 2007; National Council of State Legislatures [NCSL], 2008). Texas governor Rick Perry signed an executive order on February 2, 2007, requiring all sixth-grade girls to receive GARDASIL® (NCSL, 2008). Nursing needs to be a part of health policy discussions and should conduct research on legislative issues in order to promote and protect the public's health.

Similarly, nurse staffing ratios are a legislative issue that many states have been debating for decades. On January 1, 2008, California upgraded its staffing ratios to 1:3 on Step Down units; 1:4 on Telemetry units; and 1:4 in other specialty areas such as oncology. Other mandated ratios are 1:2 in Critical Care, 1:4 in Pediatrics, and 1:4 in the Emergency Department (California Hospital Association, 2003). Further research will be needed to determine whether these ratios improve patient care and patient safety. One problem with these ratios is that the term *nurse* is defined as a Registered Nurse (RN) or a Licensed Practical Nurse (LPN). Previous research on nursing educational level and patient outcomes determined that having RNs, those with a bachelor's degree or higher, provide direct patient care improves care by decreasing mortality (Aiken, Clarke, Cheung, Sloane, & Silber, 2003). An initial study to determine how the ratios have affected outcomes concluded that there has not been a significant positive impact on nurse-sensitive quality indicators, such as pressure ulcers and patient falls (Bolton et al., 2007).

## BACKGROUND

An exhaustive review of the literature is imperative to determine what is currently known about the subject or phenomenon. Well-written studies provide insight into the implications of the findings and suggestions for future research or directions for inquiry. A review of studies related to the topic helps to summarize the findings and thereby helps the reader to develop a sense of where the next inquiry should begin. The review will also give ideas on possible research designs, along with potential leads for experts or consultants for the study. The review should give a good suggestion of theories or conceptual models that have been applied or allude to possible conceptual frameworks for future studies.

The background section of the proposal for the study should give a concise overview of the body of science under investigation and how the studies contribute to knowledge development. The background should connect the literature and define the domains of the concepts under investigation. An explanation of how the literature search was conducted should also be provided. Common research databases include the Cumulative Index to Nursing and Allied Health Literature (CINAHL) and Medical Literature Analysis and Retrieval System Online (Medline). CINAHL is primarily used by nurse scientists, but it is important not to limit oneself to only one research database as a tool for searches. Medline® is a search engine for biomedical research. It is important to use multiple search engines when exploring a topic. Limiting oneself to one database may mean that one does not find all available research on the topic. Research fields for nursing overlap with those of other disciplines, such as medicine, pharmacy, physical therapy, nutrition, and psychology.

When searching for relevant studies, one should employ a variety of methods, including searches by subject, key words, and author. A subject search is a broad search where one is looking for general information on a topic. This may be a good starting point when determining the breadth of a particular topic or phenomena. Depending on the topic, a subject search may reveal literally thousands of papers. At this point, it can be helpful to narrow the topic area by using limits. These limits may include gender, race, human subjects, or other areas. Selecting a particular article may be helpful to determine Medical Subject Headings (Mesh®) terms as created by the National Library of Medicine (NLM). Mesh® terms are developed by NLM and consist of a preferred list of medical terms. These terms are helpful in finding other studies on the topic once a good study has been found to provide an exhaustive search on a particular topic. Chapter on general searching includes ways of maximizing the effectiveness of the literature search.

When reviewing the literature, one should review primary, not secondary, sources, that is, publications written by those who conducted the study, not publications that report on and summarize studies conducted by others. Reviewing primary sources allows the reviewer to determine the validity of the study rather than relying on another's interpretation of the study. An exception to this recommendation is the systematic review, the purpose of which is to summarize all the research on a topic to determine the outcome across a number of studies, populations, and clinical settings.

## SIGNIFICANCE

Determining the significance of a study is vital to decide if the topic is worthy of investigation. Is the topic timely? Will the topic add significant information to a body of knowledge? Does it provide new information, or does it help confirm previous results by replicating a previously done study? Is the study innovative? Does it describe a new phenomenon or a new way of studying a problem? The section on significance should point out the limited amount of information currently available or determine whether no information is currently published. On the other hand, the section on significance may indicate that there is conflicting evidence on the topic and that further investigation is needed to clarify what is known or unknown. The significance of a study may be related to testing a theory or furthering scientists' understanding of how the research will help a particular patient population. Following are examples of how the significance of a study may be articulated.

Researchers conducted a qualitative study using grounded theory processes to understand how violence of adult children affected their mothers and the process the mothers used to get assistance and to access mental health treatment (Copelan & Heilemann, 2008). The investigators determined that the significance of the study was related to the fact that little information was available about the experiences of family members and how they attempt to get assistance for their mentally ill and violent children. In another example, investigators examined overall and specific symptoms in patients with multiple sclerosis (MS) and how the symptoms correlated with physical activity (Motl, Snook, & Schapiro, 2008). They presented an extensive review of previous literature investigating symptoms related to MS, followed by a discussion of why their study was significant. They determined that previous studies had evaluated the relationship between overall symptoms, rather than specific symptoms, and physical activity. Also, previous studies did not account for possible functional limitations related to patients' ability to perform physical activities. These limitations served as the foundation for determining the significance of their study.

## PURPOSE, OBJECTIVE, AND AIMS

Once researchers have identified a topic of interest and conducted a thorough review of the literature, they can define the study further through by developing its purpose, objectives, and specific aims. The purpose statement of a study is a statement of the essence of what the investigators are attempting to explore. The statement generally begins with "The purpose of this study...." This statement will guide the development of the research project by denoting what the focus of the research is. Following is an example of a purpose statement: "The purpose of this research was to describe factors that predict health outcomes in persons with sickle cell disease (SCD) by testing a modification of a theory, the theory of self care management for SCD" (Jenerette &

Murdaugh, 2008). In one qualitative study, researchers wanted to determine the experience of nurses during the Persian Gulf combat. They stated the study's purpose as follows: "The purpose of the ongoing project is to gather accounts of nurses who have served their country during wartime, on the battle front or in supportive roles" (Rushton, Scott, & Callister, 2008).

The objectives of a study are very closely related to the purpose. Although some researchers may use the terms *purpose* and *objectives* interchangeably, they are distinct components in the research protocol. Objectives are components of the study that can be measured. Although the objectives should flow from the purpose statement and are closely related to it, they are distinctly different. In the study by Rushton, Scott, and Callister (2008), the objectives of the study were "(1) to permanently archive the nurses' accounts, (2) to generate themes that elucidate their nursing experiences, and (3) to honor nurses that have served by sharing their stories." The objectives help fulfill the purpose of the study: to describe the experiences of nurses serving during the Persian Gulf war.

Similarly, the aim of a study and its purpose are interchangeable. While the purpose is the essence of what is being studied, the aim is more aligned with the goal of the study or what the researchers want to accomplish. Generally, the aim of the study is contained in a statement that begins like this: "the aim of this study...." In one qualitative study, researchers identified the need to investigate the relationships between parents and neonatal intensive care unit (NICU) nurses during the prolonged hospitalization of premature babies (Fegran, Fagermoen, & Helseth, 2008). The specific aim of the study was stated this way: "The aim of this study was to explore the development of relationships between parents and nurses in an NICU." In one quantitative study, the investigators wanted to determine how to identify depression in patients who had communication and cognitive impairments following a stroke (Lightbody et al., 2007). The specific aim was written this way: "To determine the accuracy and utility of an observational screening tool, Signs of Depression Scale (SODS), for mood problems in a population of stroke patients, and to explore the agreement between different raters."

The decision whether to use a purpose statement or to present an aim may be based on personal preference of the researcher, the audience that the researcher is presenting to, or the funding agency. For example, thesis or dissertation committees may require specific wording related to aims in a research proposal or protocol. When writing for publication in journals, one may encounter similar requirements. When one is writing a grant proposal, one may be required to provide a list of objectives for the research project. Whatever the requirements are, the researcher will need to state in some form the essence of the project and what the researcher wants to accomplish.

## RESEARCH QUESTIONS

Once the topic of inquiry has been identified and the literature review conducted, the researcher can write the research questions. Research questions are interrogatives that bring out what is being studied specifically. Not all studies have specific research questions; some studies may have a hypothesis or hypotheses, which are discussed in the following section. The research questions contain the independent and dependent variable(s), which are also discussed in another section of this chapter. Another important factor related to research questions is the way the question is stated. The wording of the question in a quantitative study drives the statistical analysis.

Research questions are often restatements of the purpose. For example, researchers wanted to examine stress among pregnant Black women (Gennaro, Shults, & Garry, 2008). In their study, they identified three purposes: "(a) compare three commonly used measures of stress during pregnancy in Black women, (b) examine changes in stress in Black women over time to determine when stress is highest, and (c) provide exploratory information as to whether any of the stress measures help to predict Black women who might be more likely to deliver preterm infants than other Black women" (pp. 538–539). The three research questions were derived from the purpose statements: "(1) What is the relationship between three measures of stress in pregnant Black women: Corticotropin-releasing hormone (CRH) (a physiological measure), Prenatal Distress Questionnaire (PDQ), and Perceived Stress Scale (PSS)? (2) After 28 weeks, is stress highest in pregnant Black women? (3) Is there a difference in stress between Black women (a) in preterm labor who deliver preterm, (b) in preterm labor who deliver term, or (c) who experience normal term labor and deliveries?" (p. 539).

Qualitative studies also have research questions. Researchers used grounded theory methods to determine how women with potential cardiac symptoms made decisions about seeking treatment (Turris & Johnson, 2008). Their purpose statement was "to explore how women seeking treatment for the symptoms of potential cardiac illness interpreted their symptoms, made decisions about seeking treatment, and understood experiences of care in the emergency department." Their primary research question was derived from the purpose and was stated this way: "In the context of the symptoms of a potential cardiac event, what is the process by which women understand and make decisions about those symptoms?" In this qualitative study, there is a relationship between the purpose and the research question, although the research question is not an exact restatement of the purpose. Some researchers may decide to use hypotheses instead of research questions; these are discussed in the following section.

## HYPOTHESES

A hypothesis is a prediction of outcomes between one or more variables (Mateo & Newton, 1999). Generally, in order to state a hypothesis, a researcher relies on previous literature or a theoretical framework to support the relationship between variables. Hypotheses can be directional, nondirectional, or null.

A directional hypothesis not only predicts the relationship between one or more variables but also states the direction of the relationship. Researchers conducted a pilot study to determine differences in temperature rhythms, rest and activity rhythms, melatonin rhythms, sleep percentages, and daytime sleepiness in older adults living in independent apartments and in nursing homes (Chaperon, Farr, & Lochiano, 2007). They had three research hypotheses. One of the hypotheses was stated as follows: "Older age will be a predictor of increased negative effects of environmental cues" (p. 22). In this hypothesis, older age suggests a direction in the relationship between the variables; with increasing age, there is an increasing negative effect. Usually, theory or past findings enable the prediction.

In contrast, a nondirectional hypothesis does not predict the direction of the relationship. One of the hypotheses from the same researchers stated: "Apartment-dwelling residents will have different axillary body temperature rhythms, rest/activity rhythms, melatonin rhythms, sleep percentages, and daytime sleepiness than nursing home residents" (p. 22). The investigators stated that there would be a difference between apartment-dwelling residents and nursing home residents in relation to the defined outcome variables, but they did not state the direction of the association. Similarly, the other nondirectional hypothesis in this study stated: "Daytime or nighttime light exposure will be associated with differences in axillary body temperature rhythms, rest/activity rhythms, melatonin rhythms, sleep percentages, and daytime sleepiness" (Chaperon et al., 2007). The researchers stated that there would be an association but did not elaborate on which direction the association would take.

A null hypothesis or statistical hypothesis is a statement that predicts that there is no relationship between variables (Mateo & Newton, 1999). The null hypothesis is not always explicitly written but can be derived from the hypotheses that are stated. The null hypothesis is what is accepted or rejected in relation to statistical procedures. In one study, researchers wanted to explore the effects of a 5-day tactile touch intervention on oxytocin levels in critical care patients (Henricson, Berglund, Määttä, Ekman, & Segesten, 2008). The directional hypotheses stated that tactile touch would increase oxytocin levels after the intervention and continue to increase the levels over a 6-day period. The null hypothesis would be stated this way: There is no difference in the levels of oxytocin in intensive care unit patients after a tactile touch intervention.

In another example, researchers investigated whether positioning of intubated infants affected the colonization of bacteria in the trachea, putting infants at risk for infections (Aly, Badawy, El-Kholy, Nabil, & Mohamed, 2008). They hypothesized that intubated infants positioned on their sides would be less likely to have bacterial colonization in their tracheas than those positioned supinely. This is an example of a directional hypothesis. The null hypothesis would be that there is no difference in the amount of tracheal bacterial colonization in those infants positioned on their sides and those positioned supinely.

## VARIABLES

A research question is written in terms of the dependent variable (DV), also known as the observed outcome, and the independent variable(s) (IV), or the variable(s) hypothesized or thought to produce the dependent variable. Dependent variable values depend upon the independent variable(s). Variables are operationally defined by what is measured, how the indicators are measured, and how the values are interpreted. In other words, an operational definition characterizes how the variable is measured.

Variables are classified according to the level or scale of measurement; the four scales are nominal, ordinal, interval, and ratio (NOIR).

Knowing the level or scale of measurement provides the necessary information for readers to interpret the data from that variable. Certain statistical analyses are used only for data measured at certain measurement levels. The level of measurement of the independent variable, the question being asked, and the number of groups of the dependent variable are key determinants for selecting the correct statistical test to analyze the research study data. In general, it is desirable to have a higher level of measurement (e.g., interval or ratio) than to use a lower one (e.g., nominal or ordinal). When in doubt as to the level of measurement, the rule of thumb is to treat the variable at the highest level of measurement that can be justified, that is, to use an interval rather than an ordinal scale and an ordinal scale rather than a nominal one. Statistics for higher levels of measurement are more powerful at detecting differences in the research data. Once the statistical test is determined, the sample size can be calculated.

## SUMMARY

In summary, identifying a focus of study can be challenging. There are multiple sources for initially determining what to study, including, but not limited to, the literature and clinically derived questions. A thorough search of the literature will help determine what is already known on the subject and further define what the topic will be. Once the literature has been scrutinized, the purpose or aim of the study can be delineated. In conjunction with the purpose, research questions and or hypotheses are then formulated. The hypothesis describes a relationship between the independent and the dependent variable(s). The independent and dependent variables determine the statistical test to be performed once the number of groups in the study and the level of measurement (nominal, ordinal, interval, or ratio) have been determined.

## SUGGESTED ACTIVITIES

1    Suppose you were interested in determining how to reduce caregiver burden in Alzheimer's disease. Write down your strategy for determining what information is currently known and formulate a research question(s).

**2** For the following research questions, write a directional, a non-directional, and a null hypothesis:

**a** Is there a difference in the effectiveness of bland mouth washes and magic mouth washes in treating chemo- and radiation-therapy induced mucositis?

**b** Does turning medical ICU patients every 2 hours decrease the incidence of decubitus ulcers?

**c** Are maternal-infant bonding behaviors affected by the performance of initial newborn infant physical examination?

## REFERENCES

Aiken, L. H., Clarke, S. P., Cheung, R. B., Sloane, D. M., & Silber, J. H. (2003). Educational levels of hospital nurses and surgical patient mortality. *Journal of the American Medical Association 290*(12), 1617–1623.

Aly, H., Badawy, M., El-Kholy, A., Nabil, R., & Mohamed, A. (2008). Randomized, controlled trial on tracheal colonization of ventilated infants: Can gravity prevent ventilator-associated pneumonia? *Pediatrics, 122*(4), 770–774.

Bennett, J. A. Y., Heather, M., Nail, Lillian M., Winters-Stone, Kerri, & Hanson, Ginger. (2008). A telephone-only motivational intervention to increase physical activity in rural adults: A randomized controlled trial. *Nursing Research, 57*(1), 24–32.

Black, J., Baharestani, M., Cuddigan, J., Dorner, B., Edsberg, L., Langemo, D., et al. (2007). National Pressure Ulcer Advisory Panel's (NPUAP) updated pressure ulcer staging system (USA). *World Council of Enterostomal Therapists Journal, 27*(2), 18–23.

Bolton, L. B., Aydin, C. E., Donaldson, N., Brown, D. S., Sandhu, M., Fridman, M., et al. (2007). Mandated nurse staffing ratios in California: A comparison of staffing and nursing-sensitive outcomes pre- and postregulation. *Policy, Politics, & Nursing Practice, 8*(4), 238–250.

California Hospital Association. (2003). Hospital minimum nurse-to-patient ratios as required by AB 394. Retrieved November 2, 2008, 2008, from http://www.calhealth.org/public/press/Article/113/Nurse%20Ratio%20chart.pdf

Chaperon, C. M., Farr, L. A., & Lochiano, E. (2007). Sleep disturbance of residents in a continuing care retirement community. *Journal of Gerontological Nursing, 33*(10), 21–28.

Copelan, D., & Heilemann, M. (2008). Getting "to the point": The experience of mothers getting assistance for their adult children who are violent and mentally ill. *Nursing Research, 57*(3), 136–143.

Dansky, K. H., Vasey, J., & Bowles, K. (2008). Impact of telehealth on clinical outcomes in patients with heart failure. *Clinical Nursing Research, 17*(3), 182–199.

Defloor, T., Bacquerb, D. D., & Grypdoncka, M. H. (2005). The effect of various combinations of turning and pressure reducing devices on the incidence of pressure ulcers. *International Journal of Nursing Studies, 42*(1), 37–46.

Dodd, M. J., Dibble, S. L., Miaskowski, C., MacPhail, L., Greenspan, D., Paul, S. M., et al. (2000). Randomized clinical trial of the effectiveness of 3 commonly used mouthwashes to treat chemotherapy-induced mucositis. *Oral Surgery, Oral Medicine, Oral Pathology, Oral Radiology & Endodontology, 90*(1), 39–47.

Ensenauer, R. E., Adeyinka, A., Flynn, H. C., Michels, V. V., Lindor, N. M., Dawson, D. B., et al. (2003). Microduplication 22q11.2, an emerging syndrome: Clinical, cytogenetic, and molecular analysis of thirteen patients. *American Journal of Human Genetics, 73*(5), 1027–1040.

Fegran, F., Fagermoen, M. S., & Helseth, S. (2008). Development of parent-nurse relationships in neonatal intensive care units from closeness to detachment. *Journal of Advanced Nursing, 64*(4), 363–371.

Gennaro, S., Shults, J., & Garry, D. J. (2008). Stress and preterm labor and birth in Black women. *Journal of Obstetric, Gynecologic, & Neonatal Nursing, 37*(5), 538–545.

Henricson, M., Berglund, A. L., Määttä, S., Ekman, R., & Segesten, K. (2008). The outcome of tactile touch on oxytocin in intensive care patients: A randomised controlled trial. *Journal of Clinical Nursing, 17*(19), 2624–2633.

Jenerette, C. M., & Murdaugh, C. (2008). Testing the theory of self-care management for sickle cell disease. *Research in Nursing & Health, 31*(4), 355–369.

Joint Commission. (2007, July). *Sentinel event.* Retrieved October 27, 2008, 2008, from http://www.jointcommission.org/SentinelEvents/

Lightbody, C. E., Auton, M., Baldwin, R., Gibbon, B., Hamer, S., Leathley, M. J., et al. (2007). The use of nurses' and carers' observations in the identification of poststroke depression. *Journal of Advanced Nursing, 60*(6), 595–604.

Martin, W. F. (2008). Is your hospital safe? Disruptive behavior and workplace bullying. *Hospital Topics, 86*(3), 21–28.

Massie, H., & Campbell, B. K. (1992). *The Massie-Campbell scale of mother-infant attachment indicators during stress: For use during the pediatric examination and other childcare situations.* San Francisco: Child Development Media.

Mateo, M. A., & Newton, C. (1999). Progressing from an idea to a research question. In M. A. Mateo & K. T. Kirchhoff (Eds), *Using and conducting nursing research in the clinical setting* (2nd ed., pp. 191–199). Philadelphia, PA: W.B. Saunders.

Motl, R. W., Snook, E. M., & Schapiro, R. T. (2008). Symptoms and physical activity behavior in individuals with multiple sclerosis. *Research in Nursing & Health, 31*(5), 466–475.

Napoli, M. (2007). How vaccine policy is made: The story of Merck and Gardasil. *Health-Facts, 32*(3), 1–3.

National Council of State Legislatures (NCSL). (2008, September 22). HPV. *NCSL Resources—HPV Vaccine Legislation 2007–2008.* Retrieved November 2, 2008, from http://www.ncsl.org/programs/health/HPVvaccine.htm

Nemeth, L. S., Wessell, A. M., Jenkins, R. G., Nietert, P. J., Liszka, H. A., & Ornstein, S. M. (2007). Strategies to accelerate translation of research into primary care within practices using electronic medical records. *Journal of Nursing Care Quality, 22*(4), 343–349.

Reddy, M., Gill, S. S., & Rochon, P. A. (2006). Preventing pressure ulcers: A systematic review. *Journal of the American Medical Association, 296*(8), 974–984.

Rosenstein, A. H. (2002). Nurse-physician relationships: Impact on nurse satisfaction and retention. *American Journal of Nursing, 102*(6), 26–34.

Rosenstein, A. H., & O'Daniel, M. (2005). Disruptive behavior & clinical outcomes: Perceptions of nurses & physicians. *American Journal of Nursing, 105*(1), 54–65.

Rushton, P., Scott, J. E., & Callister, L. C. (2008). "It's what we're here for": Nurses caring for military personnel during the Persian Gulf wars. *Nursing Outlook, 56*(4), 179–186, quotation on p. 171.

Sharp, A. J., Mefford, H. C., Li, K., Baker, C., Skinner, C., Stevenson, R. E., et al. (2008). A recurrent 15q13.3 microdeletion syndrome associated with mental retardation and seizures. *Nature Genetics, 40*(3), 322–328.

Turris, S. A., & Johnson, J. L. (2008). Maintaining integrity: Women and treatment seeking for the symptoms of potential cardiac illness. *Qualitative Health Research, 18*(11), 1461–1476.

U.S. Food and Drug Administration. (2006). *Information from CDC and FDA on the safety of Gardasil vaccine.* Retrieved October 27, 2008, from http://www.fda.gov/cber/safety/gardasil071408.htm

World Health Organization. (2008). *Unknown disease in South Africa and Zambia.* Retrieved October 25, 2008, from http://www.who.int/csr/don/2008_10_10/en/index.html

Yobb, T. M., Somerville, M. J., Willatt, L., Firth, H. V., Harrison, K., MacKenzie, J., et al. (2005). Microduplication and triplication of 22q11.2: A highly variable syndrome. *The American Journal of Human Genetics, 76*(5), 865–876.

Young, T. (2004). The 30 degree tilt position vs. the 90 degree lateral and supine positions in reducing the incidence of non-blanching erythema in a hospital inpatient population: A randomised controlled trial. *Journal of Tissue Viability, 14*(3), 80, 90, 92–96.

# 6

# Theoretical and Conceptual Frameworks

MAGDALENA A. MATEO AND MARGE BENHAM-HUTCHINS

Systematic reviews synthesize bodies of research findings to uncover the appropriate principles to be applied to practice (Coopey & Nix, 2006), but how does the advanced practice nurse (APN) critically appraise a specific research study to determine if the findings are appropriate for integration into practice? Evidence-based practice is the use of the best clinical evidence from empirical research to make patient care decisions (Goode, 2000). The APN must have the skills necessary to scrutinize research findings to determine their usefulness in clinical practice. This is done by examining the findings for both validity and clinical applicability. An important consideration when making this determination is congruence between the conceptual framework or theory guiding the study and the research design.

Research is vital to expand nursing knowledge and an important level of evidence when striving to achieve evidence-based practice. Theory or model-guided studies are necessary for the generalizability of findings and the development of new nursing knowledge. Without a theoretical framework research studies are problem based and the findings may not be applicable to another setting (Verran, 1997). Evaluation of research reports to determine appropriateness for integration of new knowledge into clinical practice should begin with an examination of the applicability of the theory or conceptual model that was used to guide the study.

This chapter includes methods useful for assessing the scientific merit of the study and the applicability of the research findings to practice.

## EMPIRICAL RESEARCH

Empirical research is a study that has a focus on objective scientific methods and collection of data to form or test theory. It is vital that APNs gain mastery of empirical research methods to be able to critique the applicability of study findings to practice. Empirical research includes the following components:

1    Research design—overall plan for methods and procedures used to conduct a study. Concepts to be used in the proposed study should be identified and defined. Background information should include definitions and an explanation of how variables were used and evaluated in both previous studies and the present one. A summary and a critique of previous studies that used the theoretical framework being used in a present study should be identified
2    Sample—data sources; subset of a population participating in a study.
3    Instruments and experimental conditions—tools and data collection; experimental intervention should be consistent with the theoretical definitions of the concepts.
4    Data collection procedures and protection of human subjects from harm—description of when data collection occurred, where it occurred, and by whom it was done; process used to protect human subjects.
5    Data analysis techniques: word (qualitative data may use content analysis) or number data (statistical analysis).

## CONCEPTUAL FRAMEWORK

Models and theories are used to help describe, explain, and predict phenomena (Peterson & Bredow, 2009). A conceptual model or framework is more abstract and "refers to global ideas about groups, situations, and events of interest to a science" (Fawcett, 1980, p. 88). Questions posed in evaluating the philosophic underpinnings of a model must include the explicit identification of biases and values and a description of how the model incorporates, describes, and links the essential concepts within the research study and of the applicability of those linkages to practice.

Conceptual activities provide the foundation for the entire research process, from defining the research focus to interpreting results of a study. Characteristics of concepts span from concrete to abstract. Planning a study using a conceptual model requires definition of concepts based on how they have been used by researchers in the area of interest; this allows the current researcher to build on the existing body of knowledge. If possible, operational definitions of variables should also be based on valid and reliable tools that have been used in previous studies.

For example, Hess and Insel (2007) developed a conceptual model of chemotherapy-related change in cognitive function that was defined as a mental process. They reported that patients undergoing chemotherapy experience decreased cognitive functions, such as increases in forgetfulness and an inability to focus when doing everyday tasks. When an understanding of the overall cognitive-related changes in patients who are receiving chemotherapy exists, it is possible to continue further development of interventions to counteract these effects through research methods. Following testing, the conceptual model can be used to evaluate intervention outcomes of patients receiving chemotherapy.

## THEORETICAL FRAMEWORK

A theory is a set of interrelated constructs (concepts, definitions, and propositions) that present a systematic view of a phenomenon by specifying relations among variables in order to explain and predict the phenomena (Peterson & Bredow, 2009). It is used to describe, explain, or predict the occurrence of a phenomenon. It is an abstraction that presents an explanation about how phenomena (concepts) are interrelated (proposition). Research studies may be designed to generate new theory or to test existing theory. Theories make research findings meaningful and interpretable. They stimulate research by providing direction and impetus for investigation of a concept.

There are three levels of theoretical conceptualizations. Theories may be grand (e.g., a description of large segments of a population, such as the entire nursing profession); middle range, more specific to a phenomenon; or situation specific or practice specific. Grand theories are abstract, focusing on phenomena of central concern to nursing, such as the meta-paradigm concepts of person, health, nursing, and environment.

A grand theory may be used to guide the selection of concepts and phenomena and to examine relationships. For example, Orem's theory of self-care deficit has been applied in the clinical setting to guide nursing practice in giving care to a patient when he or she is unable to care for himself or herself. In contrast, middle-range theories have been used by researchers to explore phenomena that are meaningful to practice. These theories have been described as less abstract, as narrower in scope, and as focusing on more specific phenomena (Peterson & Bredow, 2009). Concepts in middle-range theories are more specific and testable (Schmitt, 1999). In Pender's revised Health Belief Model, concepts include personal factors, and the perceived benefits of action affects behavioral outcome, which is the likelihood of engaging in health-promoting behaviors. Middle-range theories give a partial view of a nursing phenomenon, are more testable and generalizable, and are applicable to practice.

Theories are classified as descriptive, explanatory, or predictive and should be matched with the appropriate research study design (descriptive, correlational, or experimental). Situation-specific and practice theories focus on nursing phenomena that reflect nursing practice, are limited to specific populations or particular field or practice, and have a narrow scope. Concepts are narrowly defined and readily measured. These theories are used in evaluating current nursing practice, such as pain management following a surgical procedure (Meleis, 2005).

For example, the purpose of descriptive research is to obtain data on the extent of a phenomenon. In order to describe how common and serious the concept of adaptation (conceptual framework) is to disease and treatment outcomes, it is vital to clarify what is meant by adaptation. A researcher might define adaptation as the adult's ability to adapt to illness. Findings of the study would be limited by the definition and measurement specified in the study. On the other hand, if a researcher wants to investigate adaptation from a multidimensional perspective that encompasses a broader spectrum of responses to illness, then the concept of adaptation would be expanded. The question then would be whether adaptation varies depending on the type of illness or situation.

## EVIDENCE-BASED PRACTICE

In Chapter 2 of this book, "Overview of Evidence-Based Practice," EBP is defined as the integration of clinical expertise with the best evidence from systematic research. The use of evidence that has been acquired and that is considered to be at a high level strengthens the argument for implementing new interventions to practice. Sources of evidence range from level 1 to level 7, with the highest level of source being a systematic review of randomized clinical trials (RCTs) (Polit & Beck, 2008). Other sources of evidence are:

Level II—A single RCT; single nonrandomized trial

Level III—Systematic review of correlational or observational studies

Level IV—Single correlational or observational study

Level V—Systematic review of descriptive or qualitative/physiologic studies

Level VI—Single descriptive, qualitative, or physiologic study

Level VII—Opinions of authorities, expert committees

Searching for the best evidence in an expeditious manner may promote EBP. Fineout-Overholt, Hofstetter, Shell, and Johnston (2005, p. 208) suggest effective ways of searching for the best evidence. Their suggestions include knowing the type of evidence needed to answer the question (e.g., a search for meaning usually requires descriptive or qualitative research, whereas an intervention requires an RCT); using controlled vocabulary headings; determining inclusion and exclusion criteria; and selecting an organizing method for evidence (e.g., RefWorks [www.refworks.com]). RefWorks was selected because it allows a team working on a project to access a shared Web space. Chapter 3 provides detailed descriptions of ways to conduct literature searches.

Web site resources that provide links to guidelines, abstracts, and evidence summaries are available. Examples of useful Web sites include:

- www.health-evidence.ca
- http//healthlinks.washington.edu/ebp.ebpresources.html
- http://www.ahrq.gov/clinic/epcix.htm

## CRITIQUING THE CONCEPTUAL AND THEORETICAL FRAMEWORK IN A RESEARCH REPORT

Fawcett (2004) provides a comprehensive framework for the analysis and evaluation of conceptual models of nursing. Her goal is to provide a clear definition of conceptual models, an explanation of how they differ from theories, and a discussion of differences in the frameworks for analysis and evaluation. She observes that a conceptual model is made up of "global ideas about the individuals, groups, situations, and events of interest to science" (p. 88). These ideas are represented by global concepts, "words bringing forth mental images of the properties of things," which are linked by "propositions stating their interrelationships" (p. 88). These propositions are based on basic scientific assumptions within the field. As such, a conceptual model provides discipline-specific assumptions that tie together abstract concepts of interest and that represent "the first step in developing theoretical formulations needed for scientific activities" (p. 88). A theory, on the other hand, "contains more concrete concepts, along with their definitions, and the propositions linking them" (p. 89) and is testable.

The purpose of analyzing and evaluating a conceptual model is to first decide to "retain, modify, or discard the model" and then to determine if the model is appropriate for your own nursing activities (Fawcett, 2004a, p. 91). The analysis process begins with a nonjudgmental examination of the philosophical base of the model. Since the model is derived from the author's personal philosophy and scientific point of reference, the first steps in the analysis process is to determine the historical development of the model, what approach is used to develop nursing knowledge, and how the four essential concepts of nursing are explained.

Evaluating the theory used in a study is an essential component of research. Fawcett and Garity (2009) identify steps that constitute critique and evaluation, which they base on the conceptual, theoretical, and empirical components of the research study (C-T-E model).

Theory-generating and theory-testing research is essential to evidence-based practice. It is therefore helpful to identify components that should be included in research reports when determining whether evidence is valid for implementation in practice. In particular, internal and external criticisms of theories are important to assess. Internal criticism refers to the fit of components; external criticism considers the theory's relationships to people, nursing, and health (Peterson & Bredow, 2009).

## Internal Criticism

Questions the reviewer should ask regarding internal criticism pertain to clarity, consistency, adequacy, logical development, and level of theory development.

- Clarity: Is the theory's main component considerations clearly stated; easily understood by the reader?
- Consistency: Does the theory's description maintain definitions of the key concepts throughout the explanation?
- Adequacy: Are the topics addressed completely? Are there gaps? Does the theory require further refinement?
- Logical development: Is the development of the theory logically derived from previous work? Do the conclusions proceed logically? Are the arguments well supported?
- Level of theory development: What is the stage of development of the theory? Are its elements named? Has the theory been around for some time, and can it be used to explain or predict outcomes? How frequently have researchers applied the theory to different situations?

## External Criticism

Aspects of the theory included in external criticism are a theory's relation to the real world of persons, nursing, and health. Components to be considered include:

- Reality convergence: Does the theory build upon premises from which it was derived and then related to reality?
- Utility: How useful is it to the researcher?
- Significance: To what extent does it address nursing phenomena and further research?
- Discrimination: What is its capacity to differentiate nursing from other health-related disciplines?
- Scope: Does it have a narrow focus that can be used to identify it as a middle-range theory, thereby making it easier to use in a research setting?
- Complexity—How complex is it? This is determined by the number of variables; the fewer the number of variables, the fewer the number of relationships between concepts.

Other aspects of the report to be considered in reviewing research include these:

- The conceptual model that guided the study should be explicitly and concisely described; the linkage between the conceptual model and/or the middle-range theory and the empirical research methods should also be included in a research report.

■ The report should specify characteristics of the middle-range theory: significance; internal consistency; parsimony; and testability. Significance of a theory is the extent to which it deals with a topic that is currently important. Internal consistency means that the concepts and propositions of the theory are comprehensible. Parsimony refers to whether the content of the theory is stated concisely. Testability means that the theory can be empirically tested.

■ The amount of information on methods given in a research report should include research design, sample, instruments, experimental conditions, data collection procedures and protection of human subjects, and data analysis techniques. Pay special attention to the design of the study and determine if the design was conducted as planned (e.g., if an intervention was introduced, was there consistency in its implementation; that is, was the protocol performed consistently by trained personnel throughout the study?). Other considerations are whether the study had approval from the institutional review board (IRB) and what instruments were used for data collection. Were the psychometric properties of tools used to measure concepts and variables adequate? Were the tools designed and tested to measure the operational definitions of variables with persons having characteristics similar to those of the participants (e. g., age, ethnicity)?

■ In evaluating the empirical adequacy of the results, one should determine whether the data agree with the theory's concepts and the propositions agree with the theory. It is necessary that there be congruence between data collected from the study and the theory concepts and propositions. When there is a lack of congruence, there may be a need to modify the concepts of a theory. For example, if anxiety is one of the variables in a study, one might ask about the operational definition in a study. Is anxiety defined as a characteristic or a trait? If the concept is a characteristic, then the tool that should be used is one that measures a person's anxiety trait. On the other hand, if the operational definition used is a measure of one's anxiety at a designated time, then a tool that was developed to assess state anxiety should be used.

■ Pragmatic adequacy refers to the usefulness of the theory for nursing practice. The theory should include useful information that can be used as evidence in developing assessment tools, protocols for interventions, and practice guidelines that can be realistically and safely used in providing care.

## SUMMARY

A conceptual model or framework is made up of concepts (words or terms) that represent abstract ideas, linked in a manner that represents the relationship between the concepts. In contrast, a theory incorporates concrete ideas and provides a more detailed explanation of the phenomenon of interest. Research studies guided by a conceptual model provide only general guidelines for practice; theory-guided research studies may provide new knowledge suitable for specific guidelines (Fawcett, 2004).

Conceptual and theoretical frameworks are useful in describing, explaining, and predicting phenomena. It is therefore vital to ensure that the framework is congruent with the research design of a study in order to have findings that are applicable to practice. Without a framework, research studies are problem based, and the findings may not be applicable to another setting (Verran, 1997).

## SUGGESTED ACTIVITIES

1   Select an article that focuses on a clinical intervention that has been implemented as part of an experimental study. Identify the conceptual model that was used to guide the study. Use the guidelines presented in this chapter to determine the fit between the focus of the study and the selected conceptual framework.

2   Select a theory, and illustrate how it can be used to describe, explain, or predict a phenomenon.

## REFERENCES

Bay, E., Kreulen, G. J., Shavers, C. A., & Currier, C. (2006). A new perspective: A vulnerable population framework to guide research and practice for persons with traumatic brain injury. *Research and Theory for Nursing Practice, 20,* 141–157.

Coopey, M., & Nix, M. P. (2006). AHRQ commentary: Translating research into evidence-based nursing practice and evaluating effectiveness. *Journal of Nursing Care Quality, 21,* 195–202.

Fawcett J. (2004). Framework for analysis and evaluation of conceptual models of nursing. In P. G. Reed, N. B. C. Shearer, & L. H. Nicoll (Eds.), *Perspectives on nursing theory* (4th ed.). Philadelphia: Lippincott, Williams & Wilkins.

Fawcett, J., & Garity, J. (2009). *Evaluating research for evidence-based nursing practice.* Philadelphia: Davis.

Fineout-Overholt, E., Hofstetter, S., Shell, L., & Johnston, L. (2005). Teaching EBP: Getting to the gold: How to search for the best evidence. *Worldviews on Evidence-Based Nursing, 2,* 207–211.

Goode, C. J. (2000). What constitutes the evidence in evidence-based practice? *Applied Nursing Research, 13,* 222–225.

Hess, L. M., & Insel, K. C. (2007). Chemotherapy-related change in cognitive function: A conceptual model. *Oncology Nursing Forum, 34,* 981–994.

Meleis, A. I. (2005). *Theoretical nursing: Development & progress* (3rd ed.). Philadelphia: Lippincott.

Myers, J. S.(2009). A comparison of the theory of unpleasant symptoms and the conceptual model of chemotherapy-related changes in cognitive function. *Oncology Nursing Forum, 36,* E1–E10.

Peterson, S. J., & Bredow, R. S. (2009). *Middle range theories: Application to nursing research.* (2nd ed.). Philadelphia: Wolters Kluwer.

Pipe, T. B. (2007). Optimizing nursing care by integrating theory-driven evidence-based practice. *Journal of Nursing Care Quality, 22,* 234–238.

Polit, D. F., & Beck, C. T. (2008). *Nursing research: Generating and assessing evidence for nursing practice*(8th ed.). Philadelphia: Lippincott, Williams & Wilkins.

Rycroft-Malone, J. (2007). Theory and knowledge translation. *Nursing Research, 56,* S78–S85.

Schmitt. M. H. (1999). The conceptual framework. In M. A. Mateo & K. T. Kirchhoff (Eds.), *Using and conducting nursing research in the clinical setting* (2nd ed., pp. 213–228). Philadelphia: Saunders.

Tomey, A. M., & Aligood, M. R. (2002). *Nursing theorists and their work* (5th ed.). St. Louis: Mosby.

Verran, J. A. (1997). The value of theory-driven (rather than problem-driven) research. *Seminars for Nurse Managers, 5,* 169–172.

# 7 Quantitative Designs

KARIN T. KIRCHHOFF

In this chapter, the common designs—experimental and nonexperimental—used in quantitative research will be defined; the purposes and requirements of each will be detailed. There are considerations of competing explanations for results for the different designs; these will be detailed, and methods to attempt to compensate for them will be provided. Recommendations for decision making when designing a study will be offered.

## RESEARCH DESIGNS

The term *design* is used loosely in research textbooks and publications. Sometimes it is defined as all the elements of a study found in a proposal. Sometimes it is defined as a type of data collection, such as a survey. In this chapter, a more narrow definition is used that consists of (a) the number of groups in the study, (b) the time period covered or the number of observations over time, and (c) the presence of a treatment. A study can have a single group and be observational, or there can be one or more control groups for comparison to another group that received an event or an administered treatment. The study can occur at one point in time (cross-sectional) or over time (longitudinal). The study can be about a naturally occurring event (impact of a hurricane) and be descriptive, or it can be about a treatment that is administered as part of the study, making the study experimental.

Researchers have devised design notation that is frequently used in research textbooks. The symbols include these: O = observation or measurement of dependent variable (presumed effect), X = treatment or independent variable (presumed cause), and R = random assignment, if used. Random assignment is the process of assigning individuals to groups in the study. The process of assigning cannot depend on the investigator's choices and must be random. Processes for assigning subjects to groups include using a random numbers table, assigning an order with the random numbers and then concealing the order in sealed envelopes, and flipping a coin.

The order of the symbols, the number of Os and Xs, is also important. For example, if the notation is:

X O

there is no basis for comparing O before the intervention and after the intervention. Some studies are performed like that of necessity. Those studying the effects (O) of the hurricanes and flooding disaster (X) in the Gulf Coast might have information only after the event. This could be called an ex post facto design. The research in question is conducted after the variations in the independent variable (the hurricane) have occurred in the natural course of events. It is weak in that the investigator is not sure what was already occurring before the hurricane.

When the notation is:

O X O

the question is—what else could it be? The assumption is that nothing else was occurring between the two observations of O and O other than X, but the likelihood is low unless the second O took place almost immediately following the X.

A better design is:

R O X 1 O

R O X 2 O

where X 1 = experimental group and X 2 = control or comparison for X1. This design has a before-after comparison for each group, as well as a comparison across groups for what else might have intervened. The R means that the individuals were randomly assigned to the groups and that many alternative explanations for the outcomes have been controlled by equalizing the groups before the X occurred. X1 is then presumed to be the only difference.

## DESIGN MODIFICATIONS

Designs can be modified in several ways.

1   By extensions in numbers of measurements or length of time:

**OOOXOOO**
**OOO OOO**

2   By extensions in numbers of groups:

**OX1O**
**OX2O**
**OX3O**

3   By use of a cross-over design. In this example, the first treatment is given to the first group and then is crossed over to the second group. This might also be a delayed treatment design in which the control group gets a highly desired treatment but has to wait for it until a later time.

**OX1O O**
**O OX1O**

## SELECTING A DESIGN

In selecting a design, there are some issues to address. For example, the factors can be categorized into those related to the topic or problem, ethical issues, the setting for data collection, characteristics of study participants, and characteristics of the researcher. The nature of knowledge of the problem area requires review. Where little is known about the problem, a descriptive approach is best. If the need is to use words to describe an experience (e.g., what it is like to have a stillborn), then a qualitative approach might be preferable. Please see Chapter 8 on qualitative research methods for information. If the percentage of subjects having an event is the information being sought, a survey or a structured interview might be preferable. In both cases, the design can be expressed as X O where X is the experience that occurred and O is the response that will assessed.

The setting available also has an impact. How long are patients available at the research site? If only a short time will elapse before the patient is seen by the provider, long interviews will not be acceptable. What is the environment like? Compromises will need to be made if the setting is very noisy or busy. Perhaps it may be possible to collect fewer data points than planned, or perhaps additional data collection by telephone may be required.

Ethical issues may prevent some actions, such as random assignment to treatment or control where the control group receives a removal of care. The adequacy of a control group comparison can be limited because of these issues. Chapter 20, on ethical aspects of studies, discusses the ethical issues in general.

The subjects in the study also affect the design. When studying the chronically ill, researchers must make allowance for fatigue and may have to plan a few short sessions rather than one long session. Interviewing children requires interaction with the parents and perhaps their presence during data collection.

The characteristics of the researcher play a part in decision making about designs. Some researchers prefer to interact with patients and do not wish to do experiments where situations must be controlled and interventions must be similar to those with other subjects.

The time available to the investigator can limit what is possible. Students trying to complete requirements for an advanced degree are less likely to take on a longitudinal design with several rounds of data collection than are established researchers. The availability of funds also limits the time dimension.

With intact groups, one cannot randomize individuals to groups. Thus, the researcher's ability to conduct a true experiment is compromised. In such cases, perhaps work groups could be randomized, rather than individuals. However, without randomization of individuals, what one has is not a true experiment but only something "like" an experiment, or a quasi-experimental design.

It is usually recommended that researchers obtain baseline measures on the subjects. One exception includes baseline measures that may affect later measures. When the subject is aware of what will be asked later, or when the baseline measures sensitize the subjects to the treatment and cause a different response than would have been obtained if they hadn't been given the baseline measures, the research can be compromised.

Sometimes the control group is upset by the random assignment. Perhaps its members signed up for the study because they wanted the intervention. In this case, consider using delayed treatment in the control group. This kind of adjustment allows for a comparison at the time of the intervention and with a second intervention group.

## AMOUNT OF CONTROL

The amount of control used in the study—low, moderate, high—is a design decision that has implications for what conclusions can be drawn from the study. In low-control studies, the generalizations that can be made from those results will be limited. Typical data collection methods might be called *retrospective surveys* (collecting data about past events), *prospective surveys* (collecting data as events are occurring), *observational studies* (recording data by taking notes or using equipment without intervening), *field studies* (collecting data in real-life events rather than in a laboratory), *participant observational studies* (interviewing and intermingling with subjects as part of the group observed), *interviews*, and *questionnaires* (tools used to collect data).

In moderate-control studies, the studies are called *lab* or *field experiments*. These are studies in which as much control as possible has been exerted. The results offer a stronger basis for assigning causation than is possible with descriptive studies that have no controls. These studies may have a control group but perhaps not random assignment of individuals.

At the highest level of control, three conditions of experiments exist: random assignment of individual subjects to groups, manipulation of the independent variable, and use of a control group or comparison group. In addition, it is also important to have constancy of conditions for the experiment; thus, the time of day when the experiment is conducted, the interaction between researcher and subject (different researchers should wear similar clothes, and possibly should be of the same gender), and the stimulus from the research should be the same.

When sample size is either slow to accumulate or is inadequate, one strategy frequently used is to include subjects from more than one institution. The caution is that there may be differences between patients in different settings; a check for interinstitutional differences will be necessary before the planned analysis can proceed. One hopes that there will be no differences between sites so that both the experimental patients and the controls across sites can be combined.

## EXPERIMENTAL DESIGNS

The purpose of an experimental design is to help the researcher answer a question with few concerns about possible alternative explanations for the study results. The experimental design controls for possible rival hypotheses that could be projected to have caused the results.

Experiments are designed to detect causation. There are three necessary (each must be present) and sufficient (when all together there is nothing else needed) conditions of causation. These are (1) temporal precedence (X must precede Y to have caused it), (2) covariation (an increase in X must lead to an increase or decrease in Y), and (3) all other variables must be eliminated. The investigator must ensure that extraneous independent variables are not associated with causation in the situation under study. For example, is it possible that the experimental group experienced a historical event that the control did not and that the outside historical event explains why they scored higher on some variable?

### Internal Validity

In order to decide whether X caused Y in an experiment, a number of questions must be addressed. One must be able to answer the question "Did the independent variable influence the dependent variable?" One of the first questions is: Are there unaccounted-for extraneous variables? These include alternative explanations for the findings that are not the independent variable. For example, when a patient's blood sugar is lowered after the patient is placed on a new drug, did this occur because the patient changed his diet as well as start on the new medication between the first reading and the second reading? Information on diet will need to be collected to answer this question.

Extraneous variables are those that can have an impact on the dependent variable but are not the independent variable or the presumed cause in the study. As a study is designed, these extraneous variables should be identified and controlled so that when the study is finished there is only one interpretation of the findings—that the independent variable of interest caused the dependent or outcome variable, and not some other factor. There are five methods of controlling extraneous variables: (1) eliminate it as a variable—for example, use subjects from just one age group or one gender into the study, (2) build the extraneous variables into the design (e.g., by comparing results by gender), (3) randomize the subjects, as a way to spread the effect of extraneous variables evenly across the groups, (4) match subject characteristics—but only on significant variables and then assign subjects randomly, and (5) use analysis of covariance (ANCOVA) to evaluate the study results. This statistical technique can be part of the initial plan or it can be used if one of the other methods fails to control extraneous variables. Randomization is not as effective with smaller sample sizes, since the number of subjects is not sufficient to allow for balance. If there is a significant age difference between the groups, for example, ANCOVA can be used to take out the effect on the outcome that is due to age.

## RANDOMIZATION

There are two techniques that use randomization or chance to make decisions. One is random selection. In this technique, every person in the population has a known chance of being selected and the chance is not zero. The sample represents the population because chance determines who was selected as subjects. Although some textbooks recommend the use of random sampling before random assignment, this is seldom done in practice. Few studies have more patients than they need, preventing the use of random sampling.

Random assignment of subjects to conditions or groups is the usual way randomization is achieved. In this case, chance determines the assignment of individuals to treatment. The intent in random assignment is to ensure the equivalence of groups except for the influence of the independent variable or treatment. The difference in the results obtained for the two groups on the dependent variable is then presumed to be caused by the independent variable because that is the only difference between the groups.

There are several ways to do random assignment. It is usually done with a random numbers table when all the subjects are known. Common methods are coin toss, shuffled cards, and roll of a die (one of a pair of dice). For a two-group assignment, a coin toss will work, with a decision made ahead of time about whether heads is for the experimental or the control group. In clinical experiments where the patients frequently trickle in, a strategy for achieving randomness and equal group size is needed. In this case and in order to have equal groups, the researcher might randomize ahead of time with equal numbers of assignments. The assignments could be placed in sealed envelopes and opened as the patients arrive.

## QUASI-EXPERIMENTAL DESIGNS

What distinguishes an experiment from a quasi-experiment? Both types of design include a manipulation of the independent variable, since that is what makes it an experiment. Quasi-experiments are missing either random assignment of individuals or the use of a control group or both. Sometimes nurses in work groups (e.g., at clinics) find that it is better to assign subjects to experimental conditions in groups than as individuals. That makes the research a quasi-experimental study, a weaker design but probably the only way to do the study. Sometimes individuals are used as their own control and then there is no control group per se.

## THREATS TO INTERNAL VALIDITY

There are a number of threats to the validity of conclusions drawn from experiments. An understanding of them is vital for if one is to be able to read experiments critically. These threats are also good for researchers to know so that they can design better studies. The way to use this list is to ask, "Is this threat plausible in my study?" If not, it can be ignored. If it is, then additional data should be collected to show why the threat was not operating and to prove that the conclusions planned are not called into question (Shadish, Cook, & Campbell, 2002).

1    History
History is a threat when an observed effect might be due to an event that takes place between the pretest and the posttest, and when this event is not the treatment of interest. An example commonly understood is that studies in hospitals should avoid the time interval around or just after July 1. Medical residents change assignments at that time, and this can alter some outcomes of interest.

**2** Maturation

This is a threat when an observed effect might be due to the respondents growing older, stronger, more experienced, more skilled, or more knowledgeable between pretest and posttest and when this maturation is not the treatment of research interest. Studies on children should plan for this threat, especially if the study will be conducted over a long time period. The longer the study is conducted, the more likely that a developmental change will occur in the population. The same notion can be true for studies that look at time to heal or length of time the patient has had a disease.

**3** Testing

This threat can occur when the outcome is affected by the number of times particular responses are measured. Familiarity with a test can sometimes enhance performance, since answers are more likely to be remembered at later testing sessions. This threat is also a concern when the same test is given more than once or the measurement of an outcome can cause the outcome to change.

**4** Instrumentation

This is a threat when an effect might be due to a change in the measuring instrument between pretest and posttest and not to the treatment (e.g., a scale that is not balanced). Another issue is the so-called ceiling or basement effect, which occurs, for example, when a number of people are already normotensive and we are trying to get all the clinic patients to a lower blood pressure. The basement effect of already having low blood pressure reduces the amount of lowering that is possible.

**5** Statistical regression

This is a threat when an effect might be due to the ways respondents are classified into experimental groups following the pretest on the basis of their pretest scores. Let's assume we want to measure patient anxiety. If those with high anxiety are put in a group and given an intervention, it is highly likely that at the next measurement, their anxiety will be lower, regardless of the treatment used, just on the basis of regression to the mean. Extreme values will tend to be less extreme on the next measurement. For example, those who were doing well at time 1 may be sleepier or preoccupied at time 2, and the change they demonstrate may be due not to treatment but to regression to the mean.

**6**   Selection

This is a threat when an effect measured may be due to the difference between the kinds of people in one experimental group as opposed to another. Is one group more highly motivated than another, just because of how the group members were selected? This threat is of great concern in quasi-experimental research where individuals have not been randomly assigned to groups.

**7**   Attrition

This is a threat when an effect may be due to the different kinds of persons who dropped out of a group during the course of an experiment. While random assignment might have made the groups approximately equal, attrition from the groups might have changed the distribution of important characteristics, so that the groups are no longer comparable at the posttest even if they were at pretest. Although coercion may not be used to keep people in a study, those who leave should be assessed on how they might be different from those left behind. The best prevention is to keep all individuals in the study and to keep the study short to avoid attrition.

**8**   Additive and interactive effects of threats to internal validity

Threats can operate simultaneously; their net bias will depend on the magnitude and direction of each. Selection-history threats occur when different groups come from different settings and have different local histories. When that history is related to the outcome variable, the researchers may be led to false conclusions.

**9**   Ambiguous temporal precedence

This threat is most likely in correlational studies that are cross-sectional. Because only one time point is studied, the variables measured are not in a time order. It is difficult to know if the parental response caused the child's behavior or if the response was the result of the child's behavior. It is impossible to identify the independent variable in this instance without additional information. This threat is not salient in most experiments, where the order of temporal precedence is usually clear.

The remaining threats discussed here were listed by Cook and Campbell (Cook & Campbell, 1979) as threats to internal validity. In the latest version of this work by Shadish, Cook, and Campbell (Shadish et al., 2002), these threats were still included but were listed as threats to a different form of validity, namely construct validity. That form of validity is concerned with the match between the way the study is operationalized and the constructs used to describe the operations. The construct of aggression (Shadish et al., 2002), for example, includes both the intent to harm others and a harmful result; studies that look at ways to decrease aggression need to include both these aspects. The following four threats were included under outcomes and treatments as they relate to the construct.

**10**  Diffusion or imitation of treatment

When treatments involve informational programs and when the various experimental (and control) groups can communicate with each other, respondents in one treatment group may learn the information intended for others. This threat can cause a lack of differences between experimental and control groups, since both groups, in effect, received the treatment. The control group, which should have been "sheltered" from the intervention, either heard about it or saw it and then adopted it. This is a common threat in many clinical studies where patients are in close proximity or share a waiting room. If nurses or patients find out that something works, they will spread the news. This threat is another reason for randomizing intact groups, rather than individuals. It is easier to keep the groups separated from each other than to keep the individuals separated.

**11**  Compensatory equalization of treatments

In this scenario, the experimental treatment provides a situation seen as a desirable benefit; administrators or others may try to compensate the control group for missing out on the benefit. The net effect is that the groups might appear to be similar in a measured outcome but the cause is really the compensation offered to the control group, not the lack of effectiveness of the intervention.

**12**  Compensatory rivalry

In this condition, those in the less desirable condition try harder because they know they did not get the desired treatment. Where the assignment of persons or organizational units to experimental and control conditions is made public, conditions of social competition may be generated. The control group, as the natural underdog, may be motivated to reduce or reverse the expected difference. This is also known as the John Henry effect, after a strong pile-driver who did not give up.

Compensatory rivalry—affecting those in the less desirable condition—sounds like #11, compensatory equalization of treatments.

What's the difference? Compensatory equalization involves a response of administrators, whereas compensatory rivalry is a response of those in the less desirable treatment groups.

**13**   Resentful demoralization

Those in the less desirable treatment or the control group may become upset because of their perceived lack of benefit from the study. They may not try at all, and this may exaggerate the differences between treatment and control, compromising the results. If an experiment is obtrusive, the reaction of a no-treatment control group or of groups receiving less desirable treatments can be associated with resentment and demoralization, as well as with compensatory rivalry. When this is likely, the researchers should make an assessment of the possibilities. These possible responses can be offset by offering a delayed treatment option so that the individuals stay in the study and eventually get the intervention.

## Randomization and Internal Validity

With quasi-experimental groups, the investigator has to make explicit all the threats to internal validity and then rule them out one by one. Some threats may not arise because of the nature of the study. Those can be ignored. The threats posed by the other factors to the study results should be evaluated to assess the possibility that they are operating.

Most of these threats are controlled by randomization. The power of random assignment is one reason controlled experiments are so highly valued. There are threats, however, that randomization does not rule out. Differential mortality according to groups may occur, reducing the equalization that random assignment had attempted to create. Imitation of treatments, compensatory equalization, compensatory rivalry, and demoralization in groups receiving less desirable treatments can each threaten internal validity, even when randomization has been successfully implemented and maintained over time. These are threats that should be checked with every experiment.

## SUMMARY

In summary, design decisions follow the nature of the question being asked. Descriptive studies are reports of what is. When statements are made about what should be done in caring for patients, tests of interventions are required. The strongest test, offering the most control, is the true experiment, where the treatment is manipulated (given to one group and not another), random assignment is used, and a control group for comparison purposes is included. When situations prevent all these conditions, a quasi-experiment may be all that is possible. Then, attention to all the potential threats to internal validity is paramount before making causal statements.

## SUGGESTED ACTIVITIES

1    Develop two research questions, one descriptive and one experimental. Sketch the design for each, using X and O, and discuss with another student what you would be able to conclude after the study is completed.
2    List three threats to internal validity. Describe how you might minimize the impact of these threats. What steps could you take? How would you write this up in your publication?

## REFERENCES

Cook, T. D., & Campbell, D. T. (1979). *Quasi-experimentation: Design & analysis issues for field settings.* Boston: Houghton Mifflin.

Shadish, W. R., Cook, T. D., & Campbell, D. T. (2002). *Experimental and quasi-experimental designs for generalized causal inference.* Boston: Houghton Mifflin.

# 8

## Qualitative Research for Nursing Practice

BETH RODGERS

Qualitative research makes up a vital part of nursing knowledge and provides essential information for evidence-based practice. Researchers frequently use methods of this type to address problems relevant to the holistic aspect of nursing practice. In order to accomplish the goal of using the best evidence available as a basis for nursing practice, nurses must understand the processes involved in this type of research and be able to evaluate the quality of evidence derived from qualitative studies.

When reading reports of qualitative studies, one immediately observes that the designs and procedures differ considerably from those of quantitative studies and what is typically thought of as "science." For many people, the mention of "science" conjures an image of a laboratory setting or, at least, an environment where the researcher carefully controls the situation by isolating the phenomenon being studied from other elements that might interfere with the results. The researcher, in this view of science, objectively conducts and observes the results of an experiment to arrive at the absolute "Truth" regarding the situation being studied. There is a belief that science, conducted in such a way, provides answers about cause and effect, definitive explanations about what happens in certain situations, and, in regard to clinical practice, a clear understanding of what is the best thing to do in a particular circumstance.

Compared to this idea of science, qualitative research certainly does seem quite unorthodox.

While society and educational systems, particularly at the early levels where students generally take "science" courses, perpetuate this idea of science, it becomes clear with just a little study of research that very little about research actually is consistent with this idea of "science." Finding one absolute, indisputable answer to questions is unreasonable in any context, much less where humans are involved. As humans interact with their environment, they change, the environment changes, and so does the phenomenon being studied. Objectivity, in a complete and unbiased sense, is not a reasonable expectation for any scientist. Where there is a need to be unbiased in gathering information and interpreting results, the mere identification of something as a "problem" involves judgment on the part of the researcher. The researcher's existing biases are integrated throughout the conduct of inquiry and, in fact, often are useful in the research situation as they provide the researcher with important tools for research, such as language, concepts, theories, and mechanisms for measurement and other forms of study. These are all biases in a sense, yet research would not be possible without them. Complete objectivity, therefore, is not possible without dispensing with all that has been learned through both education and development in a social context. Rather than seeing the possibility of one absolute answer or Truth, objectivity, and control as necessary ingredients for science, recent philosophers of science (those who explore what makes science work) provide a contemporary view of science as an attempt to solve problems, to generate solutions that "work," to exercise creativity and innovation in the interest of discovery and development of knowledge, and to tie research to a broad interest in the good of society (Rodgers, 2005).

This evolving idea of what constitutes science has fueled a substantial increase in the acceptance and, consequently, the volume of qualitative research being conducted in a variety of disciplines. Qualitative research, although a mainstay of inquiry in the social sciences for nearly a century, has blossomed in acceptance and use in a broad array of disciplines. In nursing, growth in this area began most clearly in the 1980s; in the relatively short period of time since, it has become an essential aspect of nursing's evidence base, providing valuable information on aspects of human health and illness that are best explored using the capabilities of qualitative methods.

## WHY QUALITATIVE RESEARCH?

Qualitative research is suitable for inquiry that addresses a number of aspects relevant to nursing and provides an important part of the evidence base essential to nursing practice. Qualitative research approaches the study of phenomena in a "natural" setting. Rather than attempt to control elements of the research situation, such as by manipulating variables (e.g., an intervention presented in a controlled setting), the qualitative study is designed to capture experiences or events as they naturally occur. Qualitative research also excels at capturing people's thoughts and feelings, which are not easily reduced to numbered responses to questions on paper-and-pencil instruments. Qualitative research offers insights important to viewing situations and people holistically and, therefore, is ideal to answer broad questions that warrant depth description. Questions for qualitative research often are stated in ways similar to the following:

- What is happening here?
- What is it like for people who experience a particular situation or condition?
- What are the experiences of people with "X" (the phenomenon of interest)?
- What is the meaning of "X" (the phenomenon of interest)?

Specific examples of such questions drawn from existing studies include:

- What are the experiences of women who have been diagnosed with a myocardial infarction? (Rodgers, 2007)
- What is it like for adults to make the decision about nursing home placement for an older family member? (Rodgers, 1997)

Answers to such questions meet several significant functions of qualitative research. Qualitative research can be used to describe, providing both a deep and rich description of a situation or experience. Qualitative research also helps to provide information about aspects that might be missed with a quantitative study. For example, quantitative research is appropriate for determining if one intervention is more effective than another in a way that is statistically significant. Such a study, however, will not provide information about what it is like for an individual to live with the intervention. In such a situation, qualitative research makes it possible to capture information that is essential to gaining a complete picture of a situation or experience. Qualitative research also can be very sensitizing, raising awareness of aspects of an experience that might not have been recognized previously. Such insights enable nurses to better anticipate patients' needs and concerns and to understand their perspectives when confronted with a health-related situation. Obviously, this type of knowledge is important for nursing practice because it allows nurses to individualize care and to work with psychological, social, and emotional aspects as well as physiologic components of health and illness situations. Qualitative research is ideal for enlarging our understanding of what people think, feel, believe, and live through as they encounter situations related to their health and well-being.

## TYPES OF QUALITATIVE RESEARCH

Qualitative research is distinguished from quantitative research most readily by its focus on words as data, rather than numbers. The qualitative researcher collects data in the form of words and reports results in that form, as well. In spite of this common characteristic among all the qualitative approaches, there are several distinct methodologies for qualitative research, each of which has its own unique philosophical underpinnings, history, and procedures for the conduct of a study.

On a very general level, there is a sort of generic form of qualitative research that often appears in the literature. A study might be described as *qualitative, descriptive, qualitative descriptive, exploratory, naturalistic, field research,* or *ethnographic.* All of these refer to the collection of data in the forms of words (typically through interviews and, occasionally, through observations, as well) without any more specific processes involved. Note that *descriptive* research can be quantitative, as well, so seeing a study characterized as *descriptive* in a report of research requires a closer look at the nature of the data and the manner or reporting results to determine if it is qualitative or quantitative. The term *ethnographic* similarly can have multiple meanings, referring most generally to research in a natural setting. There also is a distinct methodology known as Ethnography, which is discussed later.

Other specific methods for qualitative research that are found often in the nursing literature include Grounded Theory, Phenomenology, Hermeneutic (most often Hermeneutic Phenomenology), Narrative

Inquiry, and Ethnography. *Grounded Theory* research was introduced formally in the 1960s and is based on the work of the noted sociologist Anselm Strauss and his colleague Barney Glaser (Glaser & Strauss, 1967). This method is guided by the theoretical viewpoint of Symbolic Interactionism (Blumer, 1969). In general, Symbolic Interactionism holds that people create their sense of self, their reality, societies, and so on, through interaction with other people. How an individual experiences some event or process in life is heavily influenced, if not dependent on, those interactions. In a Grounded Theory study, the researcher seeks information about the overall "experience" of people in specific situations of interest to the researcher. That experience involves the thoughts, feelings, actions, interactions with others, and interpretations of events associated with the situation being studied.

Grounded Theory research has a unique end product in that it is used to construct a substantive theory that provides a detailed depiction of the experience being studied that is derived from (grounded in) the data obtained from participants. This theory is organized around a central idea, referred to as the *core variable* (Glaser, 1978; Glaser & Strauss, 1967), which represents the primary focus of the experience. This core variable represents the "basic sociopsychological process," or BSP, involved in the experience and reflects the symbolic interactionist foundation about interaction being important in the shaping of experience. Since Glaser and Strauss pioneered this method, in the late 1960s, other variations have been introduced, most recently a version by Strauss and Corbin (1998). The underlying principles are the same, although the Strauss and Corbin version imposes more structure on the data analysis process and on the reporting of results. Other adaptations have been created, as well (Charmaz, 2000, 2005, 2006), which have introduced notable differences in procedures. Reports of Grounded Theory studies can be evaluated similarly, keeping the foundations of this approach in mind and the expected outcome of a substantive theory, regardless of the specific variation a researcher used in a study. General criteria for evaluating qualitative studies are discussed later in this chapter.

The qualitative method known as *Phenomenology* also is used to study experiences but is focused on the "meaning" of the "lived experience" of the people in the study. Phenomenology was derived originally from the philosophies of Edmund Husserl (1960) and Maurice Merleau-Ponty (1962/1999), and its origins contribute to the extensive foundation in philosophy that is evident in this method. Following this beginning, modifications to the method were presented by the existentialist philosopher Martin Heidegger, and the method has been adapted further as a means of study in psychology. There are numerous variations in approaches that are all referred to as Phenomenology, including a variation called *Hermeneutic Phenomenology* (Plager, 1994), which is fairly common in nursing. All of these approaches have some elements in common, however. Whereas Grounded Theory is focused on social interaction and processes, Phenomenology is a method for studying the individual and how the individual ascribes "meaning" to an experience. A significant underpinning of this research method is the idea that humans construct their own realities and that, in turn, these realities have a strong influence on creating the individual. This idea often is referred to as *co-constitution,* capturing the notion that people, and their realities each have an influence on the construction of the other. Experiences and events have their own essence, what might be called the "facts" of the situation, or what truly happened. What is important in Phenomenology, however, are the layers of meaning or interpretation that the individual gives to the situation. While all qualitative methods are focused on people's experiences and their own individual realities, the phenomenological researcher typically goes beyond the actual words spoken by an individual to describe the experience in an attempt to interpret these words and identify underlying meaning. For that reason, phenomenology sometimes is referred to as an *interpretive* method (Van Manen, 1990), rather than a "descriptive" one. The product of phenomenological research is a discussion of significant ideas or meaning statements derived through analysis of the participants words and interpretation of the meanings the experience being studied has for the individual.

Narrative Inquiry is another form of qualitative research that is common in nursing. Narrative Inquiry (Labov & Waletsky, 1967; Riessman, 1993) is grounded in the premise that people typically construct "stories" about their various life experiences. These stories represent the individuals' way of weaving together elements of the event into their "story" of their experience. According to Riessman (1993), the purpose of Narrative Inquiry is to see how respondents in interviews impose order on the flow of experience to make sense of events and actions in their lives" (p. 2). These stories involve all the typical aspects of a story, including players, supporting players, settings, sequencing of events, and outcomes. Using the techniques of narrative analysis, the researcher examines these stories to uncover an underlying narrative that characterizes the stories associated with an experience (Riley & Hawe, 2005).

The final form of qualitative research that is discussed here is Ethnography. Ethnography as a specific method (in contrast to the more generic use of the term *ethnographic* to refer to research that takes place in a natural setting or "in the field") originated in the discipline of anthropology. Ethnography is focused on the study of culture. For purposes of this type of research, a culture can be made up of any group or setting in which people share ideology, values, attitudes, customs, rules, norms, or rituals (Wolf, 2007). In conducting Ethnography, the researcher typically spends extensive time in the setting being studied, identifying "key informants" or people who are particularly familiar with the setting or experience and whose perspectives are important to understanding the workings of the setting. The researcher observes the group and interactions among group members, keeping extensive notes and talking with individuals in addition to the key informants whose input is particularly important to the study. Ethnographies are found much less frequently in the nursing literature than are examples of the other methods, perhaps because of the extremely time-intensive nature of the research. In addition, ethnographies typically are so extensive and detailed that they can be reported only partially through the usual format of a journal article.

## CONDUCTING A QUALITATIVE STUDY

Before attempting the critical evaluation of qualitative studies, it is necessary to understand how qualitative research is conducted. In spite of the differences in foundation and development of the various traditions, the overall procedures for conducting all types of qualitative studies are quite similar. Those procedures differ considerably from those used in conducting quantitative studies, and a review of the steps in the process, comparing qualitative and quantitative, can be helpful to identify important differences.

It is important to remember that the intent in any type of qualitative research is to capture the individual "realities" of the participants and to provide a detailed description of those realities and the experiences of the people studied. Therefore, elements of research that involve ideas such as control, theory or hypothesis testing, reliability, and generalizability, for example, are either inappropriate or take on an entirely different meaning in the context of this type of study. To gain an understanding of how qualitative research functions, the steps in conducting a qualitative study are presented, along with ideas for what to look for in the critique of such research.

## Research Problem and Question

As with any type of research, the process of qualitative inquiry begins with identification of a problem and a research question. Problems result when there are new ideas or situations to explore and where little is known about the phenomenon, so that studies aimed at broad discovery are appropriate. A change in a treatment modality might warrant a study that explores the experiences of people who receive that treatment; changes in staffing patterns for nurses might be explored with regard to the experiences of the nurses who live with the new pattern on a regular basis or to the impact of the change on other aspects of the care delivered by the nursing staff. Problems appropriate for qualitative research also exist when there are significant gaps in knowledge. A long-standing procedure might have been studied extensively regarding its effectiveness, yet there may be very little information about what patients think or feel about the treatment and how it affects their daily lives. A problem amenable to qualitative research can be just about anything that can be answered through in-depth discovery and descriptions of the experiences, thoughts, and feelings of people who have encountered the situation being studied.

The questions for qualitative studies appear to be quite similar in spite of the specific tradition of inquiry that underlies the research. There are subtle differences in wording, however, that clue the reader into the specific tradition being explored. Phenomenology, for example, often involves the phrase *lived experience* or the word *meaning* as a specific focus of the research question. Beyond seemingly minor variations in wording, questions for a qualitative study in general addresses the broad experience or the thoughts and feelings regarding a life encounter. It is common for researchers to not provide a specific question statement in their report of qualitative studies; the absence of an actual question is not a weakness in a research report. The purpose of the study and the problem situation that led to the development of the research, however, should be clear to the reader; ideally, these are presented early in the published report. The question or problem should be one that is appropriate to qualitative inquiry, as well. Questions about what "should" be done in a situation or what is "better" are not amenable to any type of research, as they call for judgments that go beyond the actual data gained through the study. A researcher can, however, address a question about what people report, what characteristics are identified, how people describe their feelings, and how they live with some situation or experience as a step toward developing conclusions about what is "better" and why that is the case.

## Review of Literature

Another step in the qualitative research process typically involves a review of the literature. It is a bit misleading to consider this a separate step; as with any type of study, the review of the literature can be very helpful in refining the original problem. The iterative process of reviewing the literature and rethinking the original problem helps to provide clarity and important perspectives that give direction to the subsequent research. In a quantitative study, the literature review typically provides an important foundation for the research by revealing what is already known about the situation of interest. On this basis, the researcher can determine the appropriate next steps for inquiry and, depending on the type of research, develop a theoretical foundation for the study and possible hypotheses. At this point, qualitative and quantitative studies differ considerably. The qualitative researcher does not intend to build on existing research but typically embarks on an attempt to explore, discover, and describe areas and experiences about which little already is known. In this spirit, the researcher wants to remain as open as is plausible to the many possibilities that can exist in any situation. Using the literature review to frame the study would put some boundaries around what is to be explored and what might be "seen" in the data that are collected.

Some discussions of qualitative research argue against the need for any type of literature review prior to embarking on qualitative study. Avoiding contact with existing information is believed to enable the researcher to be more open and unbiased about what might be encountered through the study. While the idea of being as unbiased as possible is appealing, it is faulty on a couple of levels. First, it is never possible to be completely open and unbiased about anything. The researcher is making judgments from the very beginning of a study by identifying something as a "problem" and by naming phenomena, in other words, by using certain words to label what is being studied. The researcher also inherently possesses some bias because of the researcher's own experience as a human interacting with others and with the knowledge he or she already has accumulated. Diminishing bias in a study is a desirable goal to the extent possible, and typically the researcher does not want to skew the study in any particular direction in order to avoid placing limits on what might be discovered. In qualitative studies; therefore, there often is a literature review, though it takes on a different form from that of quantitative studies. The qualitative researcher typically does a thorough literature review prior to the start of the study, but it is oriented toward substantiating the view that a problem does exist and that qualitative methods are appropriate to address that problem, as well as, in some cases, to gain direction and support for the methods chosen for the study. Rather than provide a foundation for the research, the literature review in a qualitative study provides justification for the research and the chosen form of qualitative inquiry.

The literature review section that appears relatively early in a report of a qualitative study should be thorough and give good background information about the problem. Since the researcher usually is not building on this existing information to further inquiry in an area, the literature review sometimes is more broad, discussing a wide variety of studies that have been done and often identifying gaps in knowledge, rather than focusing on a select few to provide underpinnings for the current research. Ultimately, the researcher uses the literature review to make a clear case for the fact that a researchable problem exists and that it is important to generate information that will fill this gap. As noted before, the appropriateness of qualitative methods to address the problem should be apparent, as well.

The use of the initial literature review for substantiating the problem and methods rather than for providing a foundation for the research presents an interesting situation with regard to the literature review in qualitative studies. Rather than use the literature review to tie the study to previous work, showing how the study presented in a published report relates to other research, the researcher makes this connection to existing work near the end of the study, rather than at the beginning. As themes and patterns are identified in the data obtained during the study, the researcher will conduct an extensive literature review late in the conduct of the study to determine how the ideas that have been discovered relate to current knowledge. For example, in a study of women's experiences with myocardial infarction (MI) (Rodgers, 2007), the researcher returned to the literature to gather information about several aspects of the experience that arose during the study. While gender roles could be expected to be an issue in this study, the researcher did not anticipate that so many of the participants would refuse to be taken to the hospital by ambulance even when they finally acknowledged that they probably were having a heart attack. This raised questions about the interconnections of age, socioeconomic status, and gender and led to an extensive literature review to examine associations among these concepts as a means of connecting the findings from the study to existing knowledge.

When reading published reports of qualitative research, the researcher needs to evaluate the literature review component with connection with the initial phase of substantiating the problem, as well as in the discussion section at the end of the report. In this latter section, the researcher discusses the findings of the current study in the context of previous research and the theoretical literature. This use of the literature provides additional clarification of the findings of the study as well as a means to tie the findings to what is already known. As a result, there are benefits to the current research, and the knowledge base is expanded, as well. The researcher can compare findings to the literature as a step toward expanding and enriching the findings as well as to demonstrate how the research contributes to what has been presented previously in the literature. The elements of a good literature review are appropriate for use in evaluating this component of a qualitative study. Primary sources, evidence of a thorough search, and use of current sources, which are appropriate in any literature review, are appropriate criteria here, as well. The results of the literature review that is done later in the study to expand findings and to make connections with existing knowledge are presented in the discussion section of the research report. In this section, the researcher is expected to use relevant literature in discussion of major findings as a means to enhance understanding of the findings and to demonstrate a clear connection to prior theory and research.

## DESIGN OF QUALITATIVE STUDIES

In qualitative studies, the researcher has a broad problem of interest, and specific variables are not identified in advance. As a result, working with the problem and the initial literature review, the researcher can proceed to develop the design for the study. The typical form of design for a qualitative study is referred to as an *emergent design*—the design actually "emerges" as the study proceeds. In qualitative studies, the researcher not only is free to make changes in the design but, in the course of doing the study, actually is expected to make changes in the design in order to pursue new ideas and areas of inquiry as they are determined to be important. All of the elements of the research design cannot be planned in advance, and, in fact, the design usually needs to change in some respects if the researcher is to do a thorough investigation of the phenomenon being studied. This is in stark contrast to how quantitative research typically is conducted. In a quantitative study, the researcher plans every element of the design in advance and then collects data according to the plan. In some instances there may be minor modifications, although, if a pilot study is conducted, any necessary changes are usually worked out at that time.

A qualitative study functions best when there is a clear starting point and purpose but there is flexibility in the path to completing that objective. New information, things that the researcher could not anticipate, often arises as data are collected from participants. As new information is obtained through data collection, the astute researcher will realize that there are new avenues to be explored, people with different characteristics that should be investigated, and new questions to ask in interviews. As an example, consider the study mentioned previously about women and MI. Early in the study, it was evident, much to the investigator's surprise, that none of the women interviewed had gone to the hospital by ambulance in spite of their acknowledgment that they probably were having a heart attack at the time. This was an unanticipated finding and certainly something that had been explored in order to provide a meaningful and comprehensive description of the experiences of these women. Merely reporting this to be the case would have been interesting but would have represented a lost opportunity for full description. In response to this realization, the investigator made a couple of changes in the study. The investigator began explicitly gathering information from each woman about the actual transportation she used to get to a health care site after she realized that she was having an MI. This constituted a change in the interview process. The researcher also added a new site for subject recruitment, as those interviewed to this point in the study had been in a comfortable position economically and the researcher was interested in determining whether this observation would be replicated among women from different socioeconomic groups. In one sense, this following of "leads" sometimes is thought of as a form of hypothesis testing (e.g., do the means of transportation to the hospital differ with socioeconomic status, or age, or living situation?). The ability to follow a relevant path wherever it may lead in the inquiry is important to achieving the depth and scope of understanding of the situation that is sought in qualitative research and accounts for the need for elements of design to *emerge* in the course of a study.

## Sample Selection

Qualitative researchers often view their research as an interactive process between them and the people who are being studied. Rather than view them as "subjects" of study, researchers see the people interviewed as being active in their role in the research; this active role often involves sharing sensitive aspects of their lives and is recognized in the fact that researchers commonly refer to interviewees as participants or informants, rather than subjects. Participants help to construct the study in a way by offering information about their experiences, and this information, in turn, is used by the researcher to determine the appropriate direction of the research. Although some aspects of design can change throughout the conduct of a qualitative study, many elements can be determined in advance. The specific sample typically is not determined in advance, and probability samples usually are not appropriate for qualitative research. That does not mean, however, that the researcher simply takes into the study anyone who comes along and is willing to participate. The researcher must establish clear eligibility criteria for selection of participants, and these criteria typically involve competence to provide informed consent to participate, the ability to speak and understand the language of the researcher, and an adequate amount of engagement with the experience being studied. Other factors can be included as appropriate to determine eligibility for a study. For a study of the experiences of women with myocardial infarction, for example, obviously the participants had to have had experienced an MI. Beyond this criterion, the researcher can impose more specific requirements appropriate to the nature of the study. The MI study was focused on women's concurrent experiences, rather than on a retrospective account of their situations. Therefore, eligibility criteria included a time frame for the occurrence of the MI relative to data collection. For this study, the participant also could not have had a prior diagnosis of MI, because the researcher was interested in each woman's experience of first becoming aware that she had experienced an MI.

Because of the existence of specific criteria for eligibility, the usual sample for a qualitative study is a purposive one; there are relevant and distinct criteria that enable the researcher to purposefully recruit participants who are in the best position to provide data needed for the study. It is not uncommon for qualitative researchers to describe their samples as accidental (or convenience), and that may be an appropriate designation, depending on the specificity with which the participants are recruited for the study. Regardless of the specific type of sampling procedure employed, it is important that the qualitative researcher have participants in the study who are both willing to describe their experiences with the situation being studied and capable of doing so.

Sample size is a concern in any type of research, and qualitative research is no exception. Researchers using quantitative designs have the ability to determine appropriate sample sizes, using statistical procedures such as power analysis in many cases. In qualitative research, the researcher cannot predict in advance precisely how many participants will be needed to produce meaningful results. It is also the case that in qualitative research the amount of data that is generated has bearing on determining the appropriate sample size. One hour of an audio recorded interview generally produces as much as 30 pages of single-spaced transcribed text, an incredible amount of data. All of the data in an effectively conducted interview need to be analyzed. As a result, the amount of data available for analysis can be quite large with even a small group of participants. Qualitative research also can consume a lot of time and other resources. These factors in combination help explain why qualitative studies typically have relatively small sample sizes and also contribute to the realization that large samples are not necessary to generate meaningful and credible results because of the volume of data generated. There is no "rule" for what constitutes an adequate sample size in a qualitative study.

Determination of an adequate sample, therefore, is based on several factors, including the quantity and quality of data generated, the characteristics of the participants, the procedures employed in the study to maximize diversity in the participants and their experiences, and the ability to answer the research question with the data that are generated through the research. In planning to do a qualitative study, the researcher can anticipate approximately how many people will be needed in the sample to reach this desired outcome. Because this is not an absolute number, proposals for qualitative research often include a range for the number of participants who will be recruited for the study. Published reports may show sample sizes ranging from 10 to 30 or more. In evaluating these studies, as noted earlier, the reader must consider several factors beyond the actual number of people involved.

A common practice in qualitative research is to use the criterion of *saturation* (Morse, 1991) or *redundancy* (Lincoln & Guba, 1985; Patton, 2001) to determine when the sample size is adequate. Saturation typically is defined as the point at which the researcher is not hearing anything new in the data or, in other words, the point at which the descriptions provided by participants are sufficiently similar that there is no need to continue with subject recruitment. For reasons that should be obvious, this can be a very troublesome criterion. First, the researcher is making a fairly bold assumption that talking with additional people will not provide anything new. Second, the failure to obtain new insights through the data collection processes that are being used could be a function of the data collection process itself and not necessarily a reflection of the experiences of the participants. If the researcher is leading when asking questions or becomes fixated on certain aspects of the experience, this can lead to a premature sense that nothing new is being learned through data collection. Finally, the researcher has to avoid the development of bias by interpreting things in a particular way rather than being open to new ideas and insights that might arise through data collection and analysis. Such bias could give the false impression that there is nothing new in the data.

## Data Collection for Qualitative Research

Any nonnumerical data can be used for purposes of qualitative research. This can include notes about observations, a review of existing documentation, and records such as patient medical records, or video recordings. The majority of data collection for qualitative studies occurs through the use of interviews with individuals or in focus groups. Typically, interviews are conducted on a face-to-face basis, although telephone and even e-mail or Web-based interviews with individuals have been used in qualitative research. Interviews can have any degree of structure, ranging from specific questions that are asked consistently of each participant to very open-ended and nonstructured interviews. The amount of depth and the "richness" of the data vary with the degree of structure imposed on data collection: More structure generally leads to less richness and depth, whereas less structure provides greater depth. This may seem counterintuitive at first. In a nonstructured interview, the researcher starts with an overriding question of interest (e.g., what is it like for women to learn they have had a heart attack?). After starting with a broad opening question, the researcher allows the participant to talk, presenting his or her experience in whatever way is comfortable so that the conversation flows naturally for the participant. This allows the participant to reveal things that are of greatest concern or interest regarding the experience without the researcher providing too much direction or imposing restraint on the conversation. The researcher focuses on listening, delicately guiding the conversation to ensure that relevant aspects are covered but without abruptly redirecting the interview or otherwise imposing constraints on the conversation. The researcher will have some specific questions that he or she wants to address with each participant concerning topics such as symptoms, timeline of events, treatments received, and family history. Questions about these aspects of the experience can be incorporated into the interview at appropriate times. The emphasis on listening and on facilitating the participants' elaboration of their experiences can be challenging for nurses, who are accustomed to collecting information from patients or clients relevant to a health situation. Nurses are very skilled at eliciting specific information and then formulating conclusions and determining the actions that are appropriate. It is easy for the novice qualitative researcher to interject suggestions, make decisions, or prematurely assume that he or she understands the participant's situations. In an interview for qualitative research, however, the investigator must learn to listen very attentively, returning to significant items in the conversation and gently redirecting when appropriate. It is important to keep in mind that participants cannot be allowed to ramble completely off topic. If the interview turns into a rambling conversation, the participant (not to mention the researcher) can become fatigued and the quality of the interview may be compromised. In addition, people also have busy lives and typically cannot dedicate unlimited time to an interview. The typical in-depth interview lasts about 90 minutes to two hours, and the researcher should make sure that the interview is sufficiently on track that the desired information is obtained within a reasonable time frame.

An interesting feature of qualitative research is that some of the data in the study actually come from (or are generated by) the researcher. Data usually are thought of as information that is collected from the people who are being studied, in other words, from the subjects of the study. In qualitative studies, however, it is important that the researcher generate some of the data. Such data includes notes about the researcher's actions, thought processes, and decisions made throughout the course of the investigation. The researcher also prepares documentation that is helpful to understanding and, later, analyzing the interview data.

Notes about the setting or context for an interview, as well as observations made during the process of data collection, such as notes about a participant's behaviors or nonverbal communication, are referred to as *field notes.* These notes provide insights that are valuable in the analysis of data because they facilitate understanding the situation being studied (Rodgers & Cowles, 1993).

Evaluating the quality of data collection procedures in a qualitative study involves looking at a number of factors related to the subjects, as well as factors related to the researcher. The researcher must have gathered data from participants who have had the experience being studied, who are able to articulate their experiences, who feel comfortable and unconstrained in sharing their experience, and who have an adequate opportunity to share their experiences of interest. Accomplishing this places a considerable burden on the researcher, who must develop effective rapport with participants, ensure the confidentiality necessary to protect participants' identity when discussing matters that can be sensitive to the individual, and use effective interviewing techniques to obtain comprehensive and clear data that can be analyzed appropriately to answer the research question. In reading a qualitative study, it is important to consider the situation in which the data collection took place, for example, provisions for privacy during the interview; the amount of time allowed for an interview; efforts made by the researcher to establish rapport; and other factors, such as gender, culture, ethnicity, language, or age, that might affect the researcher-participant relationship; steps taken to ensure accuracy of the data collected, such as audio recording of interviews; and any other information the researcher provides about strategies used to enhance the quality of the data collected. The researcher also should provide an account of notes that were taken during the data collection session and describe how these were used to supplement the data collection process and enhance the quality of the data.

## Data Analysis in Qualitative Research

Data analysis can be an intimidating process in any study. In qualitative research, the volume of information, along with the lack of any prescribed structure for organizing and analyzing it, can be overwhelming, particularly for investigators new to the process. It is also the case that this process can be the most enjoyable part of the research. This is the part of the research process where the inquisitive mind, the puzzle-solver, the curiosity and the creativity of the nurse, is allowed to grow and thrive.

There are many approaches to the analysis of qualitative data with some specific guidelines that are unique to each tradition of research. Grounded Theory, for example, involves a process of analysis that leads toward the identification of a *core variable,* a central concept that describes the experience being studied, and of categories of information or themes that contribute to that core of the experience. Phenomenology involves a search for "significant statements" and "meaning" in the data, and narrative research focuses on "stories." In spite of these variations, however, all qualitative procedures have in common a similar process of reducing the data to manageable units and then constructing a description of the experience being studied by putting the pieces of the data back together into a coherent whole.

The process of analysis begins with a stage of general data reduction. Typically, the researcher reads through the data (assume an interview transcript here for this purpose), identifying statements or parts of statements that carry a unique idea, and then labels or "codes" those statements, using some term that captures the essence of that statement. This process of coding, carried out with all of the data collected in the study (including data generated by the researcher), reduces the large volume of data in the transcripts to smaller segments that then become the focus of further analysis. Working with these codes, the researcher begins to organize the codes into a meaningful structure, with common ideas grouped together. The researcher is looking for patterns or recurrent ideas in the data (sometimes called themes), and the data are organized and reorganized into categories until clear patterns or themes can be identified. This process of organizing and categorizing continues until the researcher can identify the particular themes or categories that account for and reflect the data that have been gathered without leaving any gaps in the resulting cluster of categories (Knafl & Webster, 1988). It is not necessary to account for every element of data in identifying themes or patterns. There will always be more questions, new avenues to explore, new ideas about where research is needed. There should not, however, be major pieces of data that are ignored or left out of this categorizing process or major gaps in the themes that are identified.

The physical management and organization of data is accomplished using a technique that is best described using the metaphor "cut and paste." Historically, researchers would make multiple photocopies of the data (typically the interview transcripts) and cut the transcript into small segments, each segment containing a distinct idea relevant to the focus of the study. The researcher then would paste the segment onto a card (specific cards were developed just for this purpose) and sort those cards according to patterns that were identified in the data. Researchers made various adaptations in this approach to reflect their own style of data organization and analysis: word processing software could be used, researchers could write or paste the data into large spreadsheet-type formats, or different categories could be identified directly on the transcript pages and coded using unique colors. Since the early 1980s, specific software has been developed for use in qualitative data analysis. Some of the currently popular programs are NVivo (QSR International, 2008) and an earlier version of this software named NUD*IST, ATLAS/Ti (Scientific Software Development, 2008), HyperResearch (Researchware, 2008), among many others. In reviewing a report of qualitative research, the software used will be mentioned by the researcher, and the nurse reading the report should recognize that these are simply software programs that help with aspects of data management and organization. Software programs do not analyze the data for the researcher, but they are very useful in organizing data and facilitating the researcher's cognitive processes of data analysis. The use of software does not enhance the quality of the study, nor does the absence of it detract. While there are considerable benefits to the use of software when used by a researcher skilled in the program, the process of analysis ultimately depends on the diligence and cognitive effort of the researcher.

## Reporting the Results of a Qualitative Study

The results of a qualitative study are presented in a manner appropriate to the specific method employed. Grounded Theory research, for example, produces a type of theoretical construction that presents a substantive description of the experience that was studied. Regardless of the specific approach, results generally consist of a detailed discussion of patterns that were evident in the data collected in the study. Patterns can be organized around a specific concept, such as the core variable in Grounded Theory research, in a hierarchical manner with themes and subthemes, or as categories of descriptive ideas.

A well-written report of a qualitative study reads like a good story regardless of the specific approach employed in a qualitative study. Acknowledging this characteristic of qualitative studies initially may seem to minimize the importance of this type research. Quite the contrary, however; the fact that a well-written study reads a bit like a good "story" points out the richness of this type of research. A well-written report captures the reader's attention and draws the reader into the experiences presented in the report of the study. The subjects come alive, and the reader may begin to feel as if he or she actually knows the participant or at least can relate to their experiences. As the researcher is presenting results based on the analysis of the data, quotations using the actual words of the participants provide examples that support the researcher's conclusions. The reader, therefore, does not merely have to rely on the interpretations of the researcher but is presented with evidence that supports these conclusions. Reading these examples not only adds considerable credibility to the findings but also increases the richness of the study and provides detail that is not evident in other types of research. The researcher may use some quantitative data to present demographic information, but it is the words of the participants and the researcher's weaving of these words with detailed analysis that make qualitative research so sensitizing and illustrative of individual experiences.

## TRUSTWORTHINESS AND RIGOR

The qualitative study report that is written well gives the reader a strong sense that the results are believable. The voices of the participants seem alive, and it is easy to grasp their experiences. While this can be a valuable observation in assessing the quality of a qualitative study, there are additional criteria that must be considered. In quantitative research, the criteria that are used to evaluate the quality of a study overall are referred to as validity and reliability, and these will be discussed in chapter 12 in this text. Qualitative studies are carried out to accomplish different purposes and are completed using very different procedures. Consequently, a different set of criteria, referred to using a unique vocabulary, is used to evaluate the varied aspects of a qualitative study.

Noted researchers and methodologists Lincoln and Guba (1985) presented a framework in the mid-1980s that has been accepted widely as offering appropriate criteria to ensure a quality investigation. These criteria also can also be used to evaluate the quality of studies that have been completed and reported in the literature. In order to avoid confusion with the criteria of reliability and validity that are used for quantitative research, Lincoln and Guba proposed a broad framework organized around the key concept of *trustworthiness* to evaluate the rigor and the overall quality of a study. It is interesting to note that the aspects of research addressed by these criteria could be applied to any type of research, although the terminology here is most commonly used in the context of qualitative research.

The terminology and ideas adopted from Lincoln and Guba (1985) include the essential concerns of *truth value* or credibility, *applicability* or transferability, *consistency* or dependability, and *neutrality* (p. 290). The first criterion, truth value, addresses an extremely important concern in any research, the concern about whether or not it is reasonable to "believe" or have faith in the results. For qualitative research, this means that there needs to be confidence that the results are an accurate reflection of the participants and the experiences that were studied. There are numerous techniques that qualitative researchers can use to increase the likelihood that results will be "credible." Researchers need, first, to spend sufficient time with participants to be able to fully understand their realities and how they describe their experiences (a technique referred to as *prolonged engagement*). Sufficient contact also is necessary to establish rapport with participants to increase their comfort with the researcher and, consequently, their willingness to share important details. A technique known as triangulation sometimes is used to enhance credibility or trustworthiness. The term *triangulation* is adopted from a process for navigation in which several location points are determined and the intersection of lines drawn from these points is determined. Using simple principles of geometry, it is possible for an individual at sea to pinpoint his or her specific location. When applied to a qualitative study, triangulation means the corroboration of information using multiple sources, multiple methods, different investigators, or even the perspective provided by different theories (Denzin, 1978). In a health-related study, participants' descriptions of their experiences might be triangulated with the accounts of nurses or family members or even with the medical record. It is worth noting, however, that whether or not a participant's description of an experience is factual is not always a concern. People construct their viewpoints, and the experiences are shaped by what they believe happened, whether or not such beliefs are based in fact. Someone who experienced major trauma and believes he or she "died" and was brought back to life will undoubtedly relate to that experience in a way that is shaped by that belief. Whether or not the described events actually took place clinically may be of little consequence. For occasions where different perspectives exist or there is a need to determine actual events, triangulation is a very effective technique.

Other techniques also can be used to enhance the trustworthiness of results. A process referred to as *peer debriefing* provides an opportunity for the researcher to talk through aspects of the study with a colleague (peer) who is not invested in the study. This simple act of talking through parts of the study can be helpful in bringing to light some of the thoughts and ideas of the researcher that might not have been recognized otherwise or that might have stayed hidden in the recesses of the researcher's mind. The peer debriefer asks probing questions, challenges assumptions, encourages exploration, and, overall, helps the researcher become aware of any potential misinterpretation, missed clues in the data, and personal value orientation or bias. Complete objectivity in any study is not possible; yet, while it is not possible to be completely devoid of bias in any study, peer debriefing helps the researcher to recognize what bias exists and how it might affect the study. Through this awareness, the researcher can make a conscious effort to limit the influence of bias in the research.

Occasionally, researchers use a technique known as a *member check* to ensure the credibility of their findings. In doing a member check, the researcher returns to the participants or to a subset of participants and shares findings with them so that they can verify that the researcher correctly understands the views and experiences presented in the interview. A member check also can be done at the conclusion of an interview, with the interviewer giving the participant a brief summary of the interview for their feedback. It can also be done near the conclusion of a study by taking the study results back to some of the participants for their consideration and review. Using this technique, the researcher is able to verify with study participants that the results accurately reflect the experiences that were described to the researcher. In other words, the researcher knows the results are credible because he or she asked the participants themselves to ensure that they are. Member checks are not possible in all studies and research situations. When appropriate, however, they can be a very useful means to ensure that the results of a study are credible or trustworthy.

The second criterion is referred to as *applicability* and addresses an issue similar to generalizability. As noted previously, there is no expectation or desire on the part of qualitative researchers that their results will be, in fact, generalizable. Generalizability always has to be considered with great caution; in qualitative studies, where the emphasis is on depth and richness, it minimizes the role of each unique individual to assume or stipulate that results actually will be generalizable simply by virtue of some feature of how the study was conducted. In contrast, the researcher in a qualitative study acknowledges that the consumer of the research is in the best position to evaluate whether or not results are applicable in other settings. For nurses in practice settings, this means that the nurse is in the best position to determine to what extent the results are likely to be useful for clients in the setting in which the nurse works with these individuals. How similar are the contexts and the individuals in the study to those with whom the nurse works? Rather than stipulate that results are generalizable, the qualitative researcher is obligated only to provide a sufficiently detailed description of the research situation to enable the reader of the research to make the determination whether the results are likely to "transfer" to other settings.

The two remaining criteria for conducting rigorous qualitative inquiry (and for evaluating the rigor of studies that have been reported in the literature) are *consistency* (dependability) and *neutrality* (confirmability). Consistency is similar to the concept of reliability for quantitative studies. In a quantitative study, there is an expectation that repeated use of an instrument will provide comparable results with each administration. In a qualitative study, however, things cannot be expected to be the same with repeated episodes of data collection or with repeated collection of information from different groups. As people talk about their experiences, their perspective changes. Similarly, a different investigator might elicit different descriptions from people because of the focus of the interview, whatever cognitive or emotional processing has gone on within the individual, changes in the context for data collection, and other factors that can influence what is obtained in a qualitative study. Consequently, it is unreasonable to expect an occurrence comparable to stepping repeatedly on a bathroom scale and receiving the same results each time. What is important, however, is that all aspects of a qualitative study, including the collection of data and the analytic techniques that are employed and the insights generated, are conducted in a way that is "dependable" or "confirmable." The process must be rigorous and comprehensive, and the product must be supported by appropriate data. The question, therefore, is not whether another researcher would find the same thing by replicating the research. The appropriate question is whether the results obtained by the researcher who did the study are appropriate and reasonable and whether the processes can be traced and documented so that the results are defensible.

Both of these aspects of quality can be assessed using an *audit trail* (Halpern, 1983; Rodgers & Cowles, 1993). Qualitative researchers keep records of all the steps in the process of conducting the study, including procedures, methodological changes that are instituted, insights generated during data analysis, and observational or field notes. These records can be reviewed by other investigators who serve as auditors to ensure that the processes and procedures are carried out in a rigorous manner. All of the steps in the conduct of the study can be retraced and evaluated for quality. While audits can be conducted on a large-scale basis just as a financial audit of a large company might be conducted, more often a researcher will engage a colleague to serve as a peer reviewer to evaluate aspects of the study on an ongoing basis while the research is being conducted and results are being prepared for dissemination.

## SUMMARY

Qualitative research contributes vital information necessary to effective work with human beings. It is valuable in exploring areas about which little is known, in developing theory, and in generating rich and detailed descriptions about the lives of people with whom nurses work. Understanding the human element of health situations, the thoughts, feelings, and perceptions of individuals, is essential to providing sensitive care in a manner appropriate to the people with whom nurses work. This aspect of human experience also contributes essential information for evidence-based practice, illuminating the personal experience associated with various health situations and events. The ability to recognize the roles and contributions of qualitative research and to understand and critique published studies is an important one for nurses who strive to base their practice on quality evidence relevant to the populations with whom nurses work.

## SUGGESTED ACTIVITIES

1   Discuss with a classmate a clinical problem of interest. Describe how you could approach it using a qualitative research question and with a quantitative question. What would be the differences in the findings?

2   Write questions that could be used in an interview in a qualitative study of the losses experienced with a chronic illness.

## REFERENCES

Blumer, H. (1969). *Symbolic interactionism: Perspective and method.* Englewood Cliffs, NJ: Prentice-Hall.

Charmaz, K. (2000). Grounded theory: Objectivist and constructivist methods. In N. Denzin & Y. Lincoln (Eds.), *Handbook of qualitative research* (2nd ed., pp. 509–535). Thousand Oaks, CA: Sage.

Charmaz, K. (2005). Grounded theory in the 21st century: Applications for advancing social justice studies. In N. Denzin & Y. Lincoln (Eds.), *Handbook of qualitative research* (3rd ed., pp. 507–535). Thousand Oaks, CA: Sage.

Charmaz, K. (2006). *Constructing grounded theory.* London: Sage.

Davies, D., & Dodd, J. (2002). Pearls, pith, and provocation. Qualitative research and the question of rigor. *Qualitative Health Research, 12,* 279–289.

Denzin, N. K. (1978). *Sociological methods.* New York: McGraw-Hill.

Glaser, B. (1978). *Theoretical sensitivity.* Mill Valley, CA: Sociology Press.

Glaser, B., & Strauss, A. (1967). *The discovery of grounded theory.* Chicago: Aldine.

Halpern, E. S. (1983). *Auditing naturalistic inquiries: The development and application of a model.* Indiana University. University Microfilms International AAT 8317108.

Husserl, E. (1960). *Cartesian meditations: An introduction to phenomenology* (D. Cairns, Trans.). The Hague: Martinus Nijhoff.

Knafl, K. A., & Webster, D. C. (1988). Managing and analyzing qualitative data: A description of tasks, techniques, and materials. *Western Journal of Nursing Research, 10,* 195–210.

Koch, T. (1995). Interpretive approaches in nursing research: The influence of Husserl and Heidegger. *Journal of Advanced Nursing, 21,* 827–836.

Labov, W., & Waletsky, J. (1967). Narrative analysis: Oral versions of personal experience. In J. Helm (Ed.), *Essays on the verbal and visual arts* (pp. 12–44). Seattle, WA: American Ethnological Society.

Lincoln, Y. S., & Guba, E. G. (1985). *Naturalistic inquiry.* Beverly Hills, CA: Sage.

Merleau-Ponty, M. (1999). *The phenomenology of perception.* London: Routledge. (Original work published 1962)

Morse, J.M. (1991). Strategies for sampling. In J. M. Morse (Ed.), *Qualitative nursing research: A contemporary dialogue.* Newbury Park, CA: Sage.

Patton, M. Q. (2001). Qualitative research and evaluation methods (3rd ed.). Thousand Oaks, CA: Sage.

Plager, K. A. (1994). Hermeneutic phenomenology: A methodology for family health and health promotion study in nursing. In P. Benner (Ed.), *Interpretive phenomenology: Embodiment, caring, and ethics in health and illness* (pp. 65–83). Thousand Oaks, CA: Sage.

QSR International Pty Ltd. (2008). NVivo [Computer software]. Doncaster, Victoria, Australia.

Researchware. (2008). HyperResearch [Computer software]. Randolph, MA.

Riessman, C.K. (1993). *Narrative analysis.* Newbury Park, CA: Sage.

Riley, T., & Hawe, P. (2005). Researching practice: The methodological case for narrative inquiry. *Health Education Research, 20,* 226–236.

Rodgers, B. L. (1997). Experiences of family members in the nursing home placement of an older adult. *Clinical Nursing Research, 10,* 57–63.

Rodgers, B. L. (2005). *Developing nursing knowledge: Philosophical traditions and influences.* Philadelphia: Lippincott, Williams & Wilkins.

Rodgers, B.L. (2007). *Experiences of women with myocardial infarction.* Report to the Wisconsin Women's Health Foundation, Madison, WI.

Rodgers, B. L., & Cowles, K.V. (1993). The qualitative research audit trail: A complex collection of documentation. *Research in Nursing and Health, 16,* 219–226.

Scientific Software Development. (2008). Atlas.Ti [Computer software]. Berlin, Germany.

Strauss, A., & Corbin, J. (1998). *Basics of qualitative research: Techniques and procedures for developing grounded theory.* Thousand Oaks, CA: Sage.

Van Manen, M. (1990). *Research lived experience: Human science for an action sensitive pedagogy.* Albany: State University of New York.

Wolf, Z. R. (2007). Ethnography: The method. In P. L. Munhall (Ed.), *Nursing research: A qualitative perspective* (4th ed., pp. 293–330). Sudbury, MA: Jones & Bartlett.

# 9 Sampling Methods

KARIN T. KIRCHHOFF

Sampling can be viewed from two perspectives, that of a research consumer and that of an investigator. As a research consumer, one might have the following questions: What knowledge is necessary to critique the sample section of a research article? How should a sample be constructed for a quality improvement project in a clinic? Which type of sample should be used for a comparison of two methods of encouraging patients to increase their level of exercise? From an investigator perspective, one would consider the following: How is the number of persons from whom to collect data determined? Sample size is important in engendering confidence in the results of studies. A small sample size might provide a conclusion that is not substantiated when a larger sample is used. The characteristics of the sample also help in the generalizability of the result to the broader population. All of the cardiovascular research conducted on white males has not given adequate information about how to treat minorities and women with heart disease. This chapter distinguishes among the types of samples, discusses how to choose a sample depending on the purpose of the study and how to conduct that type of sample, offers some considerations in selecting a sample size, and distinguishes these issues from response rates and random assignment.

A sample is created when individuals are selected from a population in some manner, randomly (with the intent of generalizing back to the population) or nonrandomly. The sample is used in a study, and findings about the sample are sometimes applied to the population from which it was drawn.

The major purpose of sampling is to be economical, since it is more costly to test a nursing intervention on all eligible patients. A sample is used to "stand in for" or represent the full population. Statistics are used to summarize sample characteristics, such as the average height or the median income of the clinic patients, and a relationship is projected to the parameter of the population that is not measured.

## TERMS RELATED TO SAMPLES

A number of terms are used in the discussion of research samples. Among the most important are these:

*Population:* Entire aggregation of cases that meet a designated set of criteria. Population statistics are usually designated by Greek letters, such as $\mu$, the population mean, which is estimated from the sample.

*Accessibility:* Availability of patients who meet criteria and who might participate in the study. It may refer, for example, to all the adult patients that come to a clinic with Type 2 diabetes

*Target:* The entire aggregation about which generalizations are to be made, for example, all adult patients with Type 2 diabetes in the country.

*Stratum:* A subpopulation of mutually exclusive segments, such as male and female. You might decide to sample within strata or divide your sample into strata for analysis purposes.

*Sample:* The portion of population selected in some manner to represent the entire group. Statistics for the sample are usually designated by letters of the alphabet, such as M for the mean or average in the sample.

*Census:* A count of *all* the elements in a population and/or a determination of the distributions of their characteristics. In the United States, a census of all the people is taken every 10 years. In this example, each person is an element. Because of cost, this process is done infrequently. If a survey is to be taken of hospitals and all hospitals (elements) listed by the American Hospital Association are included in the research, the study will be a census.

## SAMPLING PROCEDURES

A *sampling design* is a combination of the sampling process (selecting parts from the whole) and the estimation (making inferences about the total group from the sample data). Decisions about sample design relate to how much error can be tolerated and the costs involved. If you need to measure something very accurately, such as a laboratory sample, you can tolerate little if any error. Patients will be treated with drugs or undergo other costly interventions if the error rate in the laboratory tests places their values in the abnormal range. Issues such as risk to patient, costs of care, and extent of treatment should aim decisions toward a low error rate. If more error is tolerable, then perhaps a smaller sample will suffice. Costs of collecting data sometimes dictate how many data and which type of data we can collect and the number of people we can include in our research.

*Sampling units* are the elements or groups of elements that form the basis of sample selection. In one study, individual patients with heart disease might be the sampling unit, whereas in another study, the sampling units might be at the level of the clinics in which these patients receive care. Selection occurs at a different level in the second situation.

*Lists* are inventories of the units in a population, with a direct one-to-one correspondence between each item listed and the unit it represents. There are two types of lists: *element lists,* or lists of all the population elements (e.g., list of nurses), and *cluster lists,* lists of groups of elements in convenient natural groups (e.g., list of hospitals that employ nurses). If the plan is to sample at the level of the nurses and only a cluster list is available, sampling will be more difficult. This problem explains why studies frequently include membership lists of organizations, such as the American Association of Critical-Care Nurses (AACN), when a survey of staff nurses across settings is desired.

Problems can occur when a researcher uses lists from professional organizations or sources. Some members do not possess the attribute(s) to be placed on a particular list. In the previous example, a staff nurse who is not a member of AACN would not be included in the list of nurses from which the sample is to be drawn. Sometimes individuals intentionally keep their names off some lists. An example is the phone book, where unlisted numbers are not available for sampling. The list might be out of date, or it might include someone other than the desired respondent (e.g., when a survey mailed to a home address is received by a family who just moved into that address, rather than by the intended recipient). Sometimes an individual may appear on the list more than once. For example, when nurses work in more than one clinic, but on different days of the week, they will be listed on more than one clinic's list of employees. The biggest problem with lists is gaining access to them. With laws governing privacy and limiting access to patient health information, it has become increasingly difficult to access this kind of information.

## DEFINITIONS RELATED TO ERROR

Because a sample is seen as representing a population, there is concern about how much error is involved in generalizing from the sample to the population.

*Random error,* also called *sampling error,* is the tendency for statistics to fluctuate from one sample to another. If I have 100 patients coming to a diabetes clinic and weigh 15 successive different samples of 10 patients, I could construct a sampling distribution of 15 means for weight. The values would differ across the 15 samples and could be plotted on a graph. The various means would have some sampling error because not all 100 patients have been measured. I could then calculate a means of all 15 means. It is likely that the sample means would cluster around the grand mean of all the sample means.

A calculation of how well the sample mean represents the population mean is called the *standard error of the mean,* or SEM. The formula for the calculation involves two factors, how different the members of the sample are from one another and how large a sample was drawn. The statistic functions so that it increases as the variability of the data increases and decreases as the sample size increases. The moral here is that when the values are likely to be highly different, a larger sample will be needed.

Another type of error is *nonrandom error* or bias. For example, let's assume that I select only the patients with diabetes who come to the clinic during usual hours. The patients who come into the emergency department and are seen there instead are omitted from the sample. The sample is thereby biased toward those who have better control of their disease. Bias does not need to be planned; it can also be inadvertent if one fails to think of all the limitations imposed by decisions about how the sample design will affect the study results. Whereas random error fluctuates around the mean and can be on either side of the true mean of the population, bias falls on one side or the other. Therefore, it is more serious, since a mean of a second sample will be on the same side of the true mean (expected value is the mean for all possible sample means) and will lead to an erroneous conclusion.

## TYPES OF SAMPLES

There are two categories of samples: nonprobability and probability. The distinction is based on whether or not the selection used for the sample is random. In probability samples, different elements or individuals have an equal chance of being selected as subjects. In nonprobability samples, they do not.

### Nonprobability Samples

Nonprobability samples use a nonrandom selection to select elements for a study. The limitation is that there is no way of estimating each element's probability of being included. The selection of a second sample would likely yield different results.

There are four types of nonprobability samples: *convenience* (synonyms used include *haphazard* and *accidental*), *snowball, purposive,* and *quota.* Convenience is the most frequently used type, and when the method of selection is not given in a research report, the assumption is that the sample was a convenience sample. It is the weakest of all the types of samples since anyone available is included and no screening criteria are used.

A second type of nonprobability sample is the snowball (or network) sample. It is used when the initial contacts in the sample who meet the study criteria give information to the researcher about how to make subsequent contacts with others who also meet the study criteria. It may be necessary to use this technique when there is no list of individuals and especially when there is a reason people would not like to be on such a list. Examples might include patients who have had sexually transmitted diseases, psychiatrists who had patients who committed suicide, or other situations that might carry some stigma.

A third type of sample is the purposive sample. This might also be called a judgmental sample or a known groups sample (e.g., New Hampshire as a stand-in for the country in presidential election polling). This sample is considered typical of some characteristic. In qualitative research, theoretical sampling is used to select those who meet certain criteria and who can provide information required during ongoing data collection and analysis. The process ends when that category is saturated. For more information see Coyne (1997).

The last type of nonprobability sample is the quota sample. In this sample, the investigator identifies strata in the population, determines the proportions of elements in each stratum, and then selects a convenience sample from the stratum. The advantage is that the strata or groups can be represented in the proportion that they occur; in a simple convenience sample, in contrast, not all strata, especially those with lower counts, may be represented.

Although nonprobability samples have less stature than probability samples in terms of quality, they have a number of advantages. They are convenient to acquire. They usually cost less than probability samples, since a list does not need to be generated. At times the additional work to get a probability sample may not be warranted, especially if there is no need to generalize to a population. For example, in a quality improvement project, there might be four providers for whom chart reviews were performed to determine whether the providers ordered eye exams for their diabetic patients. These results do not need to generalize outside of the sample. Probability samples are not always possible, since lists required for sampling may not exist. Also, other studies on any given subject can and should be done and will use different samples, which will strengthen the findings over time.

Nonprobability samples have one major disadvantage. They lack representativeness of the population to which the investigator may wish to generalize.

## Probability Samples

In probability samples, the researcher is able to specify the probability that each element of the population will be included in the selection. That probability is known and must be greater than zero, known as *non-zero* chance of selection. Although the literature on sampling usually talks about equal chance of selection, only with simple random selection is the chance of selection equal for all in the population.

There are four types of probability samples: simple random, stratified, systematic, and cluster. In conducting these types of samples, the researcher must develop a sampling frame. The steps in developing a sampling frame are:

1  Develop the frame (what is to be included),
2  Enumerate all the elements in the population,
3  Select the sample in a random manner. The selection process is different for each of the probability samples.

In simple random sample (SRS), every element in the population has an equal chance of being selected. In general, the selection is usually done so that if the same person or unit comes up more than once, it is not used more than once; this is called sampling without replacement. Subjects may be chosen in one of two ways. Either a number corresponding to all the names on the list are put in a hat and randomly selected, or numbers that have been matched to names are selected from a random numbers table. In the second method, the same number can be chosen more than once, so the decision as to whether a number will be used more than once should be made before starting the process.

In stratified samples, the aim is to ensure that different segments of the population are represented. The steps in selecting a stratified sample are:

1  A decision is made *before* selection to place subjects in a particular stratum (as opposed to quota sampling in which you ask questions to determine each potential subject's eligibility for a stratum and sample as subjects appear). These strata should be mutually exclusive.

2  The population is divided into homogeneous subsets within each stratum. It is assumed that the people in the stratum are more like one another than they are like people in other strata. For example, patients may be grouped by their major illness or by the source of their medical insurance for sampling purposes.

3  The researcher then samples using the strata. The question here is whether the sample should be selected using proportional sampling within the strata or nonproportionally. For example, suppose a clinic sees only a few patients who have Medicaid as a source of insurance. A decision might be made to study a higher proportion of those patients than of the rest of the patients, who use health maintenance organizations, a more common form of insurance. Having a large enough sample in the Medicaid group would allow for some comparisons that might not be possible if simple random samples were used.

Cluster sampling is used when a list of all the elements is not available or the data collection occurs over a geographically spread-out area. The process used is successive random sampling of units, from larger to smaller groupings. First, hospitals in a region of the country might be selected, then primary care clinics within those selected hospitals. This process is usually multistage. It is more economical than working to first get a list of all primary-care clinics. The drawback is that cluster sampling increases sampling error. The way to counter this problem is to increase the sample size by sampling more clusters.

The last type of probability sample is the systematic sample. This type is used when there are large numbers of elements on a list. Let's assume there are 40,000 patients attending one of the clinics at a hospital. If the sample size desired for a satisfaction survey is 100 patients, the next step would to calculate the sampling interval (K).

If $N = 40,000$, $K = N/n = 400$. In this example, we would select a number randomly from 1 to 400 for the random start and then select every 400th case. This process would be easier than to put all these names in a hat or to number them individually and then draw 100 numbers from a random numbers table.

One shortcoming of systematic samples is that there might be a cycle in the list. In this example, the likelihood is low. If every 10th nurse on a list of nurses employed in a facility is a manager, for example, one cycle might have only nurse managers and another might have none.

The advantage of systematic samples is that they are efficient and convenient. This is the method usually used by survey centers, especially for large sample sizes.

In general, probability samples have a number of advantages. They are usually preferred to nonprobability samples but are impractical or unnecessary in some cases. They are the only way to obtain representative samples, and they allow for estimation of sampling error. If inferential statistics are to be used, probability samples are preferable. They do have some disadvantages, as well. They are expensive and inconvenient, and they are not always possible. Additionally, they are not always necessary if the attribute being studied is homogeneous. Probability samples carry an assumption of representativeness because of the nature of the sampling, but this is not guaranteed; there can be issues of refusals or nonrespondents, which weaken the representativeness, and also sample attrition over time, which changes the sample's characteristics.

Issues of response rate are also important. The idea with surveys is that giving questionnaires to large numbers and hoping that as many as 30% of recipients will respond will result in a large enough sample size. In reality, a high response rate with a small sample is preferable to a large sample size with a low response rate. The issue of bias–what separates those who responded from those who did not—should be addressed and may call the study into question, even with a larger sample size. The questionnaire should be designed so that there is at least one follow-up mailing to increase the response rate.

## SAMPLE SIZE

After the researcher decides on the type of sample, the next major decision concerns sample size. Many consultants or statisticians are approached with question about sample size as if it were a magic number that can be shared. The most frequent response is "It depends." And it does depend on a number of factors. There are advantages to large samples. They permit the principle of randomization to do the job for which it is designed—to counterbalance, in the long run, atypical values. The sample should be as large as is economical and practical.

On the other hand, there are advantages to small samples. They are more economical in terms of costs and time and can be more easily monitored. Smaller samples are appropriate for exploratory research and pilot studies.

The determining factors for sample size are the degree of precision required and the heterogeneity of the attributes under investigation. If the study must yield precise results and the variables are heterogeneous, it will be necessary to have a larger sample size than if less precision were required and the units to be sampled were more similar. If statistical testing, such as a t-test, is to be used, these factors are reflected in the statistical formula:

$$t = \frac{\text{differences between groups}}{\text{variability within groups/sample size}}$$

If there is high variability in the group and a small sample, only very large differences will be seen to be significant. If the study is to detect differences between the two groups, the groups need to be similar and the sample size needs to be larger.

Another issue to be considered in sample size relates to the analysis planned and the number of cross-classifications that will be done. If the sample consists of patients with diabetes and there are plans to compare males and females and people with Type 1 diabetes and those with Type 2, at least 40 patients will be required, since one rule of thumb is that a study should have at least 10 subjects for each cell.

The type of sample should also be considered in determining sample size. If the researcher is not using a probability sample, even having a large sample size will not eliminate all bias. The source of sampling frame is another issue. How confident are the investigators about the accuracy of the data? Also how much confidence is required for estimates back to population under consideration? If there is a need to accurately estimate the population from the sample, a larger sample size is needed to reduce sampling error.

For designs that do more than describe a sample, power analysis is used to statistically determine the needed sample size. Frequently, the information needed in the calculation is not available. One formula is the effect size (ES). This is determined from data collected previously, such as, for example, an intervention tested on two groups. The formula is:

$$ES = \frac{\text{Mean (treatment)} - \text{Mean (control)}}{\text{Standard Deviation (SD)}}$$

where SD is equal to the SD of the treatment and control groups.

Some statistics textbooks provide tables to help researchers calculate sample size. A classic textbook by Cohen (1997) offers one guideline for determining sample size. In general, these tables require the researcher to provide information about the planned statistic, the expected size of the difference between groups, and the expected variability. Perhaps the researcher can locate a published report that is similar to a proposed study and that reports a standard deviation that gives an approximation of the variance expected. There are conventions for setting other parameters; the *alpha* is usually set at .05 and the *beta* at .20 (conversely, the power to detect a change when there is one is 80%). A higher power will yield even higher and perhaps unmanageable sample sizes. At the intersection of these decisions will be a number that can be used for a sample size for each of the groups to be compared.

Another issue with sample size is the confusion between *proportional* size and *absolute* size. There is more power gained from the absolute size of the sample than from the proportional size of the sample. For example, it is more important that the sample size be 40 than that 40 is 50% of the 80 possible subjects.

## RANDOM ASSIGNMENT

Related to but different from random selection is *random assignment.* This is the process of allocating subjects to different experimental conditions on a random basis for the purpose of comparing the responses of those who have the intervention and those who do not. Since the assignment is done randomly, there is an assumption that the groups formed are approximately equivalent before the intervention. Random assignment is considered to be a close relative of random sampling. It is sometimes used with random sampling, but this is seldom done in experiments because it is rare that one has more subjects than needed. Clinical experiments usually take all eligible patients.

Huck (2000) cautions researchers about sampling. He first notes that there is frequently a mismatch between the source of data and the destination of the claims for the inferences. The sample needs to be aligned closely with the population. He also voices concerns about the nature of the sample—how restrictive is it, and how far can the results it produces be generalized. Findings from patients seen at an academic medical center may not generalize to all patients with the same disease. Sometimes the word *random* is used in a write-up, but that does not mean that the process was without investigator intrusion. This can happen, for example, when a response rate is insufficient and so another group is approached to add to the dataset.

## SUMMARY

In summary, samples are used to represent the groups to which generalizations need to be made. Aligning the characteristics of the sample with the desired group is critical. Random sampling with a large enough sample is an effective way to do this. Ensuring an adequate sample size to allow one to draw statistical conclusions is important when one is conducting a study for publication. For internal use such as quality improvement studies or outcome measurement, sample size is dependent on the number of subjects available and the size required to produce results at a sufficiently high level of confidence. For these samples, randomness is not necessary, but it can be employed when the population is large as a way to reduce the numbers used.

## SUGGESTED ACTIVITIES

1  Design a sample for a quality improvement activity at a clinic where there are 400 diabetic patients. Foot checks should be done annually on such patients, but this prevention guideline

does not seem to be followed. How many charts should be reviewed to convince practitioners to implement the guideline? Should the sample be drawn within each practitioner's panel or across the clinic?

2   The ICU nurses are concerned about how withdrawal of life support occurs in their unit. They want to know how other units do it across the country. If a national sample is to drawn, a membership list will have to be used, since there is not list of ICU nurses with contact information. Assuming the list is up-to-date and that the sampling criteria of working in an ICU and having one or more years' experience are met, what will be an adequate national sample size? Should it be stratified? If so, by which variables? If you had the printout, how would you actually do the selection?

## REFERENCES

Cohen, J. (1977). *Statistical power analysis for the behavioral sciences* (Rev. ed.). Orlando, FL.: Academic Press.

Coyne, I. T. (1997). Sampling in qualitative research. Purposeful and theoretical sampling; merging or clear boundaries? *Journal of Advanced Nursing, 26*(3), 623–630.

Huck, S. W. (2000). *Reading statistics and research* (3rd ed.). New York: Longman.

# 10

## Designing Questionnaires and Data Collection Forms

KARIN T. KIRCHHOFF

The most common tool used in data collection is the questionnaire. Because its use is so common, most individuals assume that the construction of questionnaires is easy. Those who have filled out poorly constructed questionnaires know that something is wrong but may not be aware of which rules in questionnaire construction were violated. This chapter details one approach to designing questionnaires that has been used for national and local surveys with good response rates. Comments about ease of completion are included. Although all of these suggestions may not work in one questionnaire, they can be used as guidelines for general use, with violations only for good reasons. At the same time, the seeming simplicity of a majority of these suggestions does not account for their value. When read, they may seem simple, but if they are used to critique questionnaires received in the mail, their significance will become apparent.

The purposes of questionnaire construction are many and varied. The content in this chapter can be applied to the simplest data collection purpose or to the most elegant study. Questionnaires can be used for research, quality assurance, administrative decision making, or collection of data about patients' preferences. Most situations require the development of a form specific to the topic under investigation; in other cases, there may be a standardized form available or a compilation of forms used for specific types of studies. Frank-Stromborg and Olsen (2004) have compiled a volume of instruments that can be used in clinical health care research.

This content of this chapter applies to questionnaires developed for telephone interviews, face-to-face interviews, or mailed surveys. Emphasis is placed on instances when the researcher is not present—such as mailed questionnaires—when no one is immediately available to answer a respondent's questions. In telephone interviews and face-to-face interviews, lines should be drawn on the tool to lead the eye to specific tasks. In face-to-face interviews, lists or visual aids can be shown to the respondent, but this option is not readily available in telephone interviews unless the questionnaire is mailed ahead of time. In deciding whether to use mailed questionnaires or telephone interviews, it is important to consider sample characteristics and how they work.

## GENERAL CONSIDERATIONS

Let us address some general considerations about the items included in the questionnaire and the type of data generated from them. Item types should be interesting to the intended audience. Individual items should not be embarrassing or threatening to the respondent; if they are, special care is needed to facilitate a response. The task should be easy to complete; respondents should be asked to circle an item or check a box, rather than write an answer. The cover letter, introduction, and tone of the questions should convey respect for the respondents and for their privacy and be written in a conversational tone.

The type of data needed should be carefully planned and the intended analysis should be determined before the questionnaire is finalized. Many individuals fail to make decisions about the difference between necessary and "interesting" data. The "interesting" information lengthens the questionnaire and may actually interfere with obtaining the necessary data. The novice may wallow in the data and then find that the "interesting" data may not even enter into the analysis. Such data should not have been collected.

The use of "dummy" tables is helpful in ensuring that all needed data are collected (see Exhibit 10.1 for an example). In the "dummy" table, the title, the column (e.g., Employment status), and the row labels (e.g., Yes/No) can be determined. In the cells, the proposed data (e.g., the number or percentage of the whole) can be reviewed to see if the correct

Exhibit 10.1

**DUMMY TABLE EXAMPLE**

| EMPLOYMENT STATUS | DESIRING CHILD CARE | |
|---|---|---|
| | Yes | No |
| Part-time | # or % | # or % |
| Full-time | # or % | # or % |

information was collected. For example, if age is collected by category (21–30, 31–40, and 41–50), it can form the rows of a table. However, if the actual age is not collected, the data are *not* able to be used later to determine whether there is a correlation between age and an attitude score or to calculate the average age of the respondent. When actual ages have not been obtained, the individual is placed only in a category of ages. On the other hand, by asking age in years, the researcher can calculate correlations and also compute the average age of the sample. Ages can be put into categories later if this is desirable. If the researcher does not assess the planned analysis ahead of time, some necessary data may not be collected, compromising the final report. Further discussion on level of measurement of data is provided in Chapter 13 on analyzing quantitative data.

The major reason for taking the time to properly design a questionnaire is to reduce respondent burden. The goal of a well-designed questionnaire is to engage the respondent in the process, make the respondent feel that the task is important, and encourage the respondent to complete the task readily and easily. Most of the following information is intended to achieve this goal.

## APPEARANCE

### Format

The initial appearance of the questionnaire is important. How the items are laid out and the overall format contributes to the appearance. The black-to-white ratio is critical. White should clearly predominate. When there is too much print on a page, the respondent feels that the task is difficult, even if the questionnaire is only a few pages long. The crowd-ing of black on the page, especially by reduction techniques used in photo-copying, does not fool respondents into thinking that the task is any less time-consuming than it is just because the questionnaire does not contain a lot of pages. It is more important to attend to the appearance than to the number of pages. The complexity of a questionnaire is not determined simply by the number of pages. The ease of the tasks and the spacing between items are more critical concerns. Obviously, the number of pages is *a* factor, but it is not *the* factor. Many investigators think that if they reduce a five-page questionnaire to a three-page ques-tionnaire by reducing the print size, they make it less overwhelming to respondents, but the respondents may think differently.

The cover letter and the questionnaire need to look "official." Peo-ple are not motivated to respond if the questionnaire looks like it was produced on a printer low on toner. Some software packages can give a very official appearance with little effort. Use of official letterhead for the cover letter lends an official nature to the survey.

The size of the page is also important. The default size of 8.5 x 11" is not the only possibility. If the questionnaire is to be printed profession-ally, many sizes are available. One option is to use a centerfold approach, creating the appearance of a booklet. How the questionnaire will be mailed is one consideration that will affect the researcher's decision on what size of paper to use. The size of the envelope may be another limit-ing factor.

## Color and Quality of Paper

Although white or near-white paper may give the best appearance, the researcher may choose another color for several reasons. For instance, when potential respondents need to be separated by groups, the use of different colors for each group will make the task easier. Using a color other than white also makes it less likely that the questionnaire will get lost on the respondents desk. The use of dark colors should be avoided since black print on them is hard to read. The weight of the paper can give the impression of cheapness if it is too light; on the other hand, a heavy paper may tip the scale toward more postage. Physically feel the paper stock before printing questionnaires, and weigh the number of pages required along with the envelope and the return envelope to de-termine if a slight reduction in weight will avoid the need for additional postage.

## Spacing

Spacing throughout the questionnaire is important. Spacing between questions should be greater than the spacing between the lines of each question, allowing the respondent to quickly read each question. Also, the spacing between response options should be sufficient to make it easy to determine which option was selected, especially if the task of the respondent is to circle a number. When material is single spaced, it can be difficult to determine which number was circled. Following these suggestions enhances the overall black-to-white ratio, as well.

## Respondent Code

Another consideration is the place for a respondent code number. Usually an underscore line is placed at the upper-right corner on the first page. Although code numbers are essential if follow-up is anticipated, respondents are sometimes troubled by these numbers and either erase or obliterate them. This is particularly true when respondents fear an administrator's reaction to their answers or worry about lack of privacy. An explanation for the use of a code number in the cover letter may alleviate this concern but may not be sufficient if any of the information is at all revealing. When no respondent code is used, it is not possible to follow up on the nonrespondents because they cannot be separated from the respondents. This means that everyone will need to get a second and third contact, increasing costs of the study.

When respondent codes are not used on questionnaires, different colors of paper can be used to represent separate subgroups. In this instance, response rates can still be determined for the entire sample, as well as for each subgroup. Selective follow-up without code numbers can be done on everyone in the subgroup with a low response rate if funds and time permit.

## Typeface

The typeface should be chosen carefully for readability and appearance. Script typeface should be avoided. The size of the type should be selected with the reader in mind. For example, if the questionnaire is to be read by the elderly, the typeface should be larger than would be required for a middle-aged adult. A good test is to have a few persons close to the intended respondents in age answer the planned questionnaire and describe the ease of completion.

## SECTIONS OF THE QUESTIONNAIRE

Questionnaires are structured with several components. These include the title, directions for the respondents, questions to be answered, transition statement(s) at sections change, and a closing statement. The title should relate to the content of the questionnaire. Directions for completing the questions follow the title. Specific directions may be required for each section of the questionnaire, and these should be explained in a conversational manner. The closing statement should thank the respondent for the time and effort taken to complete the tasks. Questions to be asked of respondents are addressed next.

An item consists of a question (or request for information) and possible response options. First, we discuss information about the questions; we then address response options.

## Questions

### Type of Questions

The choice between open-ended and closed-ended questions depends on several factors. The *nature of the question to be answered* by the data is one factor. Are feelings to be obtained, or facts? Feelings, especially if detail is needed, are best obtained in the respondent's own words. Therefore, open-ended questions would be the choice. Facts are more easily categorized. When detail is not required, closed-ended items can be used. If the desired outcome is a set of statements from respondents, open-ended questions should be chosen. If a quick count of responses in different categories is desired, closed-ended items will make the task easier.

Another issue in choosing between open- and closed-ended questions is *how much is known about the possible responses.* If all options are known, they can be provided in a list and the respondents can choose among them. If only some information is available, open-ended questions might be used. In instances when most of the options are known and format calls for closed-ended responses, the use of "Other (please specify) _____" gives respondents a chance to answer if their response does not match the provided responses.

One of the most important factors in selecting between the two question options is the *analysis planned.* When dealing with a small number of questionnaires (fewer than 30), the researcher can use either option. With larger surveys (e.g., an entire hospital or institution or a national survey), closed-ended questions are preferable. They can be more readily summarized.

There are tradeoffs with either choice. Richness of responses and freedom of expression are lost with closed-ended questions. Ease of analysis and time are lost when open-ended questions are used unnecessarily. The investigator's burden is different with each. The time spent on designing the closed-ended items can be significant, but their analysis is relatively quick. Open-ended items are quicker to design but may take significantly longer to analyze. Where the time is spent—up front in design or later in analysis—may be a factor in the researcher's decision making.

## Wording of the Questions

The researcher should select the words used carefully, avoiding slang, abbreviations, and words that have several meanings. When using terms that may not be familiar to the respondent, the researcher should provide a definition. One should try to avoid abbreviations altogether if possible. If that is not possible, it's a good idea to spell out the abbreviation the first time it is used and perhaps later if the second question is separated from the initial use.

The clarity of the questions and of potential responses should be ensured before the data are collected. One way to do this is to pretest the questionnaire on several people who are similar to the intended respondents. Their responses will draw out any additional meanings or potentially confusing items. These individuals should be interviewed to assess any problems they had with completing the questionnaire, to determine what they thought the questions meant, and how difficult they found it to complete the questionnaire. It is helpful to time these pretest attempts, since that information can then be included in the cover letter to the final respondents to help them estimate how long it will take them to complete the form.

## Guidelines for Well-Written Questions

1   Use a conversational tone. The tone of the questions and of the entire questionnaire should be as if the respondent were present. For example, the question:

Sex        M _____

           F _____

should be expressed:

What is your sex? Is it

Male?              1

or Female?         2

Using the word *gender* instead of *sex* in this question may be preferable since it avoids some strange responses.

2    Avoid leading questions that suggest the expected response. An example is:

Problem: Most mothers ensure that their infants receive immunizations as infants. Has your child been immunized?

Yes               1

No                2

Revision: Has your child been immunized?

Yes               1

No                2

3    Avoid double-barreled questions that ask two questions at the same time. An example is:

Problem: Do you prefer learning about your illness in a group format, or would you rather use written material?

Yes               1

No                2

Revision: Do you prefer a group format for learning about your illness?

Yes               1

No                2

Do you prefer written materials for learning about your illness?

Yes               1

No                2

4    Try to state questions simply and directly without being too wordy. For some questions, the respondent wonders, "What was the question?" after reading wordy sections. A direct approach is more likely to yield the desired information.

5    Avoid double negatives.

Problem: Should the nurse not be responsible for case management?

Yes                                   1

No                                    2

Revision: Who should be responsible for case management?

The physician                         1

The nurse                             2

An administrator                      3

Other (please specify)                4

**6**  Do not assume that the respondent has too much knowledge.

Problem: Are you in favor of care for walk-ins in the clinic?

Yes                                   1

No                                    2

Revision: In the clinic, walk-ins will be seen in short appointments on the same day they call in with questions, rather than being scheduled for appointments later in the week. There will be a block of one-hour appointments in both the morning and the afternoon left open for them.

Are you in favor of walk-ins in the clinic?

Yes                                   1

No                                    2

## Response Options

Responses are developed for close-end question. The designer of the questionnaire needs to have an idea about what the common options could be. Some options are dichotomous such as "yes" and "no." Some are more complex. When not all options are known, there should be an open-ended opportunity for the respondent to give an answer. Different types of options have common mistakes that are made in their use. These will be detailed next.

## Guidelines for Writing Response Options

There are also guidelines for the use of the response options. The most common ones are listed here.

**1**  Do not make response options *too* vague or *too* specific.
   Problem (too vague): How often do you call in sick?

Never 1

Rarely 2

Occasionally 3

Regularly 4

Revision: How often did you call in sick in the past 6 months?

Not at all 1

1–2 times 2

3–4 times 3

more than 4 times 4

Problem (too vague): Which state are you from? _____

Revision: In which state do you live? _____

In which state do you work? _____

Problem (too specific): How many total books did you read last year? _____

Revision: How many books did you read last year?

None 1

1–3 2

4–6 3

more than 7 4

2 The categories should be mutually exclusive, that is, there should be no overlap. This can become a problem when ranges are given. For example:

Problem: How old are you?

20–30 years 1

30–40 years 2

40–50 years 3

50 or more years old 4

The person who is 30 years of age does not know whether to circle a "1" or a "2."

Revision: How old are you?

20–29 years 1

30–39 years 2

| | |
|---|---|
| 40–49 years | 3 |
| 50 or more years old | 4 |

**3**  The categories must be inclusive and exhaustive.

In the previous example, only if all the respondents contacted were at least 20 years old would the categories be inclusive of all respondents. The last response, "50 or more years old," exhausts the upper age limit. The only caution in the use of such a range is that such a grouping loses detail. If only a few respondents are expected to fall into this category, then it may be adequate.

**4**  The order of options given is from *smaller* to *larger* or from *negative* to *positive*.

As an example: values for "not at all" are scored with "0" or "1" and the maximum value is scored as "5." In the analysis and explanation of the findings, it is easy to explain that higher numbers mean more of something. A mean satisfaction score that is higher than another mean satisfaction score would then be a more desirable finding.

The revised example in the next problem illustrates the correct order. If the coding were reversed, a higher score would mean less agreement (or more disagreement).

**5**  The balance of the options should be parallel.

Problem: Do you agree that nurses should receive a higher salary?

| | |
|---|---|
| Extremely strongly disagree | 1 |
| Very strongly disagree | 2 |
| Strongly disagree | 3 |
| Agree | 4 |
| Strongly agree | 5 |

Revision: Do you agree that nurses should receive a higher salary?

| | |
|---|---|
| Strongly disagree | 1 |
| Disagree | 2 |
| Agree | 3 |
| Strongly agree | 4 |

To further clarify point 4, if the order of the options were reversed, a high mean on this question would signify less agreement. That could be very confusing to those who read the write-up of the findings.

6 Limit the number of different types of response options chosen for use in the same questionnaire.

Common response options are:

approve—disapprove

agree—disagree (*alone* or with *strongly* in front of each for two additional options)

better—about the same—worse

very good—good—poor—very poor

A neutral middle can be provided if needed, such as "uncertain." Whenever possible, the use of the same response options across questions is preferred. The respondent task becomes more difficult when it is necessary to adjust to multiple types of options. The respondent feels required to constantly "change gears," and the burden is increased.

7 The number of response options per question should be minimized.

The usual recommendation is to have four or five possible responses. If a neutral middle response is desired, then five responses should be used, with the third or middle response being the neutral one. If there is an even number of responses, the respondent is forced to choose one side or the other (such as in the revision in point 5) and may find this frustrating. The respondent may feel that neither agreement nor disagreement is the right answer for him or her. Undecided respondents should be given a neutral choice that reflects their position, which avoids a negative emotional response that might result in the respondent's deciding to not answer the item or, worse, not to return the questionnaire. On the other hand, if decisions need to be made on the basis of the degree of agreement obtained, the surveyor may wish to force the respondent to choose a side. This type of forced choice should be used judiciously.

When more detail or spread-of-ratings is desired, responses can include six or seven options per question. When more than seven options are offered, the task of discriminating among them becomes difficult for the respondent.

**8**   The responses should match the question.

If the question is about how satisfied the patient is with the services, the options should not be "agree/disagree." Although this suggestion is obvious, it is easily violated if one is not careful.

## Ordering of the Questions

At the end of this book is a questionnaire (Appendix A), which was used to survey ICU nurses at several ICUs (Kirchhoff, Conradt, & Anumandla, 2003). The respondents were asked what type of information they use to prepare families for withdrawal of life support. In this case, researchers were interested in the words or phrases used, so the question was left open ended.

Opening questions are critical questions and should be related to the main topic and the title of the questionnaire. These questions serve to engage the responder to begin the task. Responders will be confused unless they are prepared for the flow of questions. This is one of the reasons that demographic questions should not be first.

Questions of similar format should be together. For example, if there are several clusters of "agree—disagree" questions, these should be grouped, unless there is some reason not to do so. Possible reasons for not grouping them include a major shift in content or a particular task that is required.

When the respondent task changes, or when a major change in topic occurs, a transitional sentence or paragraph should precede the change. In the sample questionnaire, each section asks for different information.

In the sample questionnaire, the desired respondents were ICU nurses identified by a member of the organization. If there were no local person involved in providing respondents for the study, it would have been good to establish at the outset whether the nurses were eligible for the study. The first question could be a filter question asking whether the nurse provides care to ICU patients, thereby eliminating someone who works in the ICU solely in an educator role.

If all respondents answer all questions, the logistics of the questionnaire are simple to set up. In some instances, some respondents might not answer every question, requiring a skip option. Skip patterns can become confusing; the directions should be placed close to the response option. People read from left to right; this principle is used when the response to be read precedes the response options. In the same way, the skip directions are given immediately before the option requiring an answer.

Another factor to consider in the ordering of questions is the chronology of events. If this is an issue in the questionnaire under construction, the order of questions may be partially dictated by chronology. For example, if information about the health of a child is to be obtained, the first questions should pertain to the child's birth, and later questions should focus on infancy and childhood.

Sensitive questions should be placed near the middle of the questionnaire, at a point where some rapport with the respondent has been developed. If they appear too early, this intrusion can lead some respondents to decide not to complete the entire questionnaire. On the other hand, if sensitive questions are placed too close to the end, the respondent may feel an abrupt ending in a difficult conversation. If the entire topic of the questionnaire is sensitive, the reader will be informed by reading Lee (1993), who wrote about researching sensitive topics.

Demographic questions should always appear at the end. They are the least interesting to the respondent and will be completed only if the respondent feels that a commitment has been made to finish the task. In the sample questionnaire provided, the planned analysis concerns only what nurses do with families. No analysis is planned about differences among the nurses relative to age groups or levels of experience or about whether preparation varied according to these demographics. These data were therefore not collected.

## Clinical Data Collection Forms

There are a few additional comments to be made about tools used for recording clinical data or chart information rather than for asking questions. Data collection forms are used in clinical studies to record observations or in quality-improvement activities to record compliance with standards.

In order to reduce the amount of writing, units of measurements should be written out where information is to be entered (e.g., _____mm). Hg. The use of checks or circles to complete a selection when the options are known will also reduce the amount of writing required.

When data are to be collected from various sections of a chart or in a series of steps, the data entry spaces should be placed in the order they occur, whether the data are on paper or screens. For example, if the order sheet is first in the paper chart, followed by progress notes, nursing notes, and graphs, the data collection should be ordered in that manner. When screens need to be navigated, the order of appearance can be taken into account.

The instructions about pretesting apply to data collection forms, as well. By pretesting on a real chart, one can determine whether the order has been reversed and whether placement of items is optimal.

## FOLLOWING THE DEVELOPMENT OF THE QUESTIONNAIRE

Many questionnaires are analyzed by simply counting the number of respondents for each category of response. If more complex analysis is desired, whoever is assisting with the data analysis should have some input into the process of how the data are collected. If consultation on the proposed analysis is needed, the consultant should review the questionnaire before the questionnaire is printed. Revisions may be necessary solely for analytic reasons.

Once the questionnaire has been developed, it should be pretested on subjects who are similar to the respondents who will be used. No matter how simple it seems, the pretest usually reveals areas for improvement. It is also helpful to debrief the subjects to find out what they thought about each question and the reason for the answers given. Additional areas for revision may become evident.

### Distribution of Questionnaires

Plans for obtaining an adequate response rate should be made. Some researchers recommend that one obtain at least a 50% response rate; others might suggest at least a 70% response rate. Different groups of respondents have different usual response rates. Nurses have a higher usual rate than do the recently bereaved, for example, who have had low rates (Kirchhoff & Kehl, 2008). Factors to be considered in achieving the desired return rate include (1) how the questionnaire is to be distributed and returned, and (2) how the researchers will be able to track and contact nonresponders. Personal delivery, along with immediate collection of the completed questionnaire, results in the highest return rate. Mailed questionnaires should include a cover letter and a return stamped and self-addressed envelope. Follow-up on mailed questionnaires requires that the researcher keep track of code numbers, checking off those returned and sending an additional mailing(s) to those who have not yet responded.

Mailed questionnaires with a cover letter and a return envelope have been the most used method historically. Obtaining an address for a respondent can pose difficulties. Mailing to the person at work when the topic is work related can be easier than mailing to a home address. Mailing to a job category at an institution, when the desired respondent is not known, adds another level of complexity—how to get the questionnaire to, for example, the APRN in Cardiology. Using a generic address may lead to the intended person if there is one.

Other methods of distribution take advantage of the Internet. The researcher can send an e-mail to the desired respondent with a link to a survey posted on Survey Monkey or another such service. E-mails are sometimes easier to find on institutional Web sites. Although Web-based surveys are cheaper to administer than those that use regular mail and returns are faster, they also have lower response rates than mailed surveys. There is also the issue of higher rates of nondelivery to e-mail addresses than to postal addresses (McDonald & Adam, 2003). Sending a post card as a surface mail notification before sending an e-mail increases the Internet response, bringing it closer to the response for the postal method, but an e-mail only method of delivery yields the lowest rate (Kaplowitz, Hadlock, & Levine, 2004).

Follow-up plans for all methods include developing a timeline for one or more additional contacts or telephone calls. When tracking returns, the investigator can plot the cumulative returns by day. When the return line plateaus, it signals that it is a good time to start the next wave of follow-up, whether by phone, e-mail, or regular mail. A cogent follow-up letter explaining the need for replies from all study respondents is helpful.

Phone follow-up has the advantage of permitting the respondent to clarify his or her reasons for not responding. The first mailing might not have been received, for example, especially in a complex organization. Questions that are answered in the phone call may permit the respondent to reply.

## CODING THE RESULTS

This section considers issues in coding quantitative data resulting from surveys. Directions for coding qualitative data are found in Chapter 7, on qualitative designs.

The plans for analysis need to be made according to the amount of the data, the intended level of analysis, and the method planned. If there will be a large data set or if a complicated analysis is anticipated, computer entry of the data is a necessity. With smaller data sets and when simple counts are planned, a manual system might be faster, although more errors are possible this way.

Entry of the data into the computer can be done in several ways. All of the responses can be entered onto a ScanTron sheet with response bubbles. Although this method is easy for the investigator, it is cumbersome for the respondent, who has to be sure the response is placed on the right numbered line. If the questionnaire is complicated and/or multiple sources of data are used, it may be easier to enter responses into an Excel spreadsheet or an Access database. These products facilitate the calculation of descriptive statistics that may be sufficient for analysis purposes without the researcher's having to export the data to a statistics program.

If the questionnaire is precoded and simple, the numbers circled by the respondent may be directly entered into the appropriate Excel column. In this case, each subject will be a row and each answer will be found in one column or set of columns. One should plan to check for errors, especially if a high degree of accuracy is needed.

TeleForms v10 is a software package that can facilitate the design of forms, distribute the questionnaire by fax, receive the responses by fax, and then set up the returned data as an SPSS file. TeleForms v10 can also receive data from scanned forms when the questionnaire has been mailed. Costs of data entry, time required, and error rates are all reduced with this process. This expensive software is available from Cardiff and is probably available only in larger survey centers.

The first run of the data should include a count of all the values for each variable. That allows numbers out of the expected range, illegal values, to be detected. For example, a yes-or-no question that was coded "1" and "2" would not have response numbers from "3" to "8." A "9" might be a legitimate value if the convention of inserting a "9" where there are missing data was followed. If illegal values are found, the ID number for the questionnaire containing the incorrect value needs to be determined. Then the original questionnaire for that subject should be reviewed to look for the correct value, and the spreadsheet should be corrected. This process, called data cleaning, should be done before any meaningful statistics are calculated.

## SUMMARY

Multiple decisions about questionnaire design, the questions to be asked, and the responses that are anticipated influence the quantity and the accuracy of the data that will be collected. The response rate will partially determine the value of the results to the intended audience. Development of well-designed data collection forms is vital in collecting accurate evidence for practice.

## SUGGESTED ACTIVITIES

1   Select a topic that allows both open-ended and close-ended responses. Develop three to four questions in each format. Discuss with a partner the advantages and disadvantages of each format.
2   Select a quality improvement topic from your clinical setting. Describe how you would design a tool to collect data, the process you would use to collect the data, and how you would feed back the results to those involved.

## REFERENCES

Frank-Stromborg, M., & Olsen, S. J. (2004). *Instruments for clinical health-care research* (3rd ed.). Sudbury, MA.: Jones & Bartlett.

Kaplowitz, M., Hadlock, T., & Levine, R. (2004). A comparison of Web and email surveys. *Public Opinion Quarterly, 68*(1), 94–101.

Kirchhoff, K. T., Conradt, K. L., & Anumandla, P. R. (2003). ICU nurses' preparation of families for death of patients following withdrawal of ventilator support. *Applied Nursing Research, 16*(2), 85–92.

Kirchhoff, K. T., & Kehl, K. A. (2008). Recruiting participants in end-of-life research. *American Journal of Hospice and Palliative Care, 24*(6), 515–521.

Lee, R. M. (1993). *Doing research on sensitive topics.* Newbury Park, CA. Sage.

McDonald, H., & Adam, S. (2003). A comparison of online and postal data collection methods in marketing research. *Marketing Intelligence & Planning, 21*(2), 85–95.

## ADDITIONAL READINGS

Dillman, D. A. (1978). *Mail and telephone surveys: The total design method.* New York: Wiley.

Fowler, F. J. (1988). *Survey research methods.* Newbury Park, CA: Sage.

Harris, L. E., Weinberger, M., & Tierney, W. M. (1997). Assessing inner-city patients' hospital experiences: A controlled trial of telephone interviews versus mailed surveys. *Medical Care, 35*(1), 70–76.

Jagger, J. (1982). Data collection instruments: Sidestepping the pitfalls. *Nurse Educator, 7*(3), 25–28.

Payne, S. L. (1951). *The art of asking questions.* Princeton, NJ: Princeton University Press.

Spilker, B., & Schoenfelder, J. (1991). *Data collection forms in clinical trials.* New York: Raven.

Sudman, S., & Bradburn, N. M. (1982). *Asking questions: A practical guide to questionnaire design.* San Francisco: Jossey-Bass.

Warwick, D.P., & Linninger, C. A. (1975). *The sample survey: Theory and practice.* New York: McGraw-Hill.

# 11

# Physiological Data Collection Methods

KATHLEEN S. STONE AND SUSAN K. FRAZIER

Evidence-based practice is the application of critiqued and synthesized research findings that have been replicated in an appropriate population of patients. Therefore, it is essential that the clinician have the tools to critique and evaluate research studies to determine their scientific soundness and appropriateness for application to clinical practice. Clinicians are at the forefront of the application of biomedical instrumentation. Clinicians use biomedical instrumentation to acquire information about their patient's condition and to monitor the progress of their patients. However, the biomedical instruments used in the clinical setting and in studies must be evaluated in order to ensure that the values generated are accurate. The findings of a study may be called into question if the biomedical instrument that was used to acquire the information was not appropriate, accurate, or reliable. Because clinicians are often required to evaluate and recommend the purchase of a biomedical instrument, familiarity with the principles of biomedical instrumentation, physiological parameters that can be measured, and the characteristics of biomedical instrumentation can be useful in evaluating a biomedical instrument for purchase or for the application of research findings to clinical practice.

Biomedical instruments measure physiological variables or parameters by the application or use of electrical devices. Biomedical instrumentation extends human senses by monitoring minute changes in physiological variables and by amplifying or displaying them so that they can be sensed audibly or visually. For example, the electrocardiogram monitors millivolt changes in electrical activity occurring in the heart, amplifies the signal to volts, and displays the signal audibly as a sound, or visually as a waveform on a screen or a printout from a computer.

## CLASSIFICATION OF BIOMEDICAL INSTRUMENTS

Biomedical instruments are classified into two types, *in vivo* and *in vitro*. In vivo instruments are applied directly within or on a living organism and are subdivided into invasive and noninvasive types. *Invasive* instruments require that a body cavity be entered or the skin broken for the device to be used. The introduction of an arterial catheter with the use of a pressure transducer to monitor arterial blood pressure is an example of invasive biomedical instrumentation. A *noninvasive* biomedical instrument uses the skin surface to apply the sensing device. An electrocardiogram (ECG) is an example of a noninvasive biomedical instrument. In vitro biomedical instrumentation requires the application of a device outside the organism. For example, a blood sample removed from the patient can be analyzed for a specific DNA sequence to diagnose a genetic disease using a polymerase chain reaction technique that requires the use of a biomedical instrument.

The method of monitoring (that is, invasive or noninvasive) should be considered when measuring physiological variables. It is preferable to use noninvasive techniques because there are fewer risks to the patient (such as blood loss, compromised arterial blood flow with cannulation, and infection). Consideration must also be given, however, to the degree of accuracy of the data and whether or not continuous or intermittent data are required. A noninvasive, indirect automated oscillating blood pressure cuff that cycles every minute can be used to monitor arterial blood pressure intermittently. When direct, continuous arterial blood pressure recordings are needed to enhance accuracy, however, invasive biomedical instruments are required. Although in vitro biomedical instrumentation does not pose direct risks to the human subject, consideration must still be given to the sample needed. The question to be asked is, "Can the necessary information be obtained in a sample other than blood, such as saliva (salivary cortisol), urine, (urinary catecholamines), or exhaled breath (exhaled carbon monoxide)?" Stress levels can be physiologically monitored directly by measuring epinephrine and nor-epinephrine levels in the blood or indirectly by measuring salivary corti-sol or urinary catecholamines. Carbon monoxide levels due to cigarette smoking can be measured directly in blood by co-oximetry and indirectly in exhaled air by using an ecolyzer.

## CATEGORIES OF PHYSIOLOGICAL VARIABLES DETECTED BY BIOMEDICAL INSTRUMENTS

A variety of physiological variables can be detected by using biomedical instrumentation, and these variables are commonly measured in patients in hospitals, clinics, and community and home settings. The monitoring of physiological variables is a component of comprehensive nursing care and provides a wealth of quantitative data that can be used in nursing research. To ensure accuracy of the data when collecting physiological measures with biomedical instruments, the practitioner must consider the components of the organism-instrument system (the subject, stimulus, and biomedical instrument).

### Categories of Variables That Can Be Detected With Biomedical Instruments

1 Electrical potentials
   a Brain—electroencephalogram (EEG)
   b Heart—electrocardiogram (ECG)
   c Muscle—electromyogram (EMG)
2 Pressures
   a Arteries—systolic and diastolic arterial pressure and mean arterial pressure
   b Veins—central venous pressure
   c Lungs—intra-airway and intra-pleural pressure
   d Esophagus—esophageal pressure
   e Bladder—degree of distension determined by pressure in the bladder
   f Uterus—uterine activity determined by monitoring pressure in the uterus
   g Brain—intracranial pressure
3 Mechanical waves
   a Ears—sound waves
   b Heart—heart sounds

4 Temperature
  a  Surface
  b  Core
  c  Ear
5 Gases
  a  Lungs—oxygen, carbon dioxide, nitrogen, and carbon monoxide
  b  Blood—arterial and venous concentrations of oxygen, carbon dioxide, and carbon monoxide

## COMPONENTS OF THE ORGANISM-INSTRUMENT SYSTEM

### Subject

Components of the organism-instrument system are detailed in Figure 11.1. The majority of nursing studies deal with human subjects who have specific demographic and clinical characteristics from which the researcher makes a selection. A demographic profile might portray female subjects ages 50–70 years who have congestive heart failure with no history of pulmonary or renal disease.

Some research questions regarding human subjects frequently cannot be pursued because of potential risks and must be examined first in animal models. In choosing an animal model, the researcher must consider the similarity of responses in the animal to those of humans so that the findings will be applicable.

### Stimulus

Once the parameters for the subjects (human or animal) have been selected, the experimental stimulus is identified so that the physiological response under investigation can be elicited and measured. Various stimuli, such as electric shock (to elicit an electromyogram EMG); auditory (intensive care noise or environmental noise in decibels), tactile (touching skin), visual (trauma scene or a flashing light), or mechanical stimuli (rocking motion); or a nursing care procedure (turning, range of motion, or endotracheal suctioning) can cause changes in heart rate, blood pressure, and intracranial pressure. In these examples, the stimulus elicits a response in the dependent physiological variables (in this case, heart rate,

Stimulus   Subject   Sensing   Signal   Display   Recording &
                     Equipment   Conditioning   Equipment   Data
                                 Equipment         Processing
                                                   Equipment

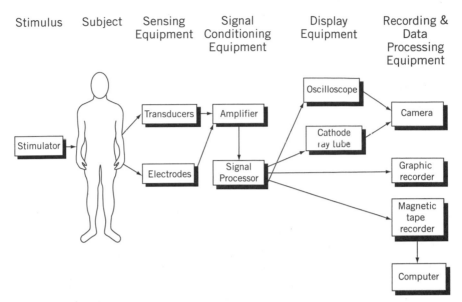

**Figure 11.1** Schema of the organism-instrument system.
From *Nursing Research: Principles & Methods* (3rd ed.), by D. F. Polit, & B. P. Hungler, 1987, p. 292. Philadelphia: Lippincott.

blood pressure, and intracranial pressure), which is then measured with biomedical instrumentation. In the experimental study, the stimulus can be altered by changing its duration, intensity, or frequency. For example, the effect of noise lasting for 5, 10, or 15 minutes (duration) can be measured at 20 and 50 decibels (intensity) every 30 minutes (frequency).

## Sensing Equipment

### Transducers

A transducer may be required to sense the change in a dependent physiological variable. This device converts one form of energy into another, measures physiological phenomena (e.g., pressure, temperature, or gases), and, at the same time, produces an electrical signal in volts proportional to the phenomenon. This conversion is required because a biomedical instrument is an electronic device and responds only to changes in electrical output.

There are many different transducers. For instance, a pressure transducer records displacement. It is placed outside the subject's body and connected to the subject by a needle or catheter inserted into the arterial or venous blood vessel. Pressurized tubing filled with fluid completes the attachment to the transducer. The tubing is connected to a fluid-filled dome that covers the surface of the sensing diaphragm on the pressure transducer. As the pressure within the blood vessel varies with pulsatile blood flow, the sensing diaphragm is displaced alternately inward and outward. The sensing diaphragm is connected by a wire to a bonded or semiconductor strain gauge.

When the wire on the strain gauge is stretched, the electrical resistance increases; conversely, when the wire is allowed to contract, the resistance decreases. As the pressure fluctuates in the blood vessel, the pressure change is transmitted to the sensing diaphragm, which bows inward and outward, changing the resistance in the wire. According to Ohm's Law, which states that the Voltage = Current x Resistance, as the resistance in the wire increases and decreases and the current remains constant, the voltage varies proportionally. Through this method, the pressure, or displacement transducer, converts pressure changes into voltage, which then can be measured by a biomedical instrument.

Temperature can be measured with a resistance thermometer or thermistor. A thermistor is a wire whose resistance increases and decreases as temperature increases and decreases. With a thermistor, changes in temperature can be converted to voltage according to Ohm's Law and measured with a biomedical instrument. A thermistor can measure skin surface, rectal temperature, and core body temperature. The small, thin, exposed wire in the tip of a Swan-Ganz catheter is an example of a thermistor.

The principles for measuring pressure and temperature can be applied to measuring the concentration of arterial blood gases. An arterial blood gas machine contains electrodes for oxygen, carbon dioxide, and pH; these electrodes are biochemical transducers that convert the concentration of gas pressure and the concentration of hydrogen ions to an electrical signal, both of which are detectable using biomedical instruments.

When using a transducer, one must address a number of issues to ensure the accuracy and reliability of the measurement. Blood pressures are measured against a specific reference plane, which is normally the right atrium of the heart. The right atrium is fixed at a point along the midaxillary line at the fourth intercostal space. This point is marked on the subject's body. The subject must be in a supine position when the reference site is determined. Then, with a level, the pressure transducer's balancing port is positioned so that it is perfectly horizontal to the subject's right atrium (Figure 11.2).

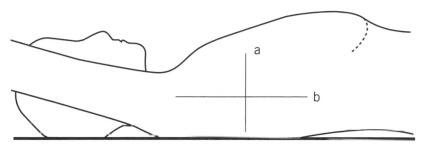

**Figure 11.2** The reference plane.
Determination of the supine measuring point by use of the phlebostatic axis. Line *a* represents the fourth intercostal space and line *b* is the midaxillary line. From "The Effects of Lateral Body Positioning on Measurements of Pulmonary Artery and Pulmonary Artery Wedge Pressure," by G. T. Kennedy, A. Bryant, & M. H. Crawford, 1984, *Heart & Lung, 13,* 157.

Leveling is important because, for each inch (2.5 cm) of difference between the balancing port and the right atrium, the blood pressure varies 2 mm Hg. If the subject's position is changed, then the position of the transducer must be releveled. The pressure transducer must then be balanced and zeroed by opening the balancing port and exposing the sensing diaphragm to atmospheric pressure. This procedure sets the strain gauge at zero voltage with respect to atmospheric pressure. Figure 11.3 illustrates this method by examining the strain gauge more closely.

To obtain the degree of sensitivity required to measure blood pressure, four strain gauges are mounted to the sensing diaphragm, and these resistances (R) are connected to form a Wheatstone bridge circuit. The gauges are attached so that as the pressure increases, two gauges stretch and two contract; the sensitivity of the transducer is then increased by fourfold. When the balancing port is exposed to atmospheric pressure, the strain gauges are balanced (equal) and the voltage output is set at zero. When the pressurized tubing from the arterial catheter is connected to the pressure transducer, the actual pressure changes occurring in the blood vessel cause the sensing diaphragm to move inward and outward, thereby changing the resistance in the wires and the voltage output. The transducer must then be calibrated against a column of mercury (Hg) or water ($H_2O$). Known values of pressure in increments of 50 to 250 mm Hg or 5 to 25 cm $H_2O$ are applied to the transducer to determine whether the output is linear and to verify that the changes in pressure in the blood vessel are proportional to the voltage output. To ensure the accuracy and reliability of the research data, the transducer should be calibrated before, during, and after data collection.

The same principles of balancing, zeroing, and calibrating apply to temperature and biochemical transducers. For example, to be zeroed,

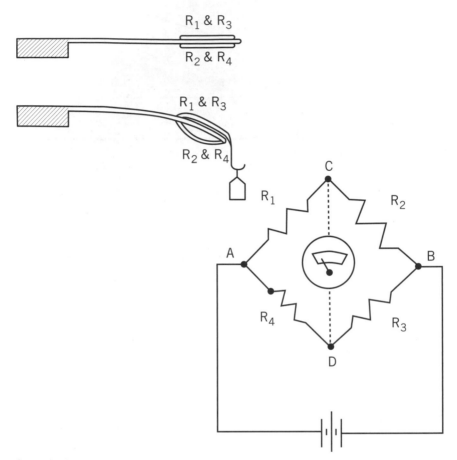

**Figure 11.3** The strain gauge transducer.

the oxygen electrode of a blood gas analyzer is exposed to a solution with no oxygen and is then calibrated against a solution of known oxygen concentration. The calibration is repeated every 30 minutes to ensure the accuracy and reliability of the data.

## RECORDING ELECTRODES

Recording electrodes used to monitor physiological variables are generally surface-type electrodes that obtain bioelectrical potentials from body surfaces. Floating silver-silver chloride (Ag/AgCl) electrodes are placed

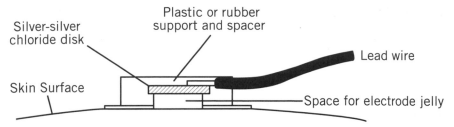

**Figure 11.4** The floating electrode.
Diagram of floating type skin surface electrode. From *Biomedical Instrumentation and Measurements* (2nd ed., p. 72), by L. Cromwell, F. J. Weibell, & E. A. Pfieffer, 1980. Englewood Cliffs, NJ: Prentice-Hall.

on the skin surface to record electrical potentials. The floating electrode is used to reduce movement artifact by eliminating direct contact between the metal in the recording electrode and the skin (Figure 11.4).

Skin contact is maintained through an electrolyte bridge of electrolyte jelly or cream applied directly to the skin surface. Electrolyte material reduces impedance of skin contact through surface oils and the outer horny layer of the skin. Needle electrodes are often used in animals but are used less frequently in humans.

## Signal Conditioning Equipment

Output signals from the transducer or the electrodes usually occur in millivolts and must be amplified. Signals are amplified from millivolts to volts to drive the display unit, which can be an oscilloscope, a computer, or a graphic recorder. Most display units require an input voltage of 5 to 10 volts. Amplification of the signal often is referred to as "increasing the gain." Once the signal has been amplified, the frequency of the signal in cycles per second is modified to eliminate noise or artifact. An example of artifact is the muscle movement seen on an electrocardiogram; another example is 60-cycle (Hz) noise from environmental electrical interference. Electronic filters control noise or artifact by rejecting the unwanted signals. Artifact can be separated, diluted, or omitted by adjusting the sensitivity control on the biomedical instrument.

## Display Equipment

After a physiological signal has been amplified or modified by signal-conditioning equipment, display equipment converts the electrical signals into visual or auditory output that our human senses can detect.

## CATHODE RAY OSCILLOSCOPE AND COMPUTERS

A cathode ray oscilloscope (CRO) displays physiological waveforms on a phosphor screen. An oscilloscope is actually a voltmeter with a rapid response time. A beam of electrons produced by an electron gun has little inertia and is, therefore, capable of rapid motion. Horizontal and vertical plates dictate whether the beam on the screen appears in the vertical or horizontal plane. A CRO is frequently used in a laboratory setting for recording data.

Different output voltages from transducers or electrodes cause the beam of electrons to be displaced proportionally. An oscilloscope can be used to display a graph of voltage against time. In the clinical setting, cathode ray oscilloscopes have been replaced by computers and computer screens that display the voltage against time changes of multiple electrical recording devices. The recording of heart rate, electrocardiogram (ECG), blood pressure, respiratory rate, airway pressure, oxygen saturation, and so on are all displayed simultaneously on the computer screen, enabling clinicians to evaluate physiological changes in their patients. These data are automatically stored and can be retrieved to compare changes in physiological parameters for different intervals of time. It is important to realize that the data recorded are only as good as the care taken to attach the electrodes in the proper location to measure ECG or to zero, balance, and calibrate the transducer to measure blood pressure. Computers with specialized software (Labview National Instruments) can be used to acquire, store, and analyze data. It is important to consider the rate at which the data are acquired to ensure that the exact values of the physiological data are captured. In addition, the software system should be evaluated to determine the ease in transferring the data to a spreadsheet format for further analysis and graphing.

## GRAPHIC RECORDERS

A permanent recording can be made by using a graphic recorder, of which there are several types. The two basic graphic recorders are the curvilinear and the rectilinear.

A curvilinear recorder has a display system in which pens move in an arc and produce a display on curvilinear paper. These recorders are relatively inexpensive and are useful for graphic data display. The curvilinear recorder is self-limiting. Because of the arc of the pen, it is not possible to obtain an exact value. In the clinical setting, graphic recorders are typically of the curvilinear variety. To determine whether or not a recorder is curvilinear, move the recording pen up and down and observe if the pen sweeps in an arc.

A rectilinear recorder has a display system in which the pens move in a linear mode and produces a display that can be used to determine an exact value. These recorders are considerably more expensive than curvilinear models but are more versatile for the collection of research data.

In addition to the instrument, the method of producing the graph should be considered. Typically, recording pens use ink to produce graphs on the surface of the recording paper. Thermal array recorders use a heat stylus pen and heat-sensitive paper. Unfortunately, a thermal graph fades with time.

## CHARACTERISTICS OF BIOMEDICAL INSTRUMENTATION

There are many issues to address in deciding whether to use clinical biomedical instrumentation or research biomedical instrumentation for data collection. These same criteria are helpful in critiquing a study for usefulness in practice. These considerations include the following:

1   *Range* of an instrument, which is the complete set of values that an instrument can measure (e.g., 0–100 grams for a scale, 1–250 beats per minute [bpm] for a cardiac monitor, 0–60 degrees centigrade for a thermometer). It is critical that the instruments chosen to record research data have the capability to measure phenomena in the ranges needed. The range of an instrument can be determined from the instrument specifications at the back of the equipment manual. Generally, the manual also provides information about the reliability of the instrument with the range specified.

2   The *frequency response* of an instrument, which indicates the capability of the instrument to respond equally well to rapid and to slow components of signals. For example, measuring the action potential of a neuron requires equipment with fast response time, because the total time for an action potential occurs in milliseconds. As a result, to record this type of physiological phenomenon, a CRO or computer is required. A graphic recorder

cannot be used to measure a neural action potential because the frequency response is too slow. The inertia of the pen as it moves across the graph paper results in a slow response time.

3   *Sensitivity* of an instrument, which is the degree of change in the physiological variable that the instrument can detect. For example, one instrument might weigh material within one tenth of a gram (0.1 gram), whereas another instrument might weigh the same material within one hundredth of a gram (0.01 gram). Obviously, the equipment that weighs the material within one hundredth of a gram is more sensitive.

4   *Stability* of an instrument, which is its ability to maintain a calibration over a given time interval. Over time, biomedical instruments frequently suffer gradual loss of calibration, called *drift*. It is important that a biomedical instrument maintain calibration because the reliability of the data is dependent on an accurate measure. The instruction manual normally specifies the stability of the instrument over time. The manual also indicates how often the manufacturer recommends recalibration. Because loss of calibration, or drift, is common among biomedical instruments, it is important to evaluate the calibration before, during, and after an experiment to ensure the reliability of the data collected.

5   *Linearity* of the instrument, which is the extent to which an input change is directly proportional to an output change. For instance, for every one degree of actual change in a subject's temperature, there is a one-degree change recorded by the thermometer.

6   *Signal-to-noise ratio* of an instrument, which indicates the relationship between the amount of signal strength and the amount of noise or artifact. The higher the signal-to-noise ratio, the fewer the artifacts.

## CHARACTERISTICS OF THE MEASUREMENTS OBTAINED BY USING BIOMEDICAL INSTRUMENTS

Different conditions call for different biomedical instrumentation. Not every piece of equipment functions equally well for all circumstances. No matter what the condition, however, there are basic characteristics that should be considered for every biomedical instrument. These features include the following:

1  *Validity*—the extent to which the biomedical instrument measures the actual parameter of interest (e.g., the validity of an arterial blood pressure measurement can be determined by the typical characteristics of the arterial pressure wave that validates the correct placement of the arterial catheter);
2  *Accuracy*—the degree to which the parameter sensed by the instrument reflects the actual value;
3  *Precision*—the discriminatory power of the instrument (i.e., the smaller the change sensed, the greater the precision of the instrument);
4  *Reliability*—the accuracy of the measurement over time.

## USING BIOMEDICAL INSTRUMENTATION FOR RESEARCH PURPOSES

A number of clinical biomedical instruments are used to evaluate patient status. An increasing number of studies use physiologic values from these instruments as research data. Several considerations require examination prior to use of these data for research. The use of bedside pulse oximetry as a data collection instrument is evaluated as an illustrative example considering the characteristics of biomedical instrumentation.

## Oxygen Saturation

Oxygen is transported to tissues either combined with hemoglobin or dissolved in plasma. Arterial blood gas evaluation of oxygen status ($PaO_2$) provides a measure of the partial pressure of oxygen dissolved in plasma; however, the $PaO_2$ represents only about 2% of the total oxygen transported. The primary means for oxygen transport is the binding of oxygen molecules with hemoglobin molecules to form saturated hemoglobin or oxyhemoglobin ($HbO_2$). Clinically, oxygen saturation can be measured by obtaining an invasive arterial blood gas sample and determined in vitro using a co-oximeter. An alternative noninvasive measure of oxygen saturation can be determined by pulse oximetry ($SpO_2$). A clear understanding of the instrumentation and technique of measurement is vital to ensure that the data obtained with a pulse oximeter are valid, accurate, reliable, and precise.

## Measurement of Oxygen Saturation

Measurement of hemoglobin saturation by pulse oximetry integrates elements of optical plethysmography with spectrophotometry. Optical plethysmography generates waveforms from pulsatile blood as the blood moves past sophisticated light-absorbance instrumentation. The presence of pulsatile blood differentiates the arterial bed from the venous to ensure that the saturation measurement is arterial in origin. Concurrently, spectrophotometry yields quantitative calculations of hemoglobin saturation based on the absorption of multiple wavelengths of light by the hemoglobin molecules. In a pulse oximeter, two light-emitting diodes (LEDs) expose the hemoglobin molecules to two wavelengths of light: a red light (~660 nm) and an infrared light (~920 nm). The oxygen binding status of hemoglobin molecules determines the absorption of the different wavelengths of light by the hemoglobin molecules. Hemoglobin can be saturated with oxygen ($HbO_2$), reduced or deoxygenated, bound to carbon monoxide called carboxyhemoglobin (HbCO), or oxidized with iron atoms called methemoglobin (Hbmet). A photodetector placed in opposition to the LEDs measures the degree of absorption of the red and infrared light by the hemoglobin molecule. Saturated hemoglobin absorbs a greater degree of infrared light, while desaturated hemoglobin absorbs a greater degree of red light. The calculation of hemoglobin saturation by the pulse oximeter is based on the relative amounts of red and infrared light transmitted through the pulsatile blood to the photodetector.

Measurement of hemoglobin saturation may be either a fractional or a functional measurement. A fractional measurement of hemoglobin saturation is performed by a co-oximeter and is obtained by analysis of an arterial blood sample. The co-oximeter uses four or more wavelengths of light. The fractional oxygen saturation is the ratio of oxygen saturated hemoglobin or oxyhemoglobin ($HbO_2$) to the *total* number of hemoglobin molecules. The total hemoglobin includes oxyhemoglobin, hemoglobin available for binding with oxygen, or desaturated hemoglobin and hemoglobin that is not capable of binding with oxygen (carboxyhemoglobin, methemoglobin). The status of total hemoglobin is evaluated with a fractional measurement.

A pulse oximeter provides a functional measurement of hemoglobin saturation. A functional measurement is the ratio of oxygen saturated hemoglobin to the total amount of hemoglobin *available for binding* to oxygen. This type of measurement does not include evaluation of hemoglobin that is not available for binding with oxygen (carboxyhemoglobin, methemoglobin). For comparison purposes, a fractional saturation value can be converted to a functional value using the following equation:

$$SaO_2\ functional = \frac{SaO_2\ fractional \times 100}{100 - (\%HbCO + \%Hbmet)}$$

## Validity of Oxygen Saturation Measurement by Pulse Oximetry

The measurement of oxygen saturation by a co-oximeter using four or more wavelengths of light is the gold standard. A number of studies have compared the values obtained by pulse oximetry with simultaneous measurement of oxygen saturation by co-oximeter. In the range of 70 to 100% oxygen saturation, there is a strong correlation between these values (range of correlation coefficients $r = 0.92$ to $0.98$). Within this range of values, pulse oximetry has been demonstrated to accurately reflect *functional* hemoglobin saturation. However, when oxygen saturation values are less than 70%, pulse oximetry may provide a falsely high value because of the calculation algorithm used in this biomedical instrument. $SpO_2$ may be a clinically useful indicator of oxygen transport; however, both the clinician and the researcher must remember that the use of a functional measurement of oxygen saturation does not reflect tissue oxygen delivery. A high oxygen saturation ($SpO_2$) value determined by pulse oximetry does not necessarily indicate adequate tissue oxygen delivery. Shifts in the oxyhemoglobin dissociation curve caused by hypothermia, alkalosis, or a decrease in 2,3 DPG can significantly alter tissue oxygen delivery even though the functional oxygen saturation value appears normal.

## Accuracy of Pulse Oximetry

Certain clinical and technical phenomena may reduce the accuracy of saturation values obtained by pulse oximetry (Table 11.1). Weak arterial pulsation produced by shock states, hypothermia with shunting of blood

Table 11.1

### FACTORS THAT ALTER ACCURACY OF PULSE OXIMETRY MEASURES

**Individual Factors**
Inadequate pulsatile arterial blood flow (hypotension, hypothermia, increased systemic vascular resistance)
Venous pulsatile flow
Dysfunctional hemoglobin (carboxyhemoglobin, methemoglobin)
Anemia
Presence of systemic dyes
Hyperlipidemia

**Technical Factors**
Motion artifact
Ambient light interference
Optical shunt
Optical cross talk
Electrical interference

flow from the periphery, and/or increased systemic vascular resistance may result in little to absent light absorption detection by the sensor. The oximeter is not capable of calculating a saturation value if pulsatile flow cannot be detected. Venous pulsation as a result of right ventricular failure or a partial obstruction to venous outflow also reduces the accuracy of $SpO_2$ values. In the presence of both arterial and venous pulsatile flow, the $SpO_2$ value may be a composite value derived from light absorbance from both arterial and venous hemoglobin. In this instance, the $SpO_2$ value provided will be lower than actual arterial saturation.

Abnormalities in the blood may produce inaccurate values of oxygen saturation. Anemia may reduce the accuracy of pulse oximetry values, particularly as saturation values decrease. The cause for this inaccuracy is not well understood but may be secondary to the scattering of light in the plasma with a shift in the degree of red light absorbed. In addition, the presence of a significant portion of hemoglobin that is unavailable for oxygen binding, like carboxyhemoglobin and methemoglobin, also reduces the accuracy of pulse oximetry measurements. For example, at a carbon monoxide partial pressure of only 0.1 mmHg, hemoglobin is 50% saturated with carbon monoxide. The functional measurement of saturation by the pulse oximeter may indicate very high oxygen saturation, since the remaining 50% of hemoglobin may be fully saturated with oxygen. This saturation value is further misleading, since the presence of high levels of carboxyhemoglobin increases the affinity of hemoglobin for oxygen and reduces oxygen unloading at the tissues.

Concentrations of certain substances in the arterial blood have been suggested to influence the accuracy of pulse oximetry. The effect of high levels of bilirubin on the accuracy of pulse oximetry is described inconsistently in the research literature. The majority of studies that compare $SaO_2$ with $SpO_2$ in the presence of hyperbilirubinemia (bilirubin up to 46.3 mg/dL) suggest that high bilirubin levels do not interfere with the accuracy of $SpO_2$ when saturation is $> 90\%$. Use of systemic dyes has also been demonstrated to affect the accuracy of pulse oximetry measurement. Indigo carmine, indocyanine green, and methylene blue absorb light at wavelengths similar to those used by the pulse oximeter (660 nm) and alter the accuracy of $SpO_2$ values. Elevated lipid levels either from endogenous lipids or administration of exogenous lipid solutions, in conjunction with total parenteral nutrition, may produce an artificially lower $SpO_2$ value.

In addition to clinical factors, technical factors may also reduce the accuracy of pulse oximetry values. Motion artifact may be interpreted by the photodetector as arterial pulsation. High-intensity, high-quantity ambient light like that found with heat lamps, surgical lights, and fluorescent lights may reduce the accuracy of $SpO_2$ values. The ambient light may be detected by the pulse oximetry photodetector. In this instance, the photodetector receives information from both the LEDs and the ambient light source. The $SpO_2$ value is then a composite value and is likely inaccurate. An optical shunt may occur when some of the light from the LEDs is transmitted to the photodetector without passing through a pulsatile vascular bed. The degree of red and infrared light received by the photodetector is again a composite of light exposed to hemoglobin and light not exposed to pulsatile blood; thus, the $SpO_2$ value is inaccurate. Optical cross-talk may occur when the pulse oximetry sensor is placed in proximity to another instrument also using red and/or infrared light. In this instance, the light emitted by the secondary instrument may be received by the pulse oximetry photodetector. The $SpO_2$ will again be a composite value that will be inaccurate. Excessive signal noise (electrical interference) may be received and interfere with signal acquisition. Signal processing may be disrupted by significant electrical interference, with resultant delayed values that may be inaccurate.

Bias is a statistical indicator of the accuracy of a measurement and is determined by calculating the mean difference between $SaO_2$ and $SpO_2$.

The greater the bias, the less accurate the measurement technique. Bias for pulse oximetry values is reported to vary depending on the degree of hypoxemia, so, as oxygen saturation decreases, bias increases. Bias for pulse oximetry measures is reported to range from less than 0.5% to as much as 10%.

Pulse oximetry values in general are reported to have a margin of error +/- 2% of the actual $SaO_2$ value. This degree of error provides a wide range of potential values if $SpO_2$ values are normally distributed. The investigator must determine whether measures with this degree of potential error provide sufficiently accurate data to address the research objectives.

## Precision of Oxygen Saturation by Pulse Oximetry

Pulse oximetry can detect a 1% change in oxygen saturation. However, the speed of response by the pulse oximeter is reported to diminish as actual $SaO_2$ values decrease. A statistical measure of the reproducibility of pulse oximetry measures is the precision. This value is obtained by calculating the standard deviation of the bias measurement and sources of error within the individual. The precision measure is analogous to the scatter of data points. Precision measures for pulse oximetry are reported to be 2% to 4% (see Table 11.2).

Table 11.2

### RANGE OF PULSE OXIMETRY VALUES IN A NORMAL DISTRIBUTION

|  | RANGE OF VALUES | RANGE IF SAO$_2$ IS 95% | RANGE IF SAO$_2$ IS 90% |
|---|---|---|---|
| Within 1 standard deviation of the mean (68% of population) | + 2% | 93% to 97% | 88% to 92% |
| Within 2 standard deviations of the mean (95% of population) | + 4% | 91% to 99% | 86% to 94% |
| Within 3 standard deviations of the mean (99.7% of population | + 6% | 89% to 100% | 84% to 96% |

## Reliability of Oxygen Saturation by Pulse Oximetry

Pulse oximetry measures are described as generally consistent over time. A majority of studies that evaluate reliability of pulse oximetry perform these studies with relationship to consistency of measurement over time using different probe types (reusable or disposable, finger, ear, and nose). The development of motion artifact appears to be the primary influence on the reliability of pulse oximetry measures. However, the development of other threats to accuracy also influences the reliability of this type of measurement.

## Guidelines to Increase the Utility of Pulse Oximetry for Research Purposes

If $SpO_2$ values are to be used as research data, the investigator must ensure these data are valid, accurate, precise, and reliable. The following guidelines improve the likelihood these data will be useful. However, the investigator must determine whether $SpO_2$ will actually provide them with the information required to answer the research questions or test research hypotheses.

- Select a pulse oximeter with indicators of signal strength and pulse waveform to ensure that adequate, appropriate signal quality is available.
- Ensure that probe type and probe position are optimal to detect arterial pulsation without technical interference from ambient light, optical shunt, or cross-talk.
- Assess the correlation between the apical heart rate and the heart rate detected by the pulse oximeter. These values must be closely correlated.
- Evaluate the individual for the presence of dysfunctional hemoglobin, hyperlipidemia, and anemia prior to data collection to ensure that these factors are not influencing $SpO_2$.
- Stabilize the probe so that motion artifact is not a significant confounding factor.
- Analyze the relationship between $SpO_2$ and $SaO_2$ regularly. These values should be highly correlated with minimal bias. Calculate the bias and precision to evaluate the accuracy and repeatability of the data.

## Measurement of Nucleic Acids in Genetic Research

Genetic testing is defined as the analysis of human DNA, RNA, chromosomes, proteins, and certain metabolites in order to detect heritable diseases. Molecular genetic testing has increased exponentially, and nurses will be increasingly involved in working collaboratively with physicians and with patients and family members. The human genome contains large amounts of deoxyribonucleic acid (DNA) that contain the code for controlling all aspects of embryogenesis, development, growth, metabolism, and reproduction. There are about 50,000 genes encoded in the DNA that make up the chromosomes in the nucleus of the cell. The double-stranded DNA serves as the code or the template for the production (transcription) of the single-stranded messenger RNA or ribonucleic acid. Messenger RNA contains the instructions for the production of proteins (translation) in the cell cytoplasm at the ribosomes of the endoplasmic reticulum. Advances in the understanding of molecular genetics have facilitated the development of revolutionary new technologies that have permitted the analysis of normal and abnormal genes and the detection and diagnosis of genetic diseases.

Molecular geneticists had to overcome two fundamental obstacles in order to study the molecular basis of hereditary disease. The first challenge was to produce a sufficient quantity of either DNA or RNA to permit analysis. Hence, molecular cloning techniques were developed. The second challenge was to purify the sequence of interest from all other segments of DNA or RNA. Polymerase chain reaction (PCR) can selectively amplify a single molecule of DNA or RNA several billionfold in a few hours. PCR is only one technique among many used in genetic research.

### *Polymerase Chain Reaction*

The polymerase chain reaction (PCR) can selectively amplify a single molecule of DNA or RNA in a few hours. PCR is an enzymatic amplification of a fragment of DNA. PCR can also be applied to the analysis of small samples of RNA in a procedure called reverse transcriptase PCR. PCR is an extremely sensitive technique. It allows for the detection and analysis of specific gene sequences. Analysis can be performed from a single cell from a hair root, from sperm obtained from a vaginal sample from a rape victim, or from a drop of dried blood found at a crime scene.

Understanding genetic testing techniques and the consequences of genetic testing will become increasingly important as nurses participate in genetic testing, counseling, and clinical trials involving genetic modification to treat and cure genetic diseases. Nurses will become increasingly challenged to evaluate genetic research studies to determine their applicability to clinic practice and to guide evidenced based practice.

## SUMMARY

When evaluating and critiquing the appropriateness of research studies to implement evidence-based practice in the clinical setting, knowledge of biomedical instrumentation is essential to determine the validity, accuracy, and reliability of the physiological data acquired. Examples of instruments used to measure physiological variables and the characteristics of these instruments and their measurements have been presented in this chapter.

## SUGGESTED ACTIVITIES

1   Select a research article in which bioinstrumentation was used to collect physiological data. Review and critique the article. Evaluate whether the data collected using the instrumentation were valid, accurate, and reliable. Determine whether the results of the reviewed study are appropriate to apply to clinical practice.

2   Select a physiological variable, such as carbon dioxide. Search the literature to determine different methods to measure carbon dioxide, including measurement from blood (blood gases in vitro) or tissue carbon dioxide ($TcPCO_2$) or exhaled carbon dioxide ($ETCO_2$). Design a study to measure carbon dioxide in a subject and provide the rationale for the choice on the basis of the method of measurement and human subject concerns (direct against indirect method and in vivo against in vitro method). Compare and contrast the validity, reliability, and accuracy of the methods.

# REFERENCES

Aston, R. (1990). *Principles of biomedical instrumentation and measurement*. Columbus, OH: Merrill.

Avant, M., Lowe, N., & Torres, A. (1997). Comparison of accuracy and signal consistency of two reusable pulse oximeter probes in critically ill children. *Respiratory Care, 42*(7), 698–704.

Batchelder, P. B., & Raley, D. M. (2007). Maximizing the laboratory setting for testing devices and understanding statistical output in pulse oximetry. *Anesthesia & Analgesia, 105*(6), S85–S94.

Bisnaire, D., & Robinson, L. (1999). Accuracy of leveling hemodynamic transducer systems. *Canadian Association of Critical Care Nurses, 10*, 16–19.

Bridges, E. J., Woods, S. L., Brengelmann, G. L., Mitchell, P., & Laurent-Bopp, D. (2000). Effect of the 30° lateral recumbent position on pulmonary artery and pulmonary artery wedge pressures in critically ill adult cardiac surgery patients. *American Journal of Critical Care, 9*, 262–275.

Carr, J., and Brown, J. M. (2001). *Introduction to biomedical equipment technology*. Upper Saddle River, NJ: Prentice-Hall.

Chulay, M., & Miller, T. (1984). The effect of backrest elevation on pulmonary artery and pulmonary capillary wedge pressures in patients after cardiac surgery. *Heart & Lung, 13*, 138–140.

Chyun, D. A. (1985). A comparison of intra-arterial and ausculatory blood pressure readings. *Heart & Lung, 14*, 223–228.

Cromwell, L., Weibell, F. J., & Pfieffer, E. A. (1980). *Biomedical instrumentation and measurements* (2nd ed., p. 72). Englewood Cliffs, NJ: Prentice-Hall.

Darovic, G. O. (2002). *Hemodynamic monitoring. Invasive and noninvasive clinical application* (3rd ed.) Saunders.

Frazier, S. K., & Skinner, G. J. (2008). Pulmonary artery catheters: State of the controversy. *Journal of Cardiovascular Nursing, 23*(2), 113–121.

Gift, A. G., & Socken, K. L. (1988). Assessment of physiologic instruments. *Heart & Lung, 17*, 128–133.

Glor, B. A. K., Sullivan, E. F., & Estes, Z. E. (1970). Reproducibility of blood pressure measurements: A replication. *Nursing Research, 19*, 170–172.

Gunn, I. P., Sullivan, E. F., & Glor, B. A. K. (1966). Blood pressure measurement as a quantitative research criterion. *Nursing Research, 15*, 4–11.

Hannhart, B., Haberer, J., Saunier, C., & Laxenaire, M. (1991). Accuracy and precision of fourteen pulse oximeters. *European Respiratory Journal, 4*, 115–119.

Kennedy, G. T., Bryant, A., & Crawford, M. H. (1984). The effects of lateral body positioning on measurements of pulmonary artery and pulmonary artery wedge pressures. *Heart & Lung, 13*, 157.

Kirchhoff, K. T., Rebenson-Piano, M., & Patel, M. K. (1984). Mean arterial pressure readings: Variations with positions and transducer level. *Nursing Research, 33*, 343–345.

Levine, S. C. (1985). A review of the use of computerized digital instrumentation to determine pulmonary artery pressure measurements in critically ill patients. *Heart & Lung, 14*, 473–477.

Matthay, R. A., Wiedemann, H. P., & Matthay, M. A. (1985). Cardiovascular function in the intensive care unit: Invasive and noninvasive monitoring. *Respiratory Care, 30*, 432–455.

McPherson, E. (2006). Genetic diagnosis and testing in clinical practice. *Clinical Medicine & Research, 4*(12), 123–129.

Mengelkoch, L., Martin, D., & Lawler, J. (1994). A review of the principles of pulse oximetry and accuracy of pulse oximeter estimates during exercise. *Physical Therapy, 74*(1), 40–49.

Moser, D. K., Frazier, S. K., Woo, M. A., & Daley, L. K. (2002). Normal fluctuations in pulmonary artery pressures and cardiac output in patients with severe left ventricular dysfunction. *European Journal of Cardiovascular Nursing, 1*, 131–138.

Nagurney, L. S. (2007). *The evolution of a bioinstrumentation course.* Paper presented at the 37th ASEE/IEEE Frontiers in Education Proceedings F1C.

Nemens, E. J., & Woods, S. L. (1982). Normal fluctuations in pulmonary artery and pulmonary capillary wedge pressures in acutely ill patients. *Heart & Lung, 11*, 393–398.

Newton, K. M. (1981). Comparison of aortic and brachial cuff pressures in flat supine and lateral recumbent positions. *Heart & Lung, 10*, 821–826.

Nussbaun, R. L., McInnes, R. R., & Willard, H. F. (2007). *Tools of human molecular genetics.* In *Thompson and Thompson Genetics in Medicine* (7th ed.). Philadelphia: W. B. Saunders.

Perkins, G. D., McAuley, D. F., Giles, S., Routledge, H., & Gao, F. (2003). Do changes in pulse oximeter oxygen saturation predict equivalent changes in arterial oxygen saturation? *Critical Care, 7*(4), R67.

Polit, D. F., & Hungler, B.P. (1987). *Nursing research: Principles and methods* (3rd ed.). Philadelphia: Lippincott.

Rice, W. P., Fernandez, E. G., Jarog, D., & Jensen, A. (2000). A comparison of hydrostatic leveling methods in invasive pressure monitoring. *Critical Care Nurse, 20*, 20–30.

Schnapp, L. M., & Cohen, N. H. (1990). Pulse oximetry. Uses and abuses. *Chest, 98*, 1244–1250.

Stone, K. S., & Frazier, S. K. (in press). Measurement of physiological variables using biomedical instrumentation (2nd ed.). In C. F. Waltz, O. L. Strickland, & E. R. Lenz (Eds.), *Measurement in nursing research*. Philadelphia: F.A. Davis.

Tittle, M., & Flynn, M. (1997). Correlation of pulse oximetry and co-oximetry. *Dimensions in Critical Care Nursing, 16*(2), 88–95.

West, R. S. (Ed.). (1981). *Using monitors nursing photobook*. Horhsam, PA: Intermed Communications.

Woods, S. L., & Mansfield, L. W. (1976). Effect of body position upon pulmonary artery and pulmonary capillary wedge pressures in noncritically ill patients. *Heart & Lung, 5*, 83–90.

# 12 Psychosocial Data Collection Methods

CAROL GLOD

Psychosocial measures are instruments that researchers and advanced practice nurses (APNs) use to measure variables related to psychological, emotional, and related areas in a study. In general, instruments focus on certain topics or content domains such as depression or anxiety. Psychosocial data collection methods are important to guide the use of evidence in nursing practice.

Where do the instruments exist, and how does a researcher or APN locate them? One place to start is with other established researchers in the field. Another source is relevant articles located and reviewed in preparation for the study. An examination of the methods and instruments section of earlier studies often gives a detailed account of which measures were used and some of their key characteristics. Since most published manuscripts do not include the actual scales, the reference list should contain a citation for the original instrument. Permission to use a new or original scale may have to be requested from the author(s). Finally, libraries and Internet sources contain compilations of standardized instruments that can be obtained by searching for key words that reflect the concept under study. There are also books that include primarily tools for measuring concepts (Frank-Stromborg & Olsen, 2004). Some instruments are copyrighted and can be purchased for a fee. The fee may be a one-time purchase fee or a per-copy or per-use fee. In order to purchase some instruments, one may have to have certain credentials, such as a Ph.D. A variety of well-established scales of different types exist to measure concepts such as depression and anxiety and to answer different research questions. These concepts may be measured using interviews, whether structured or semistructured, or questionnaires that are administered by the researcher and/or completed by the participant. Other methods, such as observation and checklists, may be used along with standardized tests to collect data on behaviors in order to validate observations. For example, a study that examines the sleep of medically ill patients may include nursing observations and an established patient self-report scale.

## SELECTION OF INSTRUMENTS

The selection of a measurement tool for psychosocial variables depends upon the research question, variables of interest, age of participant, and other factors. A general rule is that the research question dictates the broader method to be used, whether a qualitative, quantitative, or mixed method. Having a research question and key variables that are well defined helps to direct the selection of a method. Before considering various established instruments, the researcher should think about several important questions, including the study purpose, characteristics of the sample, the concept or content to be measured, and practical considerations. In order for the measure to be suitable, it should have established *reliability* and *validity* (see Exhibit 12.1).

## INSTRUMENT DEVELOPMENT

Occasionally, an investigator who is interested in a certain concept or area of study may find that there are no available scales or instruments that reflect that specific research problem. Creating new scales or questionnaires can be tempting; however, their development requires a deliberate and systematic approach. Beginning researchers may think it is a simple process to create a new scale for psychosocial variables; however, there are several steps involved. An initial step often is to bring together a group of experts in the field; these may be patients who experience a certain diagnosis or response to a problem or experienced nurses who know the topic well and can serve as content experts. For example, a

Exhibit 12.1

### FACTORS TO CONSIDER WHEN SELECTING AN INSTRUMENT

Does the instrument measure the concept being examined?
What are the psychometric properties of the instrument?
   Reliability
   Stability
   Equivalence
   Homogeneity
   Validity
   Content validity
   Criterion-related validity
   Construct validity
Is the instrument feasible?
   Instrument availability
   Costs of data-collection tools
   Nature of the study sample

From "Psychosocial Measurement," by M. A. Mateo, 1999. In M. A. Mateo & K. T. Kirchhoff (Eds.), *Using and conducting nursing research in the clinical setting* (2nd ed., pp. 256–267). Philadelphia: Saunders.

nurse researcher interested in immigrant mothers' acculturation practices may bring together 6 or 8 representative mothers to generate potential items for a questionnaire during a meeting that lasts from 1 to 2 hours. Next, content experts should review the draft questions, which should also be pretested, revised, and tested for validity and reliability. Overall, the creation of a new instrument requires extensive time and effort but is appropriate when existing measures are unavailable or inadequate for the purpose. It is generally more feasible to use existing scales. Then results can be compared across samples.

## Reliability and Validity

*Reliability* and *validity* are two important and essential concepts that relate to each potential instrument that the investigator is considering. They have specific definitions in research and can be easily confused. *Validity* refers to whether the instrument actually measures what it is supposed to measure. For example, if the nurse is interested in measuring acute stress, the instrument should measure the concept of stress and not related ones, such as anxiety or depression. There are differ-ent types of validity, detailed later in this chapter. *Reliability* refers to whether the tool conveys consistent and reproducible data, for example, from one participant to another or from one point in time to another. Several types of reliability exist, as well. In order for a scale to be valid, it must be reliable.

## Validity

Validity is the degree to which a tool measures what it is supposed to measure (Mateo, 1999). There are three types of validity; content, criterion-related, and construct.

*Content validity* relates to an instrument's adequacy in covering all concepts pertaining to the phenomena being studied. If the purpose of the tool is to learn whether the patient is anxious before taking an exami-nation, the questions should include a list of behaviors that anxious peo-ple report when they are experiencing anxiety. Content experts are vital in the development of valid and reliable tools (Mateo, 1999). Generally, "content experts," colleagues with expertise and experience in the area, are identified. Ways to identify experts include publications in refereed journals, research in the phenomenon of interest, clinical expertise, and familiarity with the dimensions being measured. It is important that an instrument be reviewed for content by persons who possess characteris-tics and experiences similar to those of the participants in a study.

*Criterion-related validity,* which can be either predictive or con-current, measures the extent to which a tool is related to other criteria (Mateo, 1999). Predictive validity is the adequacy of the tool to estimate the individual performance or behavior in the future. For example, if a tool is developed to measure clinical competence of nurses, persons who respond to the tool can be followed over time to see if this score correlates with other measures of competence, such as performance ap-praisals, commendations, or other indications of competence. If results indicate that there is a high coefficient correlation (.90), it means that the clinical competence scale can be used to predict future performance appraisals. Concurrent validity is the ability of a tool to compare the respondent's status at a given time to a criterion (Mateo, 1999). For ex-ample, when a patient is asked to complete a questionnaire to determine the presence of anxiety, results of the test can be compared to the same patient's ratings on an established measure of anxiety administered at the same time.

*Construct validity* is concerned with the ability of the instrument to adequately measure the underlying concept (Mateo, 1999). With this type of validity, the researcher's concern relates to whether the scores represent the degree to which a person possesses a trait. Since construct validity is a judgment based on a number of studies, it takes time to establish this type of validity. These studies compare results in groups that should be similar (convergent validity) or different (divergent validity). Scores on the anxiety tool should be lower among those who are receiving a massage and higher among those taking a final exam.

## Reliability

Reliability is a basic characteristic of an instrument when it is used for collecting accurate, stable, and usable research data (Mateo, 1999). The reliability of a tool is the degree of consistency in scores achieved by subjects across repeated measurements. The comparison is usually reported as a *reliability coefficient*. The reliability coefficient is determined by the proportion of true variability (attributed to true differences among respondents) to the total obtained variability (attributed to the result of true differences among respondents and differences related to other factors). Reliability coefficients normally range between 0 and 1.00; the higher the value, the greater the reliability. In general, coefficients greater than .70 are considered appropriate; however, in some circumstances this will vary. The researcher takes a chance that data across repeated administrations will not be consistent when instruments with reliability estimates of .60 or lower are used (Mateo, 1999).

Three aspects should be considered when determining the reliability of instruments: (1) stability, (2) equivalence, and (3) homogeneity (Burns & Grove, 2005; Mateo, 1999). The *stability* of a tool refers to its ability to consistently measure the phenomenon being studied; this is determined through test-retest reliability. The tool is administered to the same persons on two separate occasions. Scores of the two sets of data are then compared, and the correlation is derived. The recommended interval between testing times is 2 to 4 weeks (Burns & Grove, 2005; Mateo, 1999). The time that must lapse between the two points of measurements is important; it should be long enough so that respondents do not remember their answers on the first test, yet not so long that change in the respondents can take place. Interpretation of the test-retest correlation coefficient should be done with caution, because it might not represent the stability of the instrument; rather, it might indicate that change has occurred in those being assessed. For example, change can occur among nurses being evaluated with regard to their attitudes toward work schedules; for instance, persons who responded to the first test may have since gained seniority and now be working their preferred shifts. In this case, the second test might yield a more positive result, and the correlation coefficient obtained when the two sets of scores are compared would represent a change in the respondents rather than being an accurate measure of the stability of the tool (Mateo, 1999).

*Equivalence* should be determined when two versions of the same tool are used to measure a concept (alternative forms) or when two or more persons are asked to rate the same event or the behavior of another person (interrater reliability; Mateo, 1999). In alternative-form reliability, two versions of the same instrument are developed and administered. The scores obtained from the two tools should be similar. It is helpful for the researcher to know whether a published instrument has alternate forms; when there are, a decision must be made about which form to use. For example, the Beck Depression Inventory has a long and a short form (Beck & Steer, 1993). The researcher might decide to use the short form to test patients with short attention spans or low energy levels. Establishing interrater reliability is important when two or more observers are used for collecting data. Considerations relating to this type of reliability have already been discussed.

The *homogeneity* of an instrument is determined most commonly by calculating a Cronbach's alpha coefficient. This test is found in a number of statistical packages. This test is a way of determining whether each item on an instrument measures the same thing. Internal consistency reliability estimates are also calculated by using the Kuder-Richardson formula, described in measurement textbooks.

When more than one concept is measured in an instrument, the Cronbach's alpha is computed on the subscales, rather than the whole scale. If the scale does not attempt to measure a single concept or has subscales that measure several concepts, this test is not useful.

## TYPES AND CHARACTERISTICS OF INSTRUMENTS

In general, there are several common types of measures or instruments available to measure the selected concept under investigation. Researchers use *semistructured* or *structured* interviews with detailed questions that either guide (semistructured) the interviewer or outline a specific set of questions. The principal investigator or study staff follows the order of questions during an interview with the participant. Another option is *self-report scales* that are given to the research subject to complete; examples include scales such as the Beck Depression Inventory. Self-report instruments differ from clinician- and nurse-rated ones on the basis of who actually completes them.

Other scales may contain *open-ended* or *closed* questions. Open-ended questions allow more exploration and the opportunity for freer responses, without restraint or limitation. For example, in qualitative research, the researcher frequently asks open-ended questions, such as "what is your experience with . . ." or "tell me about. . . ." Open-ended responses allow participants to answer in their own words. Closed-ended questions, while more common, direct respondents to choose an answer from a predetermined list of possible alternatives. As a result, the participants may be pointed in certain directions that may not be appropriate or that lack uniqueness. Many of the scales used in psychosocial research have *ordinal* items, with numbers assigned to different categories that reflect increasing order, such as 0 = none, 1 = slight, 2 = mild, 3 = moderate, 4 = severe.

## Visual Analog Scales

The Visual Analog Scale (VAS) uses a 100-mm line with "anchors" at either end to explore the participant's opinion about a specific concept along a continuum. Respondents place an X on the line to mark where they stand on the continuum. For example, questions on pain prompt the respondents to describe their experience of pain level at the corresponding point on the line, which has anchors of "none" and "very much"; a mark made 80mm from the end of "none" would signify quite severe pain. Convenient and simple, the VAS is an attractive means of rating continuous measurement.

Whether structured, detailed, or open-ended, every scale has advantages as well as limitations. There are several things to consider for psychosocial tools. Many of the instruments result in a certain rating (e.g., a numerical score that indicates a moderate level of depression). These rating scales attempt to measure the underlying concept (depression) efficiently and comprehensively and to attach to it a number that then is interpreted to represent a certain range (a given score indicates a given level of depression). The researcher cannot assume that a certain score or level of score on an established scale indicates the presence of a disorder. For example, the researcher cannot assume that a total score on a depression scale means that the participant actually should be diagnosed with depression. Some people assume, incorrectly, that a scale score that results in a certain degree or severity of symptoms produces a diagnosis. These instruments are in reality only part of an evaluation for a disorder.

There are several general types of instruments that measure psychological symptoms or overall functioning. Each uses either *continuous* or *categorical* responses. Continuous variables or items usually have quantifiable intervals or values, such as weight or blood pressure. In general, categorical items contain forced and mutually exclusive choices, such as *strongly agree, agree, disagree, strongly disagree,* in contrast to continuous items, which literally contain a blended continuum of responses without specific choices. When there are two possible choices or values, such as gender, the categorical variable is termed *dichotomous.* For psychological or psychosocial ratings, the focus is generally on self-report (or parent-report for children) or clinician-rated symptoms. While these scales are most typically used for research purposes, they can also be used in clinical situations to aid in diagnostic evaluation or to help to monitor treatment response or symptoms over time. The instruments focus on particularly symptoms or concepts such as anxiety, depression, suicide, mania, suicide risk, or attention problems. Examples of commonly used instruments, along with their purpose and a general overview of their characteristics, are described.

## Clinical Global Impressions Scale

Clinical Global Impressions (CGI) is a categorical scale used for rating change from baseline over the duration of a clinical trial (Guy, 1976). The CGI consists of three global scales formatted for use with similar scoring. The scales assess global improvement, severity of illness, and efficacy index. Clinical Global Impressions-Improvement (CGI-I) is a clinician-administered scale commonly used in studies of adults and children to assess posttreatment ratings at the discretion of the researcher.

The CGI-I consists of one item ranked 0 to 7 that compares patient condition at admission to the projected patient's condition at a later time (Guy 1976). The seven levels of improvement include 0 = not assessed, 1 = very much improved, 2 = much improved, 3 = minimally improved, 4 = no change, 5 = minimally worse, 6 = much worse, and 7 = very much worse. They are most commonly rated by the clinician and the patient.

Investigators looking for at least moderate improvement on a global generic scale usually expect an improvement score of 50% or more (Bobes,
1998). Previous studies of antidepressants commonly have used the proportion of CGI-I responders, defined as patients assigned a CGI-I score
of 2 or lower by clinicians ("very much" or "much" improved).

## Brief Psychiatric Rating Scale

The Brief Psychiatric Rating Scale (BPRS) is one of the most frequently
used clinician-rated measures. It has existed for more than 40 years
(Overall & Gorham, 1962, 1976). It consists of 18 items rated on a 7-point
severity scale and is used for general overall assessment of broad psychiatric symptoms. The BPRS takes about 20 minutes to complete. Its
scoring results in an overall total score as well as scores on five major factors: anxious depression, thinking disturbance, withdrawal-retardation,
hostile suspiciousness, and tension-excitement. More specific, yet similar scales that measure positive and negative symptoms of major mental
illnesses (such as the Positive and Negative Symptoms Scale [PANSS])
are derived partly from the BPRS and have well-established validity and
reliability. Discriminant validity, a method used to validate a construct
being studied from other similar constructs, of the items and subscales
separated three homogeneous psychiatric diagnoses in patients (Lachar
et al., 2001). The ratings of each individual item were compared for different raters. Using large samples of psychiatric patients in multiple studies, individual BPRS item interrater reliability estimates ranged from .54
to .92 (median = .785), with the majority of values (10 of 18) demonstrating very good agreement (greater than .74; Lachar et al., 2001). Interrater reliability rater agreement was r = .57 for total scores and ranged
from r = .60 to .84 for the factor subscales.

## Child Behavior Checklist

The Child Behavior Checklist (CBCL) is a 118-item standardized measure that rates general behavior for children ages 4–18, drawing on
hundreds of studies of children (Achenbach, 1991). Parents (and/or
guardians) complete questions about children's social competence and
behavioral or emotional problems, reflecting either the child's current
behavior or behaviors that have occurred over the past 6 months. Items
are rated from 0 to 2, with 0 = not true; 1 = somewhat or sometimes
true; 2 = very true or often true. The 20 social competence items reflect

the child's amount and quality of participation in sports, hobbies, games, activities, organizations, jobs and chores, friendships; how well the child gets along with others and plays and works by himself or herself; and school performance (Achenbach, 1991). Two open-ended questions are included, as well.

The CBCL has well-established reliability and construct validity. Intraclass correlations for individual items equals .90 "between item scores obtained from mothers filling out the CBCL at 1-week intervals, mothers and fathers filling out the CBCL on their clinically-referred children, and three different interviewers obtaining CBCLs from parents of demographically matched triads of children" (Achenbach, 1991). Good stability of the scale exists for both behavior problems and social competencies over time, with correlations of .84 and .97, respectively. Test-retest reliability of mothers' ratings is generally .89.

## Hamilton Depression Rating Scale

For depression, there are several commonly used rating scales to measure symptoms and severity of depression. The Hamilton Depression Rating Scale (HDRS) consists of 17 or 21 items (Hamilton, 1961). It is the most widely used continuous measure to determine severity of depressive symptoms in adults and adolescents because of its comprehensive coverage of depressive symptoms. The HDRS is the standard depression outcome measure used in clinical trials presented to the U.S. Food and Drug Administration by pharmaceutical companies seeking approval of new drug applications and is the standard by which all other depression scales are measured. Although other depressive scales exist, including some developed and used for adults, the Hamilton remains the most reliable and valid. The scale takes approximately 30 minutes to complete and score.

The scale contains items defined by anchor point descriptions that increase in intensity. The rater is instructed to begin each query with the first recommended depression symptom question. Raters consider intensity and frequency of symptoms when assigning values. Total possible scores range from 0 to 63. Ten of the 21 items are rated on a scale from 0 to 4, nine items are rated from 0 to 2, and two are rated from 0 to 3. Each item score is summed to calculate total HDRS scores. Since the test's development in the 1950s, total HDRS scores have demonstrated reliability and a high degree of concurrent and discriminant validity (Carroll, Fielding, & Blashki, 1973).

## Beck Depression Inventory

The Beck Depression Inventory (BDI, BDI-II; Beck & Steer, 1993; Beck, Steer, & Garbing, 1988) is a self-report depression severity scale, designed for individuals 13 and older, that consists of 21 multiple-choice questions. It is one of the most commonly used scales in both the clinical and the research arenas. Participants are asked to rate their depressive symptoms and behaviors during the past week. The BDI assesses common symptoms of depression such as hopelessness, irritability, guilt, and self-harm, as well as physical symptoms such as fatigue, weight loss, and lack of interest in sex, with four possible forced-choice answers that range in intensity, such as:

(0) I do not feel sad.

(1) I feel sad.

(2) I am sad all the time and I can't snap out of it.

(3) I am so sad or unhappy that I can't stand it.

Values are assigned to each question and then totaled, and the total score is compared to validated scores to determine the severity of depression. Total scores between 0–9 indicate few to no depressive symptoms; 10–18 indicates mild to moderate depression; 19–29 indicates moderate to severe depression; and 30–63 indicates severe depression (Beck & Steer, 1993; Beck, Steer, & Garbing, 1988). The BDI is a copyrighted scale. Therefore, the researcher needs to request permission and actually purchase the instrument for use.

## Connors Rating Scale-Revised

The Connors Rating Scale-Revised (CRS-R) consists of several versions, with differing numbers of items, aimed specifically at parents, teachers, or adolescents, that allows them to rate childhood behaviors (Conners, Sitarenios, Parker, & Epstein, 1998). The CRS-R is a means of standardized evaluation in children and adolescents ages 3–17 for emotional, behavioral, and attentional symptoms, particularly Attention Deficit Hyperactivity Disorder. It takes several to 20 minutes to complete, depending on the version. A 10-item short version may be used to assess baseline severity of behavioral problems and to assess treatment response over time.

Short and long versions of the Connors Parent Rating Scales (CPRS), Teacher Ratings Scales (CTRS), and Adolescent Self-Report (CASS) exist; the longer versions are more comprehensive and provide a more thorough psychosocial evaluation. The parent version consists of either 80 or 27 items that focus on inattention, opposition, and hyperactive behaviors. The teacher versions, consisting of 87 or 27 items, cover similar domains. Age- and gender-based norms are available for comparison for each of the subscales and overall score.

## Instruments for Measurement of Anxiety

For anxiety, there are several rating scales available. The most common tool is the Beck Anxiety Inventory (Beck, Epstein, Brown, & Steer, 1988); 21 items are rated by the clinician. For children ages 6–19, the revised Children's Manifest Anxiety Scale consists of 37 items completed by the child (Reynolds & Richmond, 1994). Obsession symptoms or those that reflect obsessive-compulsive disorder can be measured by the Yale Brown Obsessive Compulsive Scale (Y-BOCS; Goodman et al., 1989). The adult version contains about 20 items rated by the clinician, while the child version (CY-BOCS), targeted at children ages 6–14, contains approximately 40 items (Scahill et al., 1997).

## SUMMARY

Much of what nurses do as part of daily practice can be based on systematic research. Once the research question(s) are identified and the design elucidated, APNs can focus on specific existing instruments that are valid and reliable to measure the concept of interest. Psychosocial data collection tools commonly address mood (e.g., depression, anxiety), behavior, general psychiatric or psychological symptoms, and measures of global impression. The APN or researcher may complete some instruments and the participant may complete others. Using appropriate tools to elicit psychological or behavioral content helps quantify and answer the question under investigation. Data derived using these methods can provide documentation to answer relevant clinical questions or test an intervention. As a result, the APN can use evidence to direct and guide practice and contribute to knowledge development in a given domain.

## SUGGESTED ACTIVITIES

1   Find a recent newspaper or Internet article of interest that reports the results of a study. Go to the original source (peer-reviewed article), and examine which instruments were used. For example, did the authors develop a survey, or did they use an existing measurement tool? What was the underlying concept that was being measured?

2   Next, read the description of the instrument in the journal article. What key characteristics are outlined about the instrument? What type of reliability and validity were used, and what is your interpretation of them?

## REFERENCES

Achenbach, T. M. (1991). *Integrative guide for the 1991 CBCL/4–18, YSR, and TRF profiles.* Burlington: University of Vermont, Department of Psychiatry.

Beck, A. T., Epstein, N., Brown, G., & Steer, R.A. (1988). An inventory for measuring clinical anxiety: Psychometric properties. *Journal of Consulting and Clinical Psychology, 56*(6), 893–897.

Beck, A. T., & Steer, R. A. (1993). *Manual for the Beck Depression Inventory.* San Antonio: Psychological Corporation.

Beck, A. T., Steer R. A., & Garbing, M. G. (1988). Psychometric properties of the Beck Depression Inventory: Twenty-five years of evaluation. *Clinical Psychology Review, 8,* 77–100.

Bobes, J. (1998). How is recovery from social anxiety disorder defined? *Journal of Clinical Psychiatry, 59*(Suppl. 17), 12–19.

Burns, N., & Grove, S. K. (2005). *The practice of nursing research: Conduct, critique and utilization.* Philadelphia: Elsevier Health Sciences.

Carroll, B. J., Fielding, J. M., & Blashki, T. G. (1973). Depression rating scales. *Archives of General Psychiatry, 28,* 361–366.

Conners, C. K., Sitarenios, G., Parker, J. D., & Epstein, J. N. (1998). The revised Conners' Parent Rating Scale. (CPRS–R): Factor structure, reliability and criterion validity. *Journal of Abnormal Child Psychology, 26*(4), 257–268.

First, M. B., Spitzer, R. L., Gibbon, M., & Williams, J. B. W. (1995). *Structured clinical interview for DSM-IV Axis I disorders.* New York: State Psychiatric Institute, Biometrics Research.

Frank-Stromborg, M., & Olsen, S. J. (2004). *Instruments for clinical health-care research* (3rd ed.). Sudbury, MA: Jones & Bartlett.

Goodman, W. K., Price, L.H., Rasmussen, S. A., Mazure, C., Delgado, P., Heninger, G. R., et al. (1989). The Yale-Brown Obsessive Compulsive Scale (Y-BOCS), Part I: Development, use, and reliability. *Archives of General Psychiatry, 46,* 1006–1011.

Guy, W. (1976). *Clinical Global Impression. ECDEU Assessment Manual for Psychopharmacology, revised.* Rockville, MD: National Institute of Mental Health.

Hamilton, M. (1961). Development of a rating scale for primary depressive illness. *British Journal of Social and Clinical Psychology, 6*(4), 278–296.

Lachar, D., Bailley, S., Rhoades, H., Espadas, A., Aponte, M., Cowan, K., et al. (2001). New subscales for an anchored version of the Brief Psychiatric Rating Scale: Construction, reliability, and validity in acute psychiatric admissions. *Psychological Assessment, 13*(3), 384–395.

Mateo. M. A. (1999). Psychosocial measurement. In M. A. Mateo & K. T. Kirchhoff (Eds.), *Using and conducting nursing research in the clinical setting* (2nd ed., pp. 256–267). Philadelphia: Saunders.

McLeer, S.V., Deblinger, E., Henry, D., & Orvaschel, H. (1992). Sexually abused children at high risk for post-traumatic stress disorder. *Journal of American Academy of Child & Adolescent Psychiatry, 31*(5), 875–879.

Orvaschel, H. (1982). Epidemiology of depression in young children. *Journal of Children in Contemporary Society, 15,* 79-86.

Overall, J. L., & Gorham, D. R. (1962). The Brief Psychiatric Rating Scale. *Psychological Reports, 10,* 799–812.

Overall, J. L., & Gorham, D. R. (1976). *The Brief Psychiatric Rating Scale, ECDEU Assessment Manual for Psychopharmacology.* Ed. W. Guy(pp. 157–160). Rockville, MD: U.S. Department of Health, Education & Welfare.

Reynolds, C. R., & Richmond, B. O. (1994). *Revised Children's Manifest Anxiety Scale.* Los Angeles: Western Psychological Services.

Scahill, L., Riddle, M. A., McSwiggin-Hardin, M., Ort, S. I., King, R. A., Goodman, W. K., et al. (1997). Children's Yale-Brown Obsessive Compulsive Scale: Reliability and validity. *Journal of American Academy of Child & Adolescent Psychiatry, 36*(6), 844–852.

# 13 Analyzing Quantitative Data

MARY R. LYNN

In most quantitative studies, the volumes of data need to be aggregated or reduced in scope for them to be meaningfully interpreted. It is in the data reduction that statistical methods come into play, because they facilitate the ability to make sense out of quantities of data. Statistical methods range from techniques as simple as determining the range of a set of numbers to the complex use of structural equation modeling to test elaborate conceptual and measurement models. This chapter discusses concepts and issues related to the analysis of data. For details on the use of applicability of any particular statistical method, refer to a statistics text, several of which are of particular value to health care professionals in the analysis of data (e.g., Munro, 2004).

## PURPOSE OF STATISTICS

Statistical methods are used in the analysis of data for two reasons—to describe the important *variables* in a study (descriptive statistics) and, when relevant, to make inferences about a population based on information contained in a sample (inferential statistics). It is the inferential use of statistical methods that is commonly thought of as the purpose of statistics, although the descriptive uses are equally important.

## LEVEL OF MEASUREMENT

One of the common issues in statistical analysis is the level of measurement of the study variables. The four levels of measurement, introduced by Stevens (1946), are nominal, ordinal, interval, and ratio. *Nominal* variables, from the Latin "of or belonging to a name," are measures in name only. In other words, variables that are measured on a nominal scale have numbers assigned to them for convenience only; the numbers have no mathematical meaning. In a nominal scale, a "1" is simply different from a "2" and is not seen as less than or half of the number 2. Typical nominal measures are classification variables such as gender ("Select 1 if you are female and 2 if you are male") or occupational status (1 = full-time; 2 = part-time). Nominal measures are discrete in that each value is mutually exclusive and there is no measurable interval between the values.

*Ordinal* variables are ranked in some manner. Like nominal variables, they are also discrete because the numbers are in order, but there is no consistent or measurable interval between the rankings. Using ordinal measures, distinctions between higher and lower, bigger and smaller, or even faster and slower can be made, but no other direct comparisons can be made. Questionnaire item response formats that range from "Strongly disagree" to "Strongly agree" or from "Unimportant" to "Extremely important" are examples of ordinal measures; it is known that "Extremely important" is a higher rating than "Important," but the distance between the two ratings or response points is not known.

*Interval and ratio* variables are both ordered and continuous, that is, in both scales, the interval between points on the scale can be measured, but the scales differ in the meaning of "zero." In interval variables, zero is an arbitrary point. Ratio variables are distinguished by having an absolute zero, which occurs when zero means "none of." Temperature has both an interval and a ratio counterpart. Fahrenheit or centigrade are interval scales because zero is an arbitrary point, and values below zero are both common and expected; the Kelvin scale, however, is a ratio scale because zero (0° K) is absolute zero, the coldest theoretical temperature at which the energy of motion of molecules is zero. (If the motion of molecules is zero, however, a thermometer would fall apart; nonetheless, zero in the Kelvin scale does mean "none of.") Most physiological measures are at the ratio level of measurement. The importance of the distinction between interval and ratio measures is that only with ratio level measures can we make comparative statements of proportion or ratio. To say a blood sugar of 100 is twice as high as a 50 blood sugar is accurate; to say that 100° F is twice as hot as 50° F is not, because Fahrenheit temperatures exist below zero. However, interval and ratio variables are almost always treated the same in statistical analysis, so the need to distinguish interval and ratio variables is often moot.

The importance of the level of measurement is that it is thought to dictate which statistics are to be used when describing variables and, to a great extent, which ones are used in statistical inference. There is considerable controversy about how stringently the level of measurement does, in fact, prescribe which statistical test should be used. This question most often arises when a researcher wants to use parametric statistics (those statistics that are based on the assumption that the data are normally distributed and at least interval level), in the analysis of data derived from questionnaires based on the Likert response format. The argument is that even though the Likert response format for the items is ordinal, when the items are summed for analysis, they "approach" the interval level. Purists say the connection between level of measurement of a variable and the statistic(s) to be used in its analysis is unequivocal (e.g., Stevens, 1946). Others (e.g., Armstrong, 1981; Knapp, 1990) suggest that this inextricable link is not so clear; when the researcher has items with a number of response options that are summed to create total scores for which zero is a possibility and the meaningfulness of an instrument is inferred to be interval, then the resulting data are supposed to be appropriately amenable to being analyzed using parametric statistics.

## DESCRIPTIVE VERSUS INFERENTIAL STATISTICS

*Descriptive statistics* are used to organize and summarize the information on specific variables. Most often, these statistics are used to describe the *central tendency* (where the distribution of scores or results for that particular variable is centered, or the "typical" score) and the *dispersion* (how the scores are distributed around the measure of central tendency) of variables. Because there are several methods for determining the "average" and the dispersion, knowing the level of measurement of the variable is essential in determining which measures are to be used. Table 13.1 identifies the appropriate measure of central tendency (the "average"), dispersion (variability), and correlation (relationship between two variables) for each level of measurement.

*Frequency distributions* are an additional means of describing the dispersion of a set of data. Generally, data in a frequency distribution are

Table 13.1

### APPROPRIATE MEASURES OF CENTRAL TENDENCY, DISPERSION, AND THE EXTENT OF CORRELATION FOR VARIABLES AT THE FOUR LEVELS OF MEASUREMENT

| MEASURE OF CENTRAL TENDENCY[a] DISPERSION CORRELATION | LEVEL OF MEASUREMENT | | | |
|---|---|---|---|---|
| | NOMINAL | ORDINAL | INTERVAL | RATIO |
| Mode Range Chi-square | X | X | X | X |
| Median Semi-interquartile range (SIQR) Kendall's tau, Spearman rank order | | X | X | X |
| Mean Standard deviation Pearson product-moment (PPM) | | | X[b] | X[b] |

[a]Below each "average" or measure of central tendency are the specific measures of variability (dispersion) and the statistic used to assess a relationship between two or more variables.
[b]When interval or ratio data are skewed, the median and semi-interquartile range should be used instead of the mean and standard; the Pearson product-moment correlation is still appropriate.

grouped into mutually exclusive categories, with the count of data falling within each category shown either on a table or in a graphic description such as a histogram or line graph. Occasionally, the bivariate relationship or correlation between variables is explored when describing the variables in a data set. Depending on the level of measurement of these variables, different techniques are used (see Table 13.1). When correlation or association statistics are applied for descriptive uses, the results cannot be used to make any statements or inferences about subjects other than those studied. Assertions of the existence of a relationship between these variables in the population cannot be made without assessing the significance of the correlation.

*Inferential statistics* are used when the intention is to generalize the findings from a sample to the population from which the sample was drawn. Before most inferential statistics can be used, certain assumptions must be met, such as the extent to which the data reflect a normal distribution, the level of measurement of the data to be analyzed, and the method for obtaining the sample (e.g., random, nonrandom). The two major types of inferential statistics, *parametric* and *nonparametric* statistics, differ in several ways, including the extent to which the data should reflect a normal distribution (parametric) or can be distribution-free statistics (nonparametric) and the need for specific levels of measurement for variables being analyzed—interval or ratio data (parametric) and nominal or ordinal data (nonparametric). However, they do not differ in the assumption that all data are obtained from subjects selected according to some chance (random) mechanism.

## STATISTICAL INFERENCE

Statistical inference, a formal method for drawing conclusions about populations from information obtained in samples, is based in hypothesis testing and probability theory. Whether overtly stated or not, any inferential statistical analysis is testing one or more hypotheses or questions about a population. The purest form of hypothesis is the *null hypothesis,* a statement that the researcher hopes to refute. For example, if a nurse is interested in comparing the self-care skills of patients in a new outpatient education program to those of patients not in the program, the null hypothesis might be "There is no difference in the self-care skills of patients in the outpatient education program and those of patients who are not in the outpatient program."

The convention of using a statement or hypothesis about what a researcher hopes *not* to find rather than what is thought will occur is where probability theory comes into play. In research, and therefore in statistical analysis, nothing can be definitely proved. Why? Because the researcher is not studying all persons who might fit the classifications or groupings, and the researcher is working with tools or measures that are not perfect. Although statements about populations can be refuted because a sample provides overwhelming evidence to the contrary (rejecting the null hypothesis), such statements cannot be "proved" to be undeniably true. So, in inferential statistics, the options are to reject a null hypothesis or to fail to reject it. To state that a null hypothesis, or any other hypothesis, has been "accepted," which implies that it is true, is statistically incorrect.

In reality, the null hypothesis is either true or false, and the conclusion reached from the interpretation of the data analysis either agrees or disagrees with this underlying "truth" in the population. Accordingly, when hypotheses are tested, there are four possible outcomes (Table 13.2).

In Table 13.2, no error occurs in the conclusion reached in the first and fourth scenarios, because the conclusion reached matches the "true state" of the hypothesis. Although no error is committed in the first scenario, the conclusion results in a weak statement about the hypothesis tested, because inferential statistics are used to make statements about rejection rather than to support a null hypothesis. The fourth scenario is the desired conclusion because a false hypothesis is rejected, as it should be.

Errors occur in both the second and third scenarios because the conclusion does not agree with the true state of the null hypothesis in the population. Because samples rather than populations are being studied, these errors have some likelihood of occurring. It is possible that a decision based on a sample of subjects may not represent the true nature of events; the *significance level (p)* tells how probable it is that an incorrect conclusion has been reached. *Alpha* ($\alpha$) is the probability that the second scenario's conclusion (rejecting a true null hypothesis) might occur, and *beta* ($\beta$) is the probability that the third scenario's conclusion (not rejecting a false hypothesis) might occur.

The probability of making a *type I error* is set or selected by the researcher a priori (before the fact and based on knowledge of the

Table 13.2

### POSSIBLE OUTCOMES FROM STATISTICAL TESTING OF HYPOTHESES

| SCENARIO | NULL HYPOTHESIS ($H_0$) TRUE STATE* | CONCLUSION REACHED AFTER ANALYSIS | REJECTION DECISION | TYPE OF ERROR |
|---|---|---|---|---|
| 1 | $H_0$ True | $H_0$ True | Do not reject $H_0$ | None |
| 2 | $H_0$ True | $H_0$ False | Reject $H_0$ | Type I error |
| 3 | $H_0$ False | $H_0$ True | Do not reject $H_0$ | Type II error |
| 4 | $H_0$ False | $H_0$ False | Reject $H_0$ | None |

*This is a hypothetical situation, as the "truth" about the hypothesis is never known; otherwise the research would be unnecessary.

situation in the population) on the basis of the researcher's willingness to make such an error. Traditionally, *alpha* is set at .05, meaning that the researcher is willing to conclude that a hypothesis is false when it is, in fact, true no more than 5 out of 100 times. Stated otherwise, even when a null hypothesis is true, there is a chance $(\alpha)$ that it may be concluded to be false. When concern over making such a mistake is high, such as when human life is at risk, *alpha* is set to an even more conservative value (e.g., .01 or .001). Such a high level of confidence in the conclusion (as high as 99.9%) is reserved for research with tremendous implications for the eventual recipients of the results of the research. An example is testing the tumor reduction capacity of a new oncologic agent or the ability of a medication to increase immune function in a patient population whose function has already been compromised. The researcher chooses such a conservative level of significance because she is unwilling to conclude that the medication has a positive effect unless it is almost impossible to conclude otherwise.

Occasionally, the level of significance is set at a more liberal value (e.g., $\alpha$ = .10) when the research is exploratory and nonlife-threatening, such as research being done to get a preliminary idea of the structure of events or to determine whether variables are promising enough to be included in future research. In such cases, there is no need to be more conservative or to guard against the likelihood of concluding that the null hypothesis should be rejected when it should not really be rejected.

## STATISTICAL SIGNIFICANCE

The result of a statistical test is deemed "significant" if the attained level of significance $(p)$ is less than or equal to the a priori level of significance established for the study $(\alpha)$. *Statistical significance* provides the researcher with the opportunity to say that data from the sample provide convincing evidence that what was found in the study would occur for the whole population, if studied at 1—*alpha* level of confidence.

Stated differently, a significant finding is one unlikely to have occurred by chance alone. For example, when two or more groups are being compared and are found to be "significantly different $(p < .05)$," the difference found between the groups is sufficient to warrant a conclusion that the samples come from "populations with different means (or whatever parameter)" with 95% confidence. This is often confusing to persons learning about statistical inference, who may wonder how this can occur when a single group was divided into two groups, one that received treatment and one that did not. The reason is that although the groups were similar at the outset, at the end of the study the impact of the intervention was such that the treatment group was no longer like the population represented by the untreated group *with respect to the variable for which they were found to significantly differ.* Similarly, when two variables are found to have a "significant correlation of 0.42 ($p$ < .05)," they are said to relate to each other in a moderately positive manner such that as variable A increases, variable B tends also to increase. The fact that the variables related at $r$ = .42 in the sample suggests that there will also be a systematic (nonchance) positive relationship between the variables.

Conversely, when groups being compared are found not to differ significantly, the interpretation is that whatever differences do exist are chance differences and are not large enough to the researcher to conclude that the groups are systematically or genuinely distinct. Two variables found to correlate at the level of .54 ($p$ > .05) are not significantly related to each other, so the correlation between those two variables in the population correlation should be seen as zero.

One of the most common mistakes subsequent to significance testing in which some tests resulted in significant results and some did not is for the researcher to treat all of the results as meaningful, when they are not. This most commonly occurs with correlation coefficients. When a correlation between two variables is found to be not statistically significant, *regardless of the magnitude of the calculated correlation,* the correlation between these same variables in the population is inferred to be "not different from zero," assuming that the null hypothesis was that the correlation between these two variables in the population was equal to zero. Regardless of any statistical testing, the results found for a sample do apply to the subjects or variables included in the study but, in the face of nonsignificant findings, these same results have no application to the population from whom the sample was drawn.

## CLINICAL VERSUS STATISTICAL SIGNIFICANCE

Statistical significance does not connote practical significance, and vice versa. To illustrate, consider the following two situations. In the first situation, a study is done comparing the effectiveness of iodine-based solution A to iodine-based solution B in reducing skin bacteria preoperatively.

After a tightly controlled study, solution B is found to significantly reduce bacteria ($p < .05$), with the average reduction being 1,000 colonies of usual skin flora X. In the second situation, a study of tube feeding administration is conducted with 100 subjects to determine whether there is any increase in distress when a tube feeding is administered directly from the refrigerator rather than first being warmed to room temperature. After intensive study, it is determined that there is no significant difference in distress between the tube feeding trials.

In the first case, there is statistical significance without any real clinical significance. A reduction of 1,000 colonies is of no particular clinical value because colonies are measured in the millions. Conversely, in the second situation, there is clinical significance without any statistical significance. The lack of a significant difference in distress in a solid study of temperature of administration suggests that the age-old tradition of warming tube feedings may not be necessary.

## SELECTION OF AN ANALYSIS PROGRAM

Until recently, statistical analysis was relegated to large mainframe systems; currently, a desktop personal computer can manage the analysis of most research data with one of the many analytical software programs available. Most of the commonly used programs (e.g., SPSS, SAS, SYSTAT, and STATA) offer similar arrays of procedures, although they are available at different costs and require different skills or tolerances to use. Students tend to use the program available at their educational institutions, with clinicians having fewer at-hand options. Table 13.3 provides summary information on the aforementioned commonly used programs, as well as on Epi Info (Centers for Disease Control and Prevention, 2005), the computer program mentioned in the next section. Other sources of analysis software are spreadsheet programs. For example, Microsoft Excel can perform most basic statistics (measures of central tendency and dispersion, $t$ test, correlation, regression) and is available on many home and office computer systems.

## PREPARATION OF DATA FOR ANALYSIS

Preparation of data for analysis usually proceeds from transforming the data from their raw form on a questionnaire or lab sheet to an analyzable

**Table 13.3**

## FEATURES AND PURCHASE INFORMATION FOR COMMONLY USED STATISTICAL ANALYSIS PROGRAMS

| PROGRAM | DATA ENTRY | DATA VERIFICATION | UNIVARIATE STATISTICS | MULTIVARIATE STATISTICS | MEASUREMENT/SCALE CONSTRUCTION | CFA/SEM[a] | GRAPHICS | EASE OF USE | PLATFORM | PRICE |
|---|---|---|---|---|---|---|---|---|---|---|
| SPSS[b] SPSS, Inc. Sales@SPSS.com 1-800-521-1337 Web site: SPSS.com | Y | N | Y | Y | Y | N† | Y | Easy | PC, Mac, Linux | $225 (students); $3,000 (nonstudents) |
| SAS SAS Institute, Inc. 1-800-727-0025 Web site: SAS.com | Y | Y | Y | Y | Y | Y | Y | Difficult | PC, Mac, mainframe | $60–$200/copy per computer for annual site license copy |
| SYSTAT Systat Software, Inc. Info-usa@systat.com | Y | N | Y | Y | Y | N | Y | Moderate | PC, Mac | $600 (students); $1,300 (nonstudents) |

| | | | | | | Ease of use | Platform | Cost |
|---|---|---|---|---|---|---|---|---|
| 1-312-5220-0060 Web site: SYSTAT.com | Y | N | Y | Y | N | | | |
| STATA StataCorp LP service@stata.com 1-800-782-8272 Web site: STATA.com | Y | N | Y | Y | N | Easy | PC, Mac, Unix | $48 – 100 (students); $155–$1,500 (faculty) $1,500–$1,700 (nonstudents) |
| EPI INFO Centers for Disease Control epiinfo@cdc.gov 1-404-498-6190 Web site: CDC. gov/epiinfo/ | Y | Y | Some | N | N | Difficult | PC | Free |

[a]Confirmatory factor analysis (CFA)/structural equation modeling (SEM) included in the program.
[b]SPSS produces a variety of stand-alone programs for specific applications such as AMOS (for SEM), which can be purchased separately.

form. The steps involved in the data preparation include data entry, data verification, and data cleaning. Precision in the execution of each of these steps helps ensure that one obtains a data set that is an accurate as possible.

## Data Entry

It is rare that the data from any study are analyzed without some form of computer interface, with the raw data (e.g., questionnaire responses) converted to a form amenable to analysis using the selected software program. Data entry can be conducted by manual or electronic means. Manual data entry usually includes direct entry of the data into the analysis program or indirect entry by first entering the data into a database, spreadsheet, or even a word processing program and then exporting the data file to the analysis program. The data from most small-scale projects are entered directly into the statistical analysis program, although the method of data entry varies from one program to another. For example, SPSS (Statistical Package for the Social Sciences, 2006) has a data entry screen that emulates a traditional spreadsheet, with the columns representing the variables to be entered and the rows representing the study participants. Data from each participant are entered on a single line, with data entry continuing from the first to the last relevant variable for each person.

Direct data entry or importation of a data set created outside an analysis program requires that each variable be named and the magnitude of the data to be entered for that variable (number of digits and decimal places) be known so that sufficient space is allocated to that variable. Specification of that space can become a very detailed process for imported data, depending on the format of the data. If the data for each subject are delimited, that is, if a common delimiter (space, comma, or other character) is placed between each variable and each record, then importation of the data is relatively straightforward, and the program allocates the appropriate amount of space needed for each variable. On the other hand, if data are not delimited or are incomplete, the process of importing the data can be complicated. The program then needs to be directed to the precise location and magnitude of each variable and the convention used for missing data (e.g., putting blanks or "99" in the relevant data location). Details on conversion of such data sets are contained in the instruction manuals that accompany the specific analysis program.

Electronic data entry is usually done by means of optical mark readers (OMR), or "scanners," which are popular because they circumvent the human element in data entry errors. This method is generally limited to data collected in a multiple-choice format because the scannable sheets are usually the familiar "bubble sheets" upon which study participants record their responses. Software programs do exist that can read and directly enter text and handwritten responses, but these programs are prohibitively expensive for most researchers. The expense of an OMR machine and its accompanying software can also be prohibitive. In addition, the issue of multiple responses, partially darkened responses, and people's propensity to get "off track" (e.g., putting the answer to question 3 in the slot corresponding to question 4) when marking responses on the sheets cannot be remedied by the software that converts input data from the sheets into a data file. Even when data are electronically entered, there is usually a need for "hand-editing" the data file once it is created.

## Data Verification

Independent of the means of data entry, the activity of data entry is fraught with opportunities for errors to occur. Accordingly, the data must be assessed for accuracy, which is referred to as *data verification*. The traditional method of data verification is to print the data file and compare it, number by number, with the original data source. Although this procedure is simple, it is impractical when there are numerous subjects, variables, or both. Additionally, even for a relatively small data set, this approach is tedious, optimally done with two people participating—one reading the values in the data file while the other checks those values against the original protocols—and is not an assurance of "clean" data. More technologically advanced methods of data verification exist, which, although not necessarily easier than the "hands-on" method, do provide alternative means for ensuring the reasonable accuracy of the data set.

Many analysis programs have means of data verification; SAS and Epi Info are two programs commonly used for this purpose. Both programs require the user to enter all of the data twice in two separate files, which are then compared for discrepancies. In SAS, the PROC COMPARE procedure can be used to check the contents of two supposedly identical data files. After the data have been entered independently into two separate SAS data files, the COMPARE procedure examines the contents of each file, datum by datum, and produces a printout that identifies the discrepancies between the two files. The user must then consult the original data source to determine, for each identified mismatch, which of the two entries is the correct one. Then the proper changes are made to one of the original data files and the second file is discarded. The major requirement for running a comparison procedure is that each file must contain an identification variable that uniquely identifies each record in the file, necessary because this unique record identifier is the mechanism by which the program matches the records in the two files.

Epi Info uses a different method to verify data. In this approach, data are entered once in their entirety. The data are then entered a second time, with the first file serving as a template for the second entry. This allows each piece of data entered in the second file to be compared to its counterpart in the first file at the *exact moment* it is being entered. In the event of an inconsistency between the previously entered data and the data being entered, a signal prompts the user about the inconsistency. The advantage of this real-time feedback approach to data verification is that the user can compare his or her computer entry to that on the data source immediately to determine the proper value. If the value being entered in the current data field is incorrect, then it can be remedied immediately. However, if the error lies in the underlying template file, that file must be opened and edited before the second data entry session can continue.

These methods represent computer-based approaches to ensuring accurate data entry, but they have some limitations. First, all of the data to be analyzed must be entered twice, which can be time-consuming. Also, there is no protection against the case in which the same datum is incorrectly entered twice.

Another method to increase the accuracy of data entry is an alert that can be programmed to prevent out-of-range data being entered. Microsoft ACCESS allows the creator of the database to set parameters or boundaries on the range of data that can be entered in a given field, thereby eliminating the entry of out-of-range values. For examples, if a user enters a 5 in a for a variable (e.g., level of education) that is set up to accept only values between 1 and 3, the user is notified immediately of the error and prompted to enter a number within the proper range for that field. Of course, this entry check has no effect on errors that are within the proper range of values for any field.

## Data Cleaning

The final step before the actual analysis begins is to "clean" the data set by eliminating errors not picked up in the data entry and verification

(Barhyte & Bacon, 1985; Suter, 1987). This cleaning is an essential but often forgotten step in preparing data for analysis. One easy method used to clean data is to print the data file and examine it for obvious errors in placement of data and numbers that appear to be unusual for the variables included. Such a strategy aids in the identification of values that are out of range for the variables entered, but it does not reveal entry errors in the data if they are within range. It should be noted that "out-of-range" values have a larger impact on subsequent calculations, such as central tendency, than within-range errors. Out-of-range values are more easily seen from frequency distributions for each variable, which are easily obtained from any statistical analysis program. Another method of data cleaning is to run cross-tabulations on variables that have combinations that are not reasonable, such as opposing gender and diagnosis to be sure only women have hysterectomies and only men have transurethral resections. Not all data sets have such illogical combinations, so this procedure may be of limited value in some data sets.

## Outliers

Outliers in a data set are those observations that do not seem to belong to the same set as the others. Suppose the ages of 5 participants are 24, 27, 22, 48, and 25 years. The participant with the age of 48 years seems out of place with the other subjects, who are more than 20 years younger and have similar ages. How to determine when an outlier exists and what to do with one is not completely clear. Outliers tend to be classified as observations more than 3 or 3.5 standard deviations from the mean. When one or more outliers are identified, the options are to ignore the existence of an outlier, drop the outlier's data from the data set, transform the data in some way, or analyze the data with and without the outlier(s) to determine whether it really does have an impact on the results. The last option is probably the most legitimate, because it acknowledges the existence of the outliers but does not artificially delete or alter them in order to conduct the analysis.

For example, a master's student is conducting her thesis research by assessing the effect of touch on the self-perceptions of patients undergoing ostomy surgery for the first time. In this study, she assesses the self-perceptions of 9 control subjects before surgery and at discharge. Following collection of the control group data, she implements her intervention of deliberate, appropriate touch as a part of routine postoperative care to the 9 treatment subjects, who, like those patients in the control group, have been assessed for self-perception before surgery and at discharge. Unknown to her, the wife of one of the 9 treatment subjects has filed for divorce immediately after his surgery. His at-discharge self-perception score is several standard deviations below both his preoperative score and that of the other 8 treatment participants. When the self-perception scores of 9 control and 9 treatment subjects are compared, there is no significant difference in their self-perception scores. However, when the treatment group is reduced to 8 subjects by eliminating the data from the affected patient and the average scores of the remaining subjects are compared to those of the nine control subjects, the treatment group has a significant increase in its average self-perception score. It would be a misrepresentation of the results of the study to report only the latter result; presenting both sets of results provides the only truly accurate view of the research situation.

This example also points out the relationship between sample size and the influence of outliers. The inclusion of this one patient in the treatment group has a profound effect on the results of the study, because the sample size is so small. Had the treatment group had 50 or 100 participants, it is unlikely that his inclusion would have made much of a difference in the results. Small samples are always more sensitive to the effect of the "deviant" or outlier participant.

## SELECTING THE STATISTICAL TEST

Selection of the appropriate statistical test is based on several considerations, among them the hypotheses being tested and the level of measurement of the variables. Table 13.4 provides an overview of selected common statistical tests that are appropriate for independent and dependent variables of varying levels of measurement for each of several types of research questions.

What is not apparent from the table is that there are alternative statistical means by which many data sets can be analyzed. This occurs when, despite the original level of measurement, the data are reclassified into a different level of measurement. For example, if the goal of a researcher is to assess the relationship between the age of the subjects and their ability to cope with their diagnosis, a Pearson correlation might be calculated, because both variables are at least interval in nature. However, upon finding a positive relationship between age and coping, the question of whether older participants differ from young subjects might

# Table 13.4

## LEVEL OF MEASUREMENT AND FOCUS OF THE RESEARCH HYPOTHESIS/QUESTION FOR SELECTED STATISTICAL TESTS

| STATISTICAL TEST | VARIABLE | | FOCUS OF HYPOTHESIS/QUESTION | | |
|---|---|---|---|---|---|
| | INDEPENDENT | DEPENDENT | ASSOCIATION | DIFFERENCE | CORRELATION |
| Chi-square | N[a] | N | X | | |
| | N | N | X | | |
| | O | N | X | | |
| | O | O | X | | |
| Kendall's tau and | O | O | | | X |
| Spearman rank order | O | I | | | X |
| | I | O | | | X |
| Pearson product- | I/R | I/R | | | X |
| moment regression | I/R | I/R | | | X (and prediction) |
| Z or t-test single group | n/a | I/R | | X | |
| comparison | N | O | | X | |
| Mann-Whitney U | O | N | | X | |
| t test (two groups only) | N | I/R | | X | |
| | O | I/R | | X | |
| ANOVA (2 or more | N | I/R | | X | |
| groups) | O | I/R | | X | |

[a]Level of measurement of the variables is indicated by N = nominal, O = ordinal, and I/R = interval/ratio (combined because they share the same types of analysis).

arise. To perform this analysis, it would be necessary to categorize the participants into older and younger groups, creating an ordinal variable (e.g., 0 = younger, 1 = older). This is often done by ordering the subjects by age, dividing them into thirds, and eliminating the middle third, thereby creating an older and a younger group. Following this, a *t* test could be used to compare the (mean coping of the) younger group to the (mean coping of the) older group. The ability to manipulate the data by transforming them into other configurations is a convenient feature offered in most data analysis programs.

Multivariate statistics are frequently the extension of the bivariate statistics discussed earlier. For example, a simple correlation between two variables can be extended to the correlation between sets of variables, usually a set of independent and a set of dependent variables, as in canonical correlation. Another extension of a simple correlation is the prediction of an outcome variable from a combination of "cause" or independent variables. For example, height and weight are can be correlated using a simple correlation procedure. But if we really wanted to predict a patient population's weight, we would likely need to consider other variables in addition to height, such as exercise, caloric intake, genetics, and general state of health. The advantage of moving from a simple to a multivariate statistic is that we can include a variety of relevant variables to better understand the complexity of human behavior and that the more complex analysis allows us to obtain information about the relative contribution of each variable in the analysis.

Just as was true for correlations, simple statistics used for comparisons between groups (e.g., ANOVA) can be extended to complex groups comparisons by the use of the Multivariate Analysis of Variance (MANOVA) and to multiple points in time by the use of Repeated Measures ANOVA.


## INTERPRETATION AND PRESENTATION OF THE RESULTS

While the presentation of the results of the statistical analysis in a research report is fairly clear, it is never as simple as it seems. The text must describe what was done and what was found, using supporting tables and illustrations of the results. Texts and tables are mutually exclusive presentations; what is presented in one is not presented in the other. It takes some experience to learn what to present in which venue, but with time and practice the decision becomes fairly straightforward.

The text portion of the presentation describes the process of getting to the results; the details about the demographic variables and most of the final statistics from the inferential tests are usually presented in tables. When there are only a few results of either type, a table may or may not be necessary.

Some researchers have a tendency to present "glitz" in their results, to make the analysis *seem* sophisticated and elaborate. Rarely does this approach succeed; instead, this approach is usually interpreted as being convoluted and unnecessarily cumbersome.

Construction of tables also takes practice and is best learned by examining the tables presented in journals such as *Nursing Research* or *Research in Nursing and Health* or in a publication manual (e.g., American Psychological Association, 2001). Although the construction of a table is somewhat dependent on the purpose of the report, there are a few points to consider in all tables.

1   The title should identify all the major components of the table in terms of the variables, subjects, and statistics presented. Generally, variables are listed in the first column, with subsequent columns devoted to variables and statistics.

2   Any single column should contain only one statistic, for example, percentage, median, or *t*-test value. An exception is in the presentation of means and standard deviations in the same column, which can be handled by labeling the column for both (Mean [*SD*]) and then reporting the data in that same manner (e.g., 45.43 [5.2]). This approach saves considerably on the space needed for the table, as well as on the effort it takes to understand it.

3   For all variables presented in the results section of a report, whether they are descriptive or inferential, the appropriate measures of central tendency (typical value) and dispersion (variation) should also be presented. Demographic variables are described by a mixture of these measures, because they usually vary considerably in their levels of measurement. For example, the most common demographic variables are gender, ethnicity, marital status, socioeconomic status, age, and years of education, and, in a clinical study, often there are diagnostic variables. Gender, ethnicity, marital status, and diagnosis are nominal variables; socioeconomic status is often an ordinal-level variable; and age and years of education are ratio-level variables. As shown in Table 13.1, the appropriate measures for the variable being described are used.

A note about how demographic variables are collected pertains to their eventual analysis. It is *never* in the best interest of the analysis to collect demographic variables that are otherwise interval or ratio variables by reducing them to nominal or ordinal measures. For example, the researcher should ask each subject to give his or her age, rather than give the subject age categories from which to choose. Precision in reporting these variables is lost when they are unnecessarily categorized. The exception to this caution pertains to income, which probably needs to be categorized to encourage participants' responses to the question.

The researcher should describe the central tendency and dispersion of the variables used in the inferential analysis and present the outcome of the analysis or the final statistics. These statistics are not, however, necessarily presented in the same place within the report. For example, if several *t* tests (statistical comparisons between the means of two groups testing the hypothesis that the groups are not different) are presented, then the researcher might find any of several presentation configurations: (1) a table with means and standard deviations presented in columns, with the *t* test presented in the final column of the table, (2) a table of means and standard deviations and a separate table of *t*-test values, or (3) a table of means and standard deviations with the *t*-test results presented in the text. The level of significance attained ($p$) for significant comparisons is usually indicated by means of an asterisk placed next to the *t*-test value, with the actual $p$ level noted at the base of the table. Although it has become convention to present a variety of $p$ values at the base of the table, this seems to suggest that reviewers of the findings will see some results as "more significant" than others. This is not true. The level of significance is an a priori decision for any study, and that level is the only level against which all statistical results should be assessed. To place a single $p$ value (e.g., $*p < .05$) at the base of a table to correspond to all statistical values noted with an asterisk ($*$) should convey exactly the same thing that has become this common orchestra of $p$ values, and it does so with much less clutter and "noise" (Lynn, 1990).

## SUMMARY

Statistical analysis is a complicated subject, one that is not as black and white as some statistics professors or consultants suggest. In any situation, there are likely to be several different analytical techniques that could be applied to achieve the same or similar end. The ability to choose among techniques requires considerable experience with the techniques themselves, as well as with the data manipulations that are often required. Because statistical analysis can be complicated, it is often advisable for the researcher to consult a statistician, one with whom the researcher is comfortable and who can communicate effectively as well as "speak statistics." Few people can manage all the analysis of even a simple study without some form of assistance, and several consultants may assist with the many analysis decisions of complicated studies.

A person in charge of a study does not necessarily know all about the analysis issues and statistics being applied, but such expertise must be available to assist the researcher in understanding the data and making sense of the results. Even persons who have had statistical coursework do not necessarily recall it; however, the researcher must be willing to learn about statistics used and to know where or from whom to get help.

## SUGGESTED ACTIVITIES

1   Most surveys or questionnaires contain variables with diverse levels of measurement. Examine a survey or questionnaire you locate online, and identify the level of measurement of the items and, if included, each item in the demographic portion of the instrument.

2   Review the statistical analysis section of an article in a clinical journal, and determine the following: level of measurement of the variables, *alpha* level ($\alpha$) set before the analysis and attained level of significance after the analysis ($p$), statements made about the hypotheses (if present), appropriateness of the use of tables or other means to illustrate the analysis and results, and appropriateness of the conclusion based on the analysis presented.

## REFERENCES

American Psychological Association (2001). *Publication manual of the American Psychological Association* (5th ed.). Washington, DC: American Psychological Association.

Armstrong, G. D. (1981). Parametric statistics and ordinal data: A pervasive misconception. *Nursing Research, 30,* 60–62.

Barhyte, D. Y., & Bacon, L. D. (1985). Approaches to cleaning data sets: A technical comment. *Nursing Research, 34,* 62–64.

Centers for Disease Control and Prevention (2005). Epi InfoTM Community Health Assessment Tutorial. Atlanta: Centers for Disease Control & Prevention.

Knapp, T. R. (1990). Treating ordinal statistics as interval scales: An attempt to resolve the controversy. *Nursing Research, 39,* 121–123.

Lynn, M. R. (1990). Choosing (and sticking with) a level of significance. *Journal of Pediatric Nursing, 5,* 401–403.

Munro, B. H. (2004). *Statistical methods for health care research* (5th ed.). Philadelphia: Lippincott, Williams & Wilkins.

Statistical Package for the Social Sciences (SPSS). (2006). Base user's manual. Chicago: Author.

Stevens, S. S. (1946). On the theory of scales of measurement. *Science, 103,* 677–680.

Suter, W. N. (1987). Approaches to avoiding errors in data sets: A technical note. *Nursing Research, 36,* 262–263.

## SUGGESTED READINGS

Einspruch, E. L. (2005). An introductory guide to SPSS® for Windows® (2nd ed.). Thousand Oaks, CA: Sage.

Goodwin, L. D. (1984). Increasing efficiency and precision of data analysis: Multivariate vs. univariate statistical techniques. *Nursing Research, 33,* 247–249.

Goodwin, L. D. (1984). The use of power estimation in nursing research. *Nursing Research, 33,* 118–120.

Hays, W. L. (1994). *Statistics* (5th ed.). Boston: Wadsworth.

Jacobsen, B. S. (1981). Know thy data. *Nursing Research, 30,* 254–255.

Knapp, T. R., & Campbell-Heider, N. (1989). Numbers of observations and variables in multivariate analyses. *Western Journal of Nursing Research, 11,* 634–641.

Knapp, T. R. (1995). Regression analysis: What to report. *Nursing Research, 44,* 58–59.

Knapp, T. R. (1996). The overemphasis on power analysis. *Nursing Research, 45,* 379–381.

Lynn, M. R. (1990). Don't be fooled by statistical significance. *Journal of Pediatric Nursing, 5,* 350–351.

Lynn, M. R. (1990). Choosing (and sticking with) a level of significance. *Journal of Pediatric Nursing, 5,* 401–403.

Munro, B. H. (2004). *Statistical methods for health care research* (5th ed.). Philadelphia: Lippincott, Williams & Wilkins.

Reid, B. J. (1983). Potential sources of type I error and possible solutions to avoid a "galloping" alpha rate *Nursing Research, 00,* 100–191.

Salkind, N. J. (2007). Statistics for people who (think they) hate statistics (3rd ed.). Thousand Oaks, CA: Sage.

Shavelson, R. J. (1996). *Statistical reasoning for the behavioral sciences* (3rd ed.). Boston: Allyn & Bacon.

Upton, G., & Cook, I. (2008). *A dictionary of statistics.* Oxford: Oxford University Press.

Vogt, W. P. (2005). *Dictionary of statistics and methodology: A nontechnical guide* (3rd ed.). Thousand Oaks, CA: Sage.

# Using Available Evidence

# 14 Systematic Reviews

KATHLEEN R. STEVENS

Once a number of studies on the same topic accumulate, the challenge becomes determining whether they have implications for clinical care. The systematic review (SR) is regarded as the most scientific way to summarize research evidence in evaluating health care interventions intended to prevent and treat illness. Systematic reviews can distinguish interventions that work from those that are ineffective, harmful, or wasteful. Systematic reviews give reliable estimates about how well various options work and identify gaps in knowledge requiring further research.

The systematic review is a type of research design within the larger field of the science of *research synthesis*. Systematic reviews (SRs) have emerged as an integral part of the evolution of evidence-based practice (EBP), and are considered foundational not only to effective clinical practice but also to further research. When done well, SRs are considered the highest level of evidence for clinical decision making.

A primary value of SRs is that they generate new knowledge that is not otherwise apparent from examining the set of primary research studies. This summary is accomplished by the use of rigorous scientific methods. As in other research designs, application of research methods is central in constructing accurate and valid results.

The primary purpose of this chapter is to highlight the need for systematic reviews in research; to introduce the methodology necessary to produce rigorous, credible conclusions; and to discuss who produces SRs and where SRs may be found.

## DEFINITIONS OF SYSTEMATIC REVIEW

Early in the evolution of the design of scientific methods for conducting systematic reviews, the Cochrane Collaboration advanced the following definition: "Systematic reviews are concise summaries of the best available evidence that address sharply defined clinical questions." (Cochrane Collaboration, 1999, n.p.). SRs are further described as a review of a clearly formulated question that uses systematic and explicit methods to identify, select, and critically appraise relevant research and to collect and analyze data from the studies that are included in the review; statistical methods (meta-analysis) may or may not be used to analyze and summarize the results of the included studies." (Cochrane Collaboration, 2008a, n.p.).

In short, the SR is a type of evidence summary that uses a rigorous scientific approach to combine results from a body of original research studies into a clinically meaningful whole (Stevens, 2004).

As a scientific investigation, the SR focuses on a specific type of research question and uses explicit, transparent methods through each step of identifying, selecting, assessing, and summarizing individual research studies (Haynes, Sackett, Guyatt, & Tugwell, 2006; West et al., 2002). Essential aspects of each of these steps in the SR methodology are discussed later in this chapter. It is crucial that SR investigative methods be preplanned, transparent, and replicable, as is true in other research designs. The SRs may or may not include a quantitative analysis of the results of selected studies to develop inferences (conclusions) about the population of interest (Institute of Medicine, 2008).

## HIGHLIGHTS OF THE EVOLUTION OF SYSTEMATIC REVIEWS

Because of the nascence of SRs as a research design, the broader scientific field uses multiple terms to refer to similar, sometimes overlapping, sometimes less rigorous approaches to summarizing the science on a given topic. These terms are *review* (used in medical literature); *state- of-the-science review* (used in nursing literature); and *review of literature* (commonly used in research methods textbooks). There are, however, important distinctions to be made. Today, all terms but the systematic review are considered to be flawed and to produce biased conclusions. Even the review of literature, performed to demonstrate a gap in knowledge, and therefore a need for a research study, has come under scrutiny for lack of rigor (Chalmers, 2005).

This new level of scientific rigor in research synthesis is not yet reflected in all published SRs. In seminal research, Mulrow (1987) created a strong case for moving from the then loosely performed "review" in medicine to the more scientifically performed systematic review. Mulrow's assessment of 50 "reviews" published in medical literature showed that the rigor of the reviews was woefully lacking and that, therefore, the conclusions were not trustworthy.

The distinction between SRs and traditional literature reviews is the strict scientific design that is employed in SRs. As in other research designs, if strict methods are not employed, then the conclusion is called into question for bias and accuracy. Because clinicians rely on SRs to summarize what is known about a clinical intervention, it is crucial that we "get the evidence straight" (Glasiou & Haynes, 2005) before applying it in clinical decision making. It is equally important to understand what is known before investing additional resources to conduct primary research—perhaps over questions for which the answers are already known.

Since Mulrow (1987), several other studies have appraised the quality of reviews in medical literature. Kelly, Travers, Dorgan, Slater, and Rowe (2001) conducted a study in which they assessed the quality of systematic reviews in the emergency medicine literature. Likewise, Choi et al. (2001) conducted a critical appraisal of systematic reviews in the anesthesia literature. Dixon, Hameed, Sutherland, Cook, and Doig (2005) completed a critical appraisal study in which they evaluated meta-analyses in the surgical literature. In each case, the rigor of the published SRs was found to be lacking.

Stevens (2006) demonstrated that systematic reviews published in nursing literature also reflected a lack of rigor. In a study similar to Mulrow's (1987), SRs were located in nursing journals. Randomly selected articles classified in CINAHL as of the publication type "systematic review" were evaluated using the Overview Quality Assessment Questionnaire (OQAQ; Oxman & Guyatt, 1991), a widely used critical appraisal instrument. This study showed that "systematic reviews" are overclassified in CINAHL, with classification as SR occurring when the article did not specify that the SR methods were used. In addition, 90% of the SRs fell short of the expected level of rigor.

The poignant chiding of an early EBP leader drives home the point for rigorous SRs:

> More than a decade has passed since it was first shown that patients have been harmed by failure to prepare scientifically defensible reviews of existing research evidence. There are now many examples of the dangers of this continuing scientific sloppiness. Organizations and individuals concerned about improving the effectiveness and safety of health care now look to systematic reviews of research—not individual studies—to inform their judgments. (Chalmers, 2005)

Recognizing the poor state of rigor of SRs and the significance of "getting the evidence straight," the Institute of Medicine (IOM, 2008) assessed what is needed to move synthesis science forward. Their report acknowledged the great strides made in the new science of systematic reviews. However, it called for more methodological research to produce better SRs. The report suggested that investing in the science of research synthesis will increase the quality and value of evidence in systematic reviews. The IOM committee recommended establishment of evidence-based standards for SRs (IOM, 2008).

A primary mover in the field of SRs, the Cochrane Collaboration methodology workgroup continues to evolve methods for conducting systematic reviews. Likewise, the IOM strongly urges continued development of methodologic foundations and rigorous standards for SRs (2008a).

## THE NEED FOR SYSTEMATIC REVIEWS

Science is largely composed of two types of research: (1) primary research—original studies based on observation or experimentation on subjects; and (2) secondary research—reviews of published research that draw together the findings of two or more primary studies.

SRs offer a number of advantages to practice and in planning the next primary study. A systematic review distills a volume of data into a manageable form; clearly identifies cause-and-effect relationships; increases generalizability across settings and populations; reduces bias; resolves complexity and incongruence across single studies; increases rate of adoption of research into care; and offers basis for ease of update as new evidence emerges (Mulrow, 1994). With such advantages, the need for rigorous execution of SRs is clear.

SRs are a type of secondary research that follows highly rigorous and prescribed methods to produce an unbiased summary of what is known on a particular topic. In science, there is general agreement about a hierarchy of knowledge produced through various methods. In this hierarchy, the systematic review is considered the most robust, producing the most accurate view of objective truth. That is, SRs are deemed the most reliable form of research that provides conclusions about "what works" in health care to produce intended patient outcomes (IOM, 2008).

Moreover, given their value in determining state of the science and the rigorous scientific standards now supporting the conduct of SRs, these reviews are considered a research design worthy of specific funding and support. This point was demonstrated in a study of the relative citation impact of study designs in the health sciences (Patsopoulos, Apostolos, & Ioannidis, 2005). The investigators compared the frequency of citation across a variety of research designs (SR, true experiment, cohort, case control, case report, nonsystematic review, and decision analysis). Meta-analyses were cited significantly more often than all other designs after adjusting for year of publication, high journal impact factor, and country of origin. When limited to studies that addressed treatment effects, meta-analyses received more citations than randomized trials (Patsopoulos et al., 2005).

The purpose of an SR is twofold: (1) to indicate what we know about the clinical effectiveness of a particular health care process; and (2) to identify gaps in what is known, pointing to a need for further research. So valuable is the SR in setting the stage for further research that leaders have recommended denial of funding of proposals that are not preceded by a systematic review on the topic (Chalmers, 2005).

Three of the most important reasons for conducting SRs are (1) to reduce the volume of literature that must guide clinical decisions; (2) to reduce bias arising from several sources; and (3) to provide a resolution among single primary studies that draw conflicting conclusions about whether an intervention is effective.

## Reducing Volume of Literature

An oft-cited benefit of an SR is that it reduces a number of single research studies into one, harmonious statement reflecting the state of the science on a given topic. Literally thousands of new health research studies are published weekly. Each year, Medline indexes more than 560,000 new articles, and Cochrane Central adds about 20,000 new randomized trials to its database. This represents about 1,500 new articles and 55 new trials per day (Glaziou & Haynes, 2005). Individual readers are daunted by the challenge of reading and staying abreast of the published literature. The SR offers a solution in that it reduces the world's scientific literature to a readable summary of synthesized knowledge.

For example, a CINAHL search on "falls in the elderly" yields 1,500 articles. Even limiting the search to "research publications" reduces the list to 830 articles. Narrowing the search to "systematic reviews" yields 15 articles for review. The systematic reviews range in rigor; however, one article on the subject (Gillespie et al., 2009) was published in the Cochrane Database of Systematic Reviews, ensuring that the synthesis was conducted in a highly systematic (scientific) way. This SR report notes that, after searching multiple bibliography databases and screening studies for relevance and quality, the authors included 62 trials involving 21,668 people in the SR (Gillespie et al., 2009). Upon synthesizing effects using meta-analysis, the researchers drew conclusions about interventions that are likely to be beneficial in reducing falls and interventions whose effectiveness is unknown. Results are expressed in terms of relative risk and confidence intervals. An example of a beneficial intervention is expressed as follows: A significant pooled relative risk (0.86 with a 95% confidence interval of 0.76–0.98) from five studies representing 1,176 participants suggests the clinical effectiveness of a multidisciplinary multifactoral risk screening and an intervention program for elders with a history of falling or those at high risk to reduce falls (Gillespie et al., 2009).

SRs consolidate research results from multiple studies on a given topic to increase the power of what we know about cause and effect, making an excellent foundation for clinical decision making.

## Avoiding Bias

The term *bias* refers to a deviation in accuracy of the conclusion (Cochrane Collaboration, 2008a). An SR reduces bias and provides a true representation of the science. Common sources of bias are (1) an incomplete literature search; (2) biased selection of literature; and (3) exclusion of nonpublished literature. Conducting SRs according to a structured scientific approach ensures that a true representation of knowledge is presented.

## Resolving Conflicting Results

Rapid growth in the number of health care studies has sharpened the need for SRs to assist clinicians, patients, and policymakers in sorting through the confusing and sometimes conflicting array of available evidence. While one study may conclude that an intervention is effective, a second study may conclude that the intervention offers no advantage over the comparison. The simplistic approach of comparing the number of studies that favor an intervention and the number that do not yields an erroneous conclusion. Some studies have larger sample sizes or higher-quality methodologies and therefore carry more weight. Some studies of poor quality may be excluded by using preset criteria.

The growth and maturation of methods and expertise for conducting and using systematic reviews have increased the reliability of evidence for use in making health care decisions. It is crucial that nurses engage in conducting rigorous systematic reviews and critically appraise those that are presented in the literature.

## FUNDAMENTALS OF SYSTEMATIC REVIEWS

Whether they are serving as the lead investigator or as a member of an interprofessional team, nurses should have knowledge and skills related to SRs. Essential competencies for nurses include locating, critically appraising, and conducting SRs (Stevens, 2005).

Two primary organizations, the Agency for Healthcare Research and Quality (AHRQ) and the Cochrane Collaboration, have established guidelines for conducting systematic reviews. The process has been adapted and renamed by others; however, there are commonly accepted principles for conducting a systematic review.

A systematic review should consist of a detailed description of the approach and parameters used to ensure completeness in identifying the available data, the rationale for study selection, the method of critical appraisal of the primary studies (evidence), and the method of analysis and interpretation. Documentation of each step is requisite and provides the necessary transparency so that the systematic review may be replicated. It is strongly suggested that persons well versed in SR methods be part of the research team for all systematic review studies.

The five basic steps listed here should be followed, and the key decisions that constitute each step of the review should be clearly documented.

Step 1: Formulate the research question.

Step 2: Construct an analytic (or logic) framework.

Step 3: Conduct a comprehensive search for evidence.

Step 4: Critically appraise the evidence.

Step 5: Synthesize the body of evidence.

## Step 1: Formulate the Research Question

Like other research designs, systematic reviews use specific methods of inquiry to yield new and valid knowledge. The aim of a systematic review is to create a summary of scientific evidence related to the effects (outcome) produced by a specific action (intervention). Therefore, the research question used in a systematic review is designed in a very specific way. A well-formulated, clearly defined question lays the foundation for a rigorous SR. The question guides the analytic framework; the overall research design, including the search for evidence; decisions about types of evidence to be included; and critical appraisal of the relevant evidence from single research studies.

The SR research question must define a precise, unambiguous, answerable research question. The mnemonic PICO was devised (Richardson, Wilson, Nishikawa, & Hayward, 1995) to reflect the four key elements of the SR question:

1   Patient population
2   Intervention
3   Comparison
4   Outcome(s) of interest

An example of a well-stated SR question is as follows:

What is the evidence that physical activity interventions, alone (I) or combined with diet modification or smoking cessation (C), are effective in helping cancer survivors (P) improve their psychosocial or physiological outcomes (O)? (Holtzman et al., 2004, n.p.)

A second question, in which the comparison condition is implied, is as follows:

> What are the effects of smoking cessation programs (I) implemented during pregnancy on the health (O) of the fetus, infant, mother, and family (P)? (Lumley, Oliver, Chamberlain, & Oakley, 2004, n.p.)

Note that, in this example, the implied comparison is the absence of smoking cessation programs.

The population characteristics, such as age, gender, and comorbidities, usually vary across studies and are likely to be factors in the effect of an intervention. In addition, a given intervention may produce a number of outcomes of interest. The SR question is formulated so that it includes beneficial and adverse outcomes. For example, while prostate cancer treatment reduces mortality, the SR should also examine harmful effects of treatment such as urinary incontinence (IOM, 2008)

Depending on the specific SR question, different types of original studies will be of interest. For example, questions about effectiveness of prescription drugs will generate searches for randomized, controlled trials. On the other hand, a question about the effects of illicit drug use will find no trials that assign one group to such drug use; in this case, the question will generate a search for observational studies that compare the health of otherwise similar groups of users and nonusers.

The SR question is typically formulated during initial literature searches and evolves as the SR team examines background literature. In addition, a broader group of stakeholders is often involved in question formulation. These may include policymakers, managers, health professionals, and consumers (AHRQ, 2005).

## Step 2: Construct an Analytic (or Logic) Framework

After stating the SR question, the researcher then constructs a framework. This framework maps the relations between the intervention and the outcomes of interest. In the case of the relations between screening and various outcomes as depicted in Figure 14.1, the analytic framework was developed by the U.S. Preventive Services Task Force to depict causal pathways (Harris et al., 2001).

The analytic framework demonstrates which factors are intermediate to the outcomes of interest and guides the construction of the search.

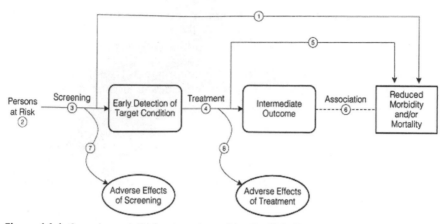

**Figure 14.1** Generic analytic framework used by the U.S. Preventive Services Task Force for topics about health screening.
From "Translating Evidence into Recommendations," Agency for Healthcare Research and Quality, Rockville, MD. Retrieved from http://www.ahrq.gov/clinic/ajpmsuppl/harris3.htm#source

## Step 3: Conduct a Comprehensive Search for Evidence

The comprehensive search for evidence is the most important—and time-consuming—step in conducting a reliable and valid SR (Cochrane Collaboration, 2008b). The search is crucial to identifying *all* relevant studies; in addition, search details must be documented so that the search can be replicated. The comprehensiveness of the search is what distinguishes a SR from a traditional narrative review (Moynihan, 2004). The question asked generates the specific search for evidence from original studies.

Constructing an adequate search strategy requires the skills of a librarian knowledgeable about evidence-based practice. The expert search strategy may consist of more than three pages of search terms, limited, for example, to human research, randomized control trials, the specific intervention, outcomes of interest, and multiple bibliographic databases. The world's literature is searched across databases such as CINAHL, Medline, EmBase, and others. Often, the initial search may yield 2,000 to 3,000 articles. In addition to these databases, other sources are searched, including review group registers (e.g., Cochrane Central Register of Controlled Trials Database), and hand searches of textbook bibliographies, citation indexes, and Web site resources are also conducted.

The inclusion of unpublished studies reduces publication bias. Because studies that find no effect are less likely to be published (Dickersin, 2005), reliance on published studies produces an overestimate of the effects of interventions. To minimize publication bias, it is important to find "fugitive" or "gray" literature—for example, conference proceedings and unpublished studies. Researchers often contact experts directly to locate articles that were not found in the literature.

## Step 4: Critically Appraise the Evidence

Once found, studies are screened to select the highest-quality studies available and to guard against selection bias. Studies are judged according to explicit criteria for design quality, strength of findings, and consistency with other studies in the set. Each study is examined to determine its applicability to the population and outcomes of interest and internal and external validity (AHRQ, 2005; Cochrane Collaboration, 2008b; Glaziou & Haynes, 2005).

Using specifically designed forms, the researcher extracts data from the studies that meet the quality criteria for inclusion. This abstraction process treats each study as a "subject" of the SR. The data extracted primarily include the effect size of the intervention on the outcome. Typically, at least two investigators independently extract data; if opinions about either quality or data extraction diverge, consensus is gained through discussion and/or third-party adjudication. (Cochrane Collaboration, 2008b)

## Step 5: Synthesize the Body of Evidence

### Summarizing Across Studies

SRs originally were developed to summarize quantitative research using statistical techniques. Summary approaches in synthesizing nonexperimental and qualitative research are also used. To synthesize a body of quantitative evidence, many systematic reviews use meta-analyses. This is an approach that statistically combines results of separate original studies into a single result, originated by Glass (1976) and advanced by the Cochrane Collaboration and AHRQ as useful in systematic reviews. The meta-analytic method provides a more precise estimate of the effect of the intervention than other methods such as vote counting, in which the number of positive studies is compared to the number of negative studies. Meta-analysis takes into account the weight of the effect of each individual study.

The results of a meta-analysis are often displayed in a forest plot (Figure 14.2). The plot provides a simple visual representation of the information from the individual studies that went into the meta-analysis. The graphical display conveys the strength of evidence in quantitative studies.

Forest plots are usually presented in two columns. The left column lists studies, and the right column is a plot of the measure of effect for each study. Effect estimates and confidence intervals for both individual studies and meta-analyses are displayed (Lewis & Clarke, 2001). Single-study estimates are represented by a square, the size of which reflects its weight in the meta-analysis. The confidence interval for that study is represented by a horizontal line extending on either side of the block. The length of the line is an indication of the width of the confidence interval around the result; the longer the line, the wider the confidence interval and the less precise the estimate of effect size. The meta-analyzed measure of effect (pooled result across all the included studies) is plotted as a diamond, with the lateral points reflecting the synthesized confidence interval (Cochrane Collaboration, 2008b).

A vertical line is also plotted, representing 'no effect.' If the confidence interval line crosses the vertical line, it cannot be said that the result was different from no effect—i.e., there was no statistically significant difference between intervention and comparison conditions. The same applies for the meta-analyzed measure of effect (the diamond) (Cochrane Collaboration, 2008b).

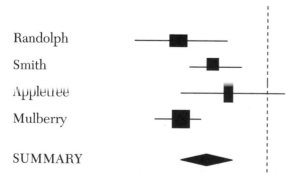

Randolph

Smith

Appletree

Mulberry

SUMMARY

              Favors Treatment       Does Not Favor Treatment

**Figure 14.2** Example of a forest plot.

## Analyzing Bias

Two primary types of bias can occur: bias in the individual studies that are incorporated into the SR and biases resulting from the selection of studies into the SR. To examine bias of individual studies, researchers use traditional design critique. Bias in study selection is examined using approaches that detect publication bias (studies that show an effect are more likely to be published), citation bias (studies that show an intervention effect are more often cited), language bias (large studies are typically published in English-language journals), and multiple publication bias (the same study results are sometimes published multiple times). All of these biases are in the same direction—indicating that the intervention was effective.

The funnel plot is the primary analytic technique employed to assess bias. The funnel plot detects publication bias by examining the range of effect sizes represented in the set of studies. If small studies are represented, then the funnel plot is asymmetric (AHRQ, 2005; Cochrane Collaboration, 2008b). In the absence of bias, the funnel plot is symmetric, as represented in Figure 14.3. Note that the points in the figure form an upside down funnel. Figure 14.4 depicts a funnel plot reflecting bias, probably arising from publication bias.

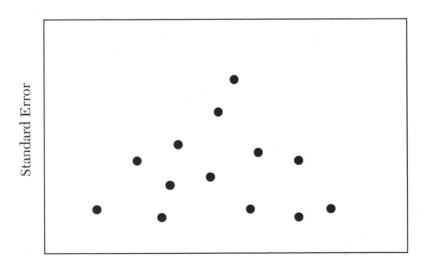

Log Odds Ratio

**Figure 14.3** Funnel plot representing no bias.

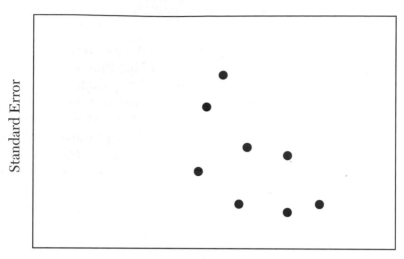

**Figure 14.4** Funnel plot representing bias.

## SUMMARY

SRs put the "science" into reviews of literature. The rigorous approach used in producing SRs ensures that the synthesis of studies is valid, representing accuracy and truth. The IOM notes, "Systematic reviews of evidence on the effectiveness of health care services provide a central link between the generation of research and clinical decision making. Systematic review is itself a science and, in fact, is a new and dynamic science with evolving methods" (IOM, 2008, p. 108).

If nursing care is to be effective in producing intended outcomes, it must be based on rigorously conducted SRs. Nurse scientists can contribute to the evolution of methodologies that match the science of nursing. High priority should be given to conducting quantitative and qualitative SRs and the methodologies that guide these processes (Cochrane Collaboration, 2008b; IOM, 2008). Nurse scientists and clinical experts are called on to engage in the conduct of SRs to guide clinical decision making in nursing and health care.

## SUGGESTED ACTIVITIES

1   Visit the Cochrane Collaboration Web site at http://www. cochrane.org/. Read the introduction. Search for "logo" in the

Web site search box, and read the explanation of the Cochrane Collaboration logo.

2   Visit the Web site for the Agency for Healthcare Research and Quality at http://www.ahrq.gov/. Under "Clinical Information," click on "Evidence-Based Practice."

a   Search the Web site for *Nurse Staffing and Quality of Patient Care* (Kane et al., 2007), and read the Structured Abstract.

   i   Did this SR find an association between nurse staffing and mortality and morbidity of patients?

   ii   Was it causal? (answer: No, it was an association)

   iii   Download the full report. View page 57, Figure 4, Flow of Study Selection for Questions 1, 2, and 4.

   1   How many total citations did the reviewers initially screen? (answer: 2,858)

   2   How many studies were included in the meta-analysis? (answer: 96)

b   Search the Web site for *Effects of Soy on Health Outcomes* (Balk et al., 2005).

   i   Download the full report. View page 97, Figure 9, Meta-analysis of the effect of soy products on triglycerides.

   ii   What is the summary statement of the meta-analysis? (answer: The black diamond does not touch the vertical line; therefore, soy is effective in reducing triglycerides.

## References for Suggested Activities

Balk, E., Chung, M., Chew, P., Ip, S., Raman, G., Kupelnick, B., et al. (2005, August). *Effects of soy on health outcomes.* Evidence Report/Technology Assessment No. 126. (Prepared by Tufts-New England Medical Center Evidence-Based Practice Center under Contract No. 290–02–0022.) AHRQ Publication No. 05-E024–2. Rockville, MD: Agency for Healthcare Research and Quality.

Kane, R. L., Shamliyan, T., Mueller, C., Duval, S., & Wilt, T. (2007, March). *Nursing staffing and quality of patient care.* Evidence Report/Technology Assessment No. 151 (Prepared by the Minnesota Evidence-Based Practice Center under Contract No. 290–02–0009.) AHRQ Publication No. 07-E005. Rockville, MD: Agency for Healthcare Research and Quality.

## Definitive Resources on Conducting Systematic Reviews

The Agency for Healthcare Research and Quality's *EPC Partner's Guide* details information on the Evidence-Based Practice Center program for current and potential partner organizations. It also presents background on the program and the roles and responsibilities of key participants, including the Agency for Healthcare Research and Quality (AHRQ), the partners, the EPCs, and the EPC Coordinating Center. Additional information is at http://www.ahrq.gov/clinic/epcpartner/

*Cochrane Handbook for Systematic Reviews of Interventions* provides guidance on how to prepare and maintain Cochrane Intervention reviews. The handbook may be found at http://www.cochrane.org/resources/handbook/

## REFERENCES

Agency for Healthcare Research and Quality. (2005). *Evidence-based Practice Centers partner's guide.* Washington, DC: Agency for Healthcare Research and Quality.

Chalmers, I. (2005). Academia's failure to support systematic reviews. *Lancet, 365*(9458), 469.

Choi, P. T-L., Halpern, S. H., Malik, N., Jadad, A. R., Tramer, M. R., & Walder, B. (2001). Examining the evidence in anesthesia literature: A critical appraisal of systematic reviews. *Anesthesia and Analgesia, 92,* 700–709.

Cochrane Collaboration. (1999). *Cochrane handbook for systematic reviews of interventions.* The Cochrane Collaboration, out of print.

Cochrane Collaboration. (2008a). *Glossary of Cochrane Collaboration and research terms.* Retrieved November 12, 2008, from http://www.cochrane.org/resources/glossary.htm

Cochrane Collaboration. (2008b). *Cochrane handbook for systematic reviews of interventions* (Version 5.0.1). Ed. J. P. T. Higgins & S. Green. Retrieved April 25, 2009, from www.cochrane-handbook.org.

Dickersin, K. (2005). Publication bias: Recognizing the problem, understanding its origins and scope, and preventing harm. In H. Rothstein, A. Sutton, & M. Borenstein (eds.), *Publication bias in meta-analysis: Prevention, assessment, and adjustments.* London: Wiley.

Dixon, E., Hameed, M., Sutherland, F., Cook, D. J., & Doig, C. (2005). Evaluating meta-analyses in the general surgical literature: A critical appraisal. *Annals of Surgery, 241*(3), 450–459.

Gillespie, L. D., Gillespie, W. J., Robertson, M. C., Lamb, S. E., Cumming, R. G., & Rowe, B. H. (2009). Interventions for preventing falls in elderly people. Cochrane Database of Systematic Reviews

Glass, G. V. 1976. Primary, secondary and meta-analysis. *Educational Researcher, 5*(10), 3–8.

Glasziou, P., & Haynes, B. (2005). The paths from research to improved health outcomes. *ACP Journal Club, 142*(2, Suppl.), A-8-A–10.

Harris, R. P., Helfand, M., Woolf, S. H., Lohr, K. N., Mulrow, C. D., Teutsch, S. M., et al. (2001). Current methods of the U.S. Preventive Services Task Force: A review of the process. *American Journal of Preventive Medicine, 20*(3, Suppl.), 21–35.

Haynes, R. B., Sackett, D. L., Guyatt, G. H., & Tugwell, P. (2006). *Clinical epidemiology: How to do clinical practice research* (3rd ed.). Philadelphia: Lipincott, Williams & Wilkins.

Holtzman J., Schmitz K., Babes, G., Kane, R. L., Duval, S., Wilt T. J., et al. (2004). Effectiveness of behavioral interventions to modify physical activity behaviors in general populations and cancer patients and survivors. Evidence Report/Technology Assessment No. 102. AHRQ Publication No. 04-E027-2. Rockville, MD: Agency for Healthcare Research and Quality.

Institute of Medicine. (2008). *Knowing what works in health care.* Ed. J. Eden, B. M. Wheatley, & H. Sox. Washington, DC: National Academies of Science.

Kelly, K. D., Travers, A., Dorgan, M., Slater L., & Rowe, B. H. (2001). Evaluating the quality of systematic reviews in the emergency medicine literature. *Annals of Emergency Medicine, 38*(5), 518–526.

Lewis, S., & Clarke, M. (2001). Forest plots: Trying to see the wood and the trees. *BMJ, 322,* 1479–1480.

Lumley, J., Oliver, S. S., Chamberlain, C., & Oakley, L. (2004). Interventions for promoting smoking cessation during pregnancy. *Cochrane Database of Systematic Reviews,* Issue 4. Art. No. CD001055. DOI: 10.1002/14651858.CD001055.pub2.

Moynihan, R. (2004). *Evaluating health services: A reporter covers the science of research synthesis.* New York: Milbank Memorial Fund.

Mulrow, C. (1987). The medical review article: State of the science. *Annals of Internal Medicine 106*(3), 485–488.

Mulrow, C. (1994). Rationale for systematic reviews. *British Medical Journal, 309,* 597–599.

Oxman, A. D., & Guyatt, G. H. (1991). Validation of an index of the quality of review articles. *Journal of Clinical Epidemiology, 4*(411), 1271–1278.

Patsopoulos, N. A., Apostolos, A. A., & Ioannidis, J.P.A. (2005). Relative citation impact of various study designs in the health sciences. *Journal of the American Medical Association, 293,* 2362–2366.

Richardson, W. S., Wilson, M. C., Nishikawa, J., & Hayward, R. S. A. (1995). The well-built clinical question: A key to evidence-based decisions. *ACP Journal Club, 123,* A12–A13.

Stevens, K. R. (2001). Systematic reviews: The heart of evidence-based practice. *AACN Clinical Issues, 12*(4), 529–538.

Stevens, K. R. (2004). *The ACE Star Model of Knowledge Transformation.* The University of Texas Health Science at San Antonio. Retrieved November 20, 2008, from www.acestar.uthscsa.edu

Stevens, K. R. (2005). *Essential competencies for evidence-based practice in nursing.* San Antonio: University of Texas Health Science Center at San Antonio.

Stevens, K. R. (2006). Evaluation of systematic reviews in nursing literature. *Proceedings of the Summer Institute on Evidence-Based Practice,* San Antonio, TX.

West, S., King, V., Carey, T., Lohr, K., McCoy, N., Sutton, S., et al. 2002. *Systems to rate the strength of scientific evidence.* Evidence Report/Technology Assessment No. 47. (Prepared by the Research Triangle Institute-University of North Carolina Evidence-Based Practice Center under Contract No. 290–97–0011.) AHRQ Publication No. 02-E016. Rockville, MD: Agency for Healthcare Research and Quality.

# Finding and Appraising Clinical Practice Guidelines

15

MARY D. BONDMASS

Nurses in all specialty areas and at all practice levels may consider a clinical practice guideline (CPG) a requisite to assist their clinical decision making. Because advanced practice nurses (APN) frequently have prescriptive privileges, they may need to be even more acutely aware of how to find and appraise CPGs for practice. Moreover, APNs need to know what CPGs are and what they are not.

This chapter focuses on defining, finding, and appraising CPGs for the APN. Information is provided from both governmental and professional organizational sources. The first half of this chapter defines CPGs and addresses ways to find them from myriad sources, but specifically from governments and professional organizations. Critical appraisal of CPGs for use in practice is the focus of most of the second half of the chapter. The chapter concludes with a brief discussion about the medical-legal literature related to the use of CPGs. Specific learning activities are provided at the end of this chapter to promote understanding of the information. The information presented here is primarily specific to the United States; however, international resources are also included.

## DEFINITION OF CLINICAL PRACTICE GUIDELINES AND THE INSTITUTE OF MEDICINE

The definition of CPGs employed in this chapter is that developed by the Institute of Medicine (IOM): "Clinical practice guidelines are systematically developed statements to assist practitioner and patient decisions about appropriate health care for specific clinical circumstances" (IOM, 1990). The IOM serves as an adviser to the U.S. government on health issues; however, its mission embraces the health of people worldwide. Established in 1970, under the charter of the National Academy of Sciences, the IOM provides independent, objective, evidence-based advice to policymakers, health professionals, the private sector, and the public. Its Web site is http://www.iom.edu/.

Some may consider the name *IOM* to be somewhat of a misnomer, because nurses and practitioners from disciplines other than medicine are part of its membership. Moreover, at least one quarter of its membership comes from outside the health professions, from such fields as the natural, social, and behavioral sciences, law, administration, engineering, and the humanities. Despite its name, the purpose of the IOM is to provide advice on issues relating to biomedical science, medicine, and health.

The publications of the IOM frequently make the case for the use of CPGs, with numerous and often-referenced IOM citations found in the scientific and economic health care literature. Two of the best-known and perhaps landmark publications of the IOM are *To Err Is Human: Building a Safer Health System* (1999) and *Crossing the Quality Chasm: A New Health System for the 21st Century* (2001).

In early 2008, the IOM published *Knowing What Works in Health Care: A Roadmap for the Nation.* The conceptual framework and central premise of this recent IOM work is that the individual patient's clinical decisions should be based on the "conscientious, explicit, and judicious use of current best evidence" (Sackett, Rosenberg, Gray Haynes, & Richardson, 1996). The IOM proposes a national clinical effectiveness assessment program (the Program) with a threefold mission: (1) setting priorities for evidence assessment, (2) assessing evidence (systematic review), and (3) developing (or endorsing) standards for trusted CPGs. This last goal, of course, is the focus of this chapter.

On the continuum of knowledge used to make clinical decisions within the evidence-based practice (EBP) paradigm, the IOM refers to CPGs and recommendations as interpretations of the strength of the overall credible evidence. This is similar to the ACE Star Model of Knowledge Transformation© (Stevens, 2004a, 2004b) and is the conceptual perspective of the author for this chapter. Stevens (2004a, 2004b) names CPG as the third "star point" in the cycle of knowledge transformation, representing the translation or interpretation of the knowledge used in clinical decision making. Figure 15.1 presents the adapted schematic

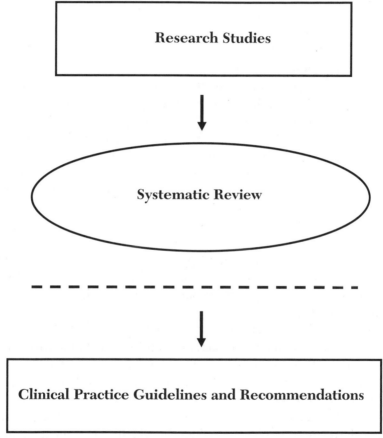

**Figure 15.1** Continuum of evidence for clinical decision making
*Note:* The dashed line is the theoretical dividing line between the systematic review of the research literature and its application to clinical decision making, including the development of clinical guidelines and recommendations. Below the dashed line, decision makers and developers of clinical recommendations interpret the findings of systematic reviews to decide which patients, health care settings, or other circumstances they relate to.
From *Knowing What Works in Health Care: A Roadmap for the Nation,* by IOM, 2008, J. Eden, B. Wheatley, B. McNeil, and H. Sox (Eds.). Washington, DC: National Academies Press. Reprinted with permission from the National Academies Press, Copyright 2008, National Academies of Sciences.

(West et al., 2002), that the IOM used to demonstrate the continuum that begins with evidence from individual or primary research studies, extends through the systematic review of the body of evidence, and culminates in the development of CPGs and recommendations that are the interpretation of the strength of the overall evidence (IOM, 2008).

## FINDING CLINICAL PRACTICE GUIDELINES

Many CPG Internet sites were evaluated in the preparation of this chapter; however, none were found to be as comprehensive as the official U.S. government site. In the past, locating or finding a CPG was considered a formidable task; now that task is relatively easy. Appraising CPGs for use in practice takes much more time and effort. It should also be noted that basic computer and Internet search skills and high-speed Internet access are essential.

In the United States, the National Guideline Clearinghouse™ (NGC), hosted by the Agency for Healthcare Research and Quality (AHRQ) of the U.S. Department of Health and Human Services is a public resource that includes a comprehensive database of evidence-based CPGs and related documents. The NGC Web site was initially launched in 1999, but, since 2003, it has been complemented by the National Quality Measures Clearinghouse™ (NQMC). The NQMC, also sponsored by AHRQ, is a public repository for evidence-based quality measures and measure sets. The respective Web site addresses for the NGC and NQMC are http://www.guidelines.gov and http://www.quality measures.ahrq.gov.

What makes the NGC the first choice of the many available databases for locating CPGs is that many national and international professional organizations' CPGs are housed within the database. The NGC includes CPGs from approximately 360 different organizations. Even though the NGC is a U.S.-sponsored Web site, the CPGs included contain data from international organizations, as well, and can be accessed by practitioners globally; however, all data are in English, which may limit their use to some international readers. Exhibit 15.1 presents key components and other features of the NGC's Internet site. Exhibit 15.2 includes the most frequently asked question related to finding CPGs on the NGC site.

Some readers may be familiar with publications from the U.S. Preventive Services Task Force (USPSTF), an organization that in the past also produced several CPGs. The USPSTF was convened by the U.S.

Exhibit 15.1

## KEY COMPONENTS AND OTHER FEATURES OF THE NATIONAL GUIDELINE CLEARINGHOUSE

### *Key components of the National Guideline Clearinghouse (NGC).*

■ Structured abstracts (summaries) about the guideline and its development.
■ Links to full-text guidelines, where available, and/or ordering information for print copies.
■ Palm-based PDA downloads of the Complete NGC Summary for all guidelines represented in the database.
■ A Guideline Comparison utility that gives users the ability to generate side-by-side comparisons for any combination of two or more guidelines.
■ Unique guideline comparisons called Guideline Syntheses, prepared by NGC staff, compare guidelines covering similar topics, highlighting areas of similarity and difference. NGC Guideline Syntheses often provide a comparison of guidelines developed in different countries, providing insight into commonalities and differences in international health practices.
■ An electronic forum, NGC-L, for exchanging information on clinical practice guidelines, their development, implementation, and use.
■ An Annotated Bibliography database that allows users to search for citations for publications and resources about guidelines, including guideline development and methodology, structure, evaluation, and implementation.

### *Other user-friendly features*

■ What's New enables users to see what guidelines have been added each week and includes an index of all guidelines in NGC.
■ Expert Commentaries are authored by the NGC/NQMC Editorial Board and/or by other experts working in conjunction with their board. The Editorial Board is diverse in terms of its clinical expertise, geographical representation, and stakeholder affiliation.
■ NGC Update Service is a weekly electronic mailing of new and updated guidelines posted to the NGC Web site.
■ Detailed Search enables users to create specific search queries based on the various attributes found in the NGC Classification Scheme.
■ NGC Browse permits users to scan for guidelines available on the NGC site by disease/condition, treatment/intervention, or developing organization.
■ PDA/Palm List provides users with information regarding the availability of full-text guidelines and/or companion documents available through the guideline developer, that can be downloaded for the handheld computer (e.g., Personal Digital Assistant [PDA], Palm, Blackberry).
■ AHRQ Evidence Reports/Technical Assessments list provides users with links to the Summaries and Full-Text Reports for evidence reports and technology assessments produced under the Agency for Healthcare Research and Quality (AHRQ) Evidence-Based Practice Center (EPC) Program. Access the list of EPC Reports, with links to summaries and/or full-text publications.
■ Glossary provides definitions of terms used in the standardized abstracts (summaries).

AHRQ = Agency for Healthcare Research and Quality; EPC = Evidence-based Practice Center; NGC = National Guideline Clearinghouse; PDA = Personal Digital Assistant. Blue text indicates available Web links on NGC web page. From http://www.guidelines.gov From http://www.guideline.gov/about/about.aspx

Exhibit 15.2

---

**MOST FREQUENTLY ASKED QUESTION: HOW TO FIND A SPECIFIC CLINICAL GUIDELINE? TO DETERMINE WEBSITE QUALITY**

---

*How can I find guidelines on a specific topic?*

- Go to NGC's How to Search and How to Browse pages to learn useful tips on how to search and browse the NGC database for guidelines of interest.
- Type your search term in the Search box accessible on all NGC Web pages to quickly search the database.
- You can also use NGC's Detailed Search feature to perform specific and refined searches of the NGC database. This feature allows you to filter your search by one or more guideline attributes, including methods used to develop the guideline, guideline developer type, and patient material available.
- NGC has also prepared a Frequent Search page to assist NGC users in finding guidelines related to frequently requested topics (Kovacs, 2000).

---

NGC = National Guideline Clearinghouse; blue text indicate available Web link. From http://www.guidelines.gov

---

Public Health Service in 1984 and has been sponsored by AHRQ since 1998. It is the leading independent panel of independent experts in prevention and primary care in the United States. The USPSTF conducts rigorous, impartial assessments of the scientific evidence for the effectiveness of a broad range of clinical preventive services, including screening, counseling, and preventive medications. Its recommendations are considered the gold standard for clinical preventive services. The mission of the USPSTF is to (1) evaluate the benefits of individual services based on age, gender, and risk factors for disease, (2) make specific recommendations about which preventive services should be incorporated routinely into primary medical care and for which populations, (3) identify a research agenda for clinical preventive care (www.ahrq.gov/clinic/uspstfab.htm).

Some researchers have asked how the USPSTF's recommendations differ from those of other professional organizations. As the USPSTF notes on its Web site, USPSTF recommendations are made by a multidisciplinary team of primary care experts that uses a systematic, evidence-based approach to focus on preventive services in the clinical setting. The USPSTF specifically bases its recommendation on a balanced look at the benefits and harms of each preventive service and on the basis of explicit criteria. Recommendations issued by the USPSTF are intended for use in the primary care setting. The USPSTF recommendation statements present health care providers with information about the evidence behind each recommendation, allowing clinicians to make informed decisions about implementation. The USPSTF is supported by an Evidence-Based Practice Center (EPC). Under contract to AHRQ, the EPC conducts systematic reviews of the evidence on specific topics in clinical prevention that serve as the scientific basis for USPSTF recommendations. The USPSTF reviews the evidence, estimates the magnitude of benefits and harms for each preventive service, reaches consensus about the net benefit for each preventive service, and issues a recommendation. The Task Force grades the strength of the evidence for an intervention either "A" (strongly recommends), "B" (recommends), "C" (no recommendation for or against), "D" (recommends against), or "I" (insufficient evidence to recommend for or against).

The USPSTF ceased publishing guidelines in 1996. Most of its existing guidelines were withdrawn from distribution as being out of date in 2000. According to the USPSTF Web site, the guidelines that have been withdrawn have not been, and will not be, updated. The reader is referred to http://www.ahrq.gov/clinic/cpgonline.htm to access the guidelines that are still considered current. The outdated guidelines are archived online at the National Library of Medicine and can be accessed via the AHRQ Internet site at http://www.ahrq.gov/clinic/cpgarchv.htm; however, the reader is cautioned that the information in these guidelines is no longer considered current for practice. For current guidelines for other sources, the reader is advised to visit the NGC Web site. Exhibit 15.3 presents some well-known worldwide resources for finding CPG.

## APPRAISING CLINICAL PRACTICE GUIDELINES

### Possible Problems With Current Clinical Guidelines

Since the late 1980s and early 1990s, CPGs have become increasingly popular and practical tools to assist practitioners, policymakers and payers make clinical and administrative management decisions about patients. So popular and plentiful are CPGs that clinicians may have difficulty choosing from the plethora of available documents of varying quality. The challenge is to select a CPG that contains recommendations that are valid, useful, and based on the best available evidence and that were

Exhibit 15.3

### NATIONAL AND INTERNATIONAL CLINICAL GUIDELINES ORGANIZATIONS AND DATABASES

■ U.S. National Guideline Clearinghouse™ (listing of national and international guideline development organizations); www.guideline.gov/browse/browseorgsbyLtr.aspx?Letter=*
■ National Guideline Clearing House™ (USA) (a public resource for evidence-based clinical practice guidelines); www.guideline.gov/
■ Clinical Practice Guidelines Online, Agency for Healthcare Research and Quality (AHRQ); www.ahrq.gov/clinic/cpgonline.htm
■ Behave Net (directory of guidelines from professional organizations); www.behavenet.com/guidelines.htm
■ Canadian Medical Association Clinical Practice Guidelines Infobase; www.cma.ca/index.cfm/ci_id/121/la_id/1.htm
■ Centres for Health Evidence, Canada, Guideline Advisory Committee ("a joint body of the Ontario Medical Association and the Ontario Ministry of Health and Long-Term Care"); www.cche.net/
■ Registered Nurses' Association of Ontario; www.rnao.org/bestpractices
■ Kementerian Kesihatan Malaysia (Malaysia Ministry of Health); www.moh.gov.my/MohPortal/index.jsp

developed with a sound scientific methodology (Cote & Hayden, 2001). While there is some evidence that guideline-driven care in nursing is effective in improving some processes and outcomes (Thomas et al., 2000), the IOM noted that "Unfortunately, the current processes underlying guideline development are often vulnerable to bias and conflict of interest. Overall, the quality of a CPG is often poor" (IOM, 2008).

Keeping in mind the conceptual framework, which places CPGs within the translation or interpretation domain in the EBP paradigm (IOM, 2001; Stevens, 2004a, 2004b), appraising their value for use should be straightforward, but, as noted by the IOM, it is not. The development of CPG is a highly decentralized process. In the United States, many public and private organizations, such as medical and nursing professional societies, patient advocacy groups, payers, and government agencies, develop CPGs. When multiple groups and multiple processes are used to develop CPGs, there can be inherent problems in the final products available. For example, the NGC currently has 475 guidelines related to hypertension, 408 for heart failure, 298 related to stroke, 221 related to smoking cessation, and 107 for alcohol withdrawal. It is rational to assume that with so many CPGs for similar topics, there probably are variations in the quality and the recommendations included in them. Even considering the multifactorial problems involved with many clinical syndromes, why are so many guidelines needed? More important to the individual practitioners might be this question: How do I appraise the quality of a CPG for my practice?

While much progress has been made regarding strategies to improve the reliability and trustworthiness of the information contained within the available CPGs, is it still not possible to say that there is a standard, scientifically validated process that serves as the basis for the development of CPGs. In its most recent publication, the IOM has recommended that groups developing CPGs or recommendations only use scientifically validated standards, developed and evaluated by the IOM's proposed Program (IOM, 2008). Despite the creditability of the IOM and its *Roadmap for the Nation,* it is anticipated that its Program, if approved, will not be instituted before subsequent editions of this text are available; therefore, tools and strategies currently available for appraising the value of CPGs are presented here.

## Tools for Appraising the Quality of Clinical Practice Guidelines

### Appraisal of Guidelines Research and Evaluation (AGREE)

The first formal and probably most recognized tool available for appraising the quality of CPG is the AGREE instrument. AGREE stands for "Appraisal of Guidelines Research and Evaluation." It originates from an international collaboration of researchers and policymakers who work together to improve the quality and effectiveness of CPGs by establishing a shared framework for their development, reporting, and assessment. Canada, New Zealand, and the United States are AGREE Collaboration participants, as is a core of European countries, including Denmark, Finland, France, Germany, Italy, the Netherlands, Spain, Switzerland, and the United Kingdom. When using the word *quality* regarding CPG, the AGREE collaboration is referring to "the confidence that the potential biases of guideline development have been addressed adequately, and that the recommendations are internally and externally valid, and are feasible for practice" (AGREE Collaboration, 2001).

The AGREE instrument consists of 23 key items within six domains. Each item is rated on a 4-point scale as to the extent to which an item (criterion) has been fulfilled. The responses include 4, "Strongly Agree"; 3, "Agree"; 2, "Disagree"; and 1, "Strongly Disagree." Each domain score is calculated by summing the domain's items and standardizing the total as a percentage of the maximum possible score for that domain. While this may sound a bit complicated at first reading, it is quite simple. Examples of how to calculate domain scores are provided in the AGREE instrument handbook, which may be downloaded at no cost to a computer or personal digital assistant (PDA) or viewed online (AGREE Collaboration, 2001). See Exhibit 15.4 for a description of the AGREE instrument's structure and content domains.

Limitations of the AGREE instrument include the inability to obtain an overall or single quality score. The six domain scores are independent and should not be aggregated into a single quality score. It could be very time consuming to compare scores for several same-topic CPGs, because each CPG would have to be compared across each of the six AGREE domains. The AGREE instrument guide also indicates that it is not possible to set thresholds for the domain scores that might determine a "good" or "bad" guideline. There is, however, a section at the end of the instrument for overall assessment with a series of options, including "Strongly Recommend," "Recommend (with provisos or alterations)," "Would not Recommend," and "Unsure." After considering all the appraisal criteria, the appraiser must then make a judgment as

Exhibit 15.4

### STRUCTURE AND CONTENT DOMAINS OF THE AGREE INSTRUMENT

(1) *Scope and Purpose:* addresses the overall aim of the guideline, the specific clinical questions and the target patient population (3 items).

(2) *Stakeholder Involvement:* focuses on the extent to which the guideline represents the views of its intended users (4 items).

(3) *Development Rigor:* addresses the process used to gather and synthesize the evidence and the methodology used to formulate the recommendations and to update them (7 items).

(4) *Clarity and Presentation:* relates to the language and format of the guideline (4 items).

(5) *Applicability:* Refers to the likely organizational, behavioral and cost implications of applying the guideline (3 items).

(6) *Editorial Independence:* related to the independence of the recommendations and acknowledgement of possible conflict of interest from the guideline development group (2 items).

From The AGREE Collaboration. *Appraisal of Guidelines for Research & Evaluation (AGREE) Instrument* (www.agreecollaboration.org).

to the quality of the guideline in order to complete an overall appraisal. Additionally, a team of two to four appraisers is suggested for each CPG under consideration (AGREE Collaboration, 2001).

## NGC's Brief Summary Feature

Another known CPG appraisal strategy is the use of the NGC's *Brief Summary* feature. The NGC includes structured summaries for each guideline to assist the user in assessing the guideline's quality and explains the rating and levels of evidence used. Similar to quality attributes addressed in the AGREE collaboration instrument (2001) and by Lohr and Field (1992), these NGC Summaries describe a particular guideline's attributes. Referring to the *Criteria for Inclusion of Clinical Practice Guidelines* and the *Guideline Syntheses* feature on the NGC Web site may also be helpful.

## Critically Appraised Topics (CAT)

One last possible strategy is the use of a *Critically Appraised Topic* (CAT). A CAT can be used to evaluate particular sections or interventions addressed within CPGs. While there is no universal Web site for CATs, several sites are available. Not surprisingly, a quick Google search resulted in more than 3,200 possible CAT-related Web addresses.

Peer-to-peer networks for CAT that would allow for sharing of relevant clinical information regarding the most contemporary data on specific clinical problems have been proposed (Castro, et al., 2003). Others, such as Dong and colleagues (2004), are conducting studies to demonstrate ease of use and the validity of a meta-search engine approach related to CAT use. They found that improved clinical decision making resulting from inherent filters underlies the practical usefulness of this type of a tool for clinicians. While the use of CAT may sound appealing, perhaps because it allows someone else (a presumed expert) to appraise an issue for you, caution should be exercised until the standards for the appraisal criteria of CAT are determined. See Exhibit 15.5 for the Internet addresses for resources related to appraising CATs.

## Evidence Grading Systems

Whether or not one chooses to use any of the appraisal methods or strategies presented, it is expected that all prudent practitioners will, at the very least, want to be familiar with levels and/or categories of the

Exhibit 15.5

---

**RESOURCES AND TOOLS FOR GUIDELINE QUALITY APPRAISAL AND EVALUATION**

---

Criteria for Inclusion of Clinical Practice Guidelines in the U.S. National
Guideline Clearinghouse™ (www.guideline.gov/about/inclusion.aspx) and the
Brief Summary feature for each clinical practice guideline of interest.
AGREE Instrument for guideline quality appraisal (http://www.agreecolla
boration.org/)

- Conference on Guideline Standardization (COGS): checklist of components
  of practice guidelines; http://gem.med.yale.edu/cogs/
- Guidelines for the development and implementation of clinical practice
  guidelines (Australia): http://www.nhmrc.gov.au/publications/synopses/
  cp30syn.htm
- Protocure: Improving medical protocols by formal methods http://www.
  protocure.org/
- The G-I-N initiative (Guidelines International Network) for the development
  and implementation of clinical practice guidelines: http://www.g-i-n.net/
- GLIA: instrument for GuideLine Implementability Appraisal; http://www.
  openclinical.org/appInstrument_glia.html

---

evidence rating and grading systems used in any of the CPGs they choose
for practice. While there are no universal grading systems, many, but not
all, professional organizations adopt one evidence grading system for all
the CPGs and position statements they publish.

The American Heart Association (AHA), for example, frequently
publishes guidelines or statements together with other professional societies, such as the American College of Cardiology (ACC). All AHA's
and affiliating organizations' current guidelines adhere to the levels of
evidence and classes of recommendation established by the ACC/AHA
Guidelines Task Force (Gibbons, Smith, & Antman, 2003a, 2003b),
which determines classifications by size of treatment effect. *Class I* interventions are considered useful and effective; *Class II* interventions
have conflicting evidence and/or divergence of opinion about useful-
ness/efficacy (*Class IIa* have the weight of evidence or opinion in favor
of usefulness or efficacy, whereas *Class IIb* interventions have usefulness
or efficacy that is less well established by evidence or opinion); *Class III*
interventions are not recommended and may be harmful. Levels of evidence and estimates of certainty (precision of treatment effect) are also
used and run from level *A* (multiple population risk strata evaluated) to
*C* (very limited population risk strata evaluated).

Two other prominent evidence rating systems found in the literature are the *USPSTF system* (described earlier) and the *Grades of*

*Recommendation Assessment, Development and Evaluation* (GRADE) system (Atkins et al., 2004a, 2004b, 2005; Guyatt et al., 2006; Harris et al., 2001). The USPTF system is considered limited by some because there is no formal mechanism (e.g., a point system) that would allow end users to reproduce these judgments, even though numerous factors are listed that one should consider when making judgments (and narrative text is used to explain these judgments).

The GRADE system was developed to fill the void of a point system. The GRADE system emphasizes study design to set a starting quality grade and then considers other components that may increase or decrease the grade. Four outcome-specific grades can result including "High," "Moderate," "Low," and "Very Low." The American College of Chest Physicians Task Force recently revised the GRADE system to combined "Low'" and "Very Low" into one category, that of "Low" (Guyatt et al., 2006).

Yet another system was proposed in 2006. Treadwell and colleagues (2006) contend that previous evidence rating systems, including GRADE and USPSTF, are largely silent on the role of meta-analysis in systematic reviews. Their proposed system "uses meta-analysis and meta-regression (when clinically appropriate) to increase statistical power and employ precise study weights" (p. 10). Additionally, the system proposed by Treadwell et al. purports to be unique in incorporating the results of these analyses into evidence ratings. However, until (if ever) there is a standardized system of evidence rating, the reader is cautioned to be aware of the particular system being used by each particular guideline of interest.

Most professional organizations use some sort of grading system for their published CPGs and position statements. In almost every situation, the evidence grading system is explained as part of the methodology used in the organization's guideline development. This critical information should be in the preface or in the body of the CPG document itself or perhaps appear somewhere on the organization's Web site. If practitioners come across a guideline for which evidence is not rated (or graded) and/or the rating scheme is not explained, the suggestion is to find another guideline.

## Other Issues

Since the initial appearance of CPGs in the health care literature, aside from the methodological issues discussed earlier, concerns have been raised regarding variations in individual characteristics and clinical settings that may not be addressed in a guideline (Berg, 1998; Cook,

Greengold, Ellrodt, & Weingarten, 1997; Haynes, 1993). Moreover, it is common for there to be different recommendations on the same clinical topic, perhaps because of variations in the composition of the guideline development panels or in the organizations themselves or perhaps just a reflection of varying views on interpretation of the evidence (Berg, Atkins, & Tierney, 1997; Lohr, 1995).

Not to be overlooked is the exponential growth of information in health care that has made it virtually impossible for clinicians to keep up with new developments, even in their own specialty. So it is appropriate to ask how current the CPG being considered is. In 2001, an analysis of the then-current validity of 17 CPG published by AHRQ was conducted, and 13 were found to need updating. A time frame of 3 years for reassessment was suggested (Shekelle et al., 2001).

Another issue that APNs may need to address before implementing a CPG relates to whether the sources of evidence account for the individual patient experience, personal clinical expertise, and policy considerations at their institution. A way to examine these issues is to determine:

1   Similarities between the APN's patients and those addressed in the CPG
2   Feasibility of the treatment under consideration in the setting
3   Patients' values and expectations about the treatment and outcomes (Rycroft-Malone, 2003; Straus, Richardson, Glasziou, & Haynes, 2005).

Haynes (1993) suggested the use of the "three Rs"—*right person,* at the *right time,* in the *right way*—when considering the application of a CPG. Other considerations include ethical concerns regarding recommended treatments such as the utilization of all available resources for patients in specific age groups (Gray, 2005).

## MEDICAL-LEGAL ASPECTS OF USING CLINICAL PRACTICE GUIDELINES

The role that CPGs play in medical malpractice litigation has been a developing area of interest for practitioners and attorneys (Solomon, 2002). In the United States, the heart of clinical negligence lies with the standard of practice, or lack thereof. A central question related to CPGs is whether they can be admitted as evidence of the standard of expected practice or whether they would be considered hearsay or out-of-court statements, with the author(s) not being sworn in or available for cross-examination. Clinical practice guidelines are considered evidentiary and are admissible in U.S. courts if they are qualified as authoritative material or a learned treatise; however, a U.S. Supreme Court decision (*Daubert v. Merrell Dow Pharmaceuticals,* 1993) may encourage judges to critically evaluate the motivation and rationale behind the CPG before accepting its evidential value.

Few published data are available on the actual use of CPGs in litigation. Hyams and colleagues (1995, 1996) reviewed 259 claims from two liability insurance companies. They found only 17 cases, or 7%, involved CPGs; 12 of the CPGs were introduced by the plaintiff, 4 by the defense, and 1 was undetermined. Additionally, this study surveyed attorneys from all 50 states; 399 of 980 responded. Of those responding, 48% reported that they had at least one case per year in which CPGs played some role, but only 36% said they had only one case annually in which a CPG played an important role. Additionally, 31% reported refusing to take at least one case within the preceding 3 years because the physician (defendant) had followed established CPGs in caring for the patient (plaintiff). Last, only 22% indicated that they perceived that the judge or jury had been influenced by a CPG in at least one case in the previous year. These finding suggest that CPGs do not have, or at least have not had in the past decade, an overwhelming impact on case outcomes. Most of the responding attorneys considered the CPG as a double-edged sword, and issues surrounding CPG, for either defense or plaintiffs' arguments, remain somewhat ambiguous.

A practitioner defendant may not necessarily have an adverse outcome if he or she did not follow an established CPG. In the case of a treating physician who had arbitrarily deviated from the AHA's guideline for advanced cardiac life support (ACLS) by administering atropine rather than epinephrine, an appellate court affirmed judgment for the defendant. The defense argued that the use of CPGs was not mandatory and therefore could be overridden by clinical judgment in an individual case (*Lowry v. Henry Mayo Newhall Memorial Hospital,* 1986).

Conversely, a practitioner defendant may not necessarily be exonerated because he adhered to a CPG. Courts in the United States, although acknowledging that a CPG may be relevant, can determine the standard of practice from other sources of information, such as an institution's own policies and procedures and expert evidence (*Denton Regional Medical*

*Center v. Lacroix,* 1997). In another, much older case, the plaintiff appealed a judgment that favored an ophthalmologist, arguing that the customary standard of care that was presented was inadequate and therefore unreasonable. The Washington Supreme Court refused to be bound by the widely endorsed CPGs upon which the defendant based his standard practice defense, demonstrating that there is no absolute judicial deference to compliance with CPGs (*Helling v. Carey,* 1974).

It is not known whether the increasing medical evidence and CPGs will be a help or a hindrance to the courts. Perhaps better evidence might make it easier for juries and judges to make more accurate courtroom decisions in technically difficult cases. On the other hand, inconsistent, conflicting CPGs might muddy the water even further.

While sound professional medical and nursing judgments will always be necessary, the use of empirical evidence as to what works and what doesn't should be maximized. Synthesized available scientific data in the form of a critically appraised CPG may assist practitioners to apply their best clinical judgment. Benefits may then flow to the legal system, as well, allowing for more accurate dispute resolutions about the appropriateness of health care decisions (Roscoff, 2001).

## SUMMARY

As defined by the IOM, "clinical practice guidelines are systematically developed statements to assist practitioner and patient decisions about appropriate health care for specific clinical circumstances" (IOM, 1990). The APN should be aware that CPGs are not cookie cutter or medical/ nursing cookbooks with exact recipes for health care; they should support the conscientious, explicit, and judicious use of current best evidence by practitioners who exercise appropriate clinical judgment with regard to each individual patient.

There are multiple national and international Internet sites available to help practitioners locate clinical guidelines. One of the most comprehensive is the NGC database, at http://www.guidelines.gov. Additionally, there are multiple tools available for use by the APN to critically appraise CPGs, including the AGREE instrument and CATS. Regardless of which appraisal tool a practitioner chooses to use, the practitioner should know the evidence rating or grading system used by a particular guideline before implementing any interventions suggested in that guideline.

In the United States, the past use of CPGs in medical malpractice litigation has been considered a double-edged sword. Improvements in existing and conflicting CPGs, coupled with sound medical and nursing judgment, may positively affect medical-legal decision making in the future.

## SUGGESTED ACTIVITIES

1  Pick a clinical topic of interest to you.
2  Search the NGC Web site for a current CPG; more than likely, you will find more than one. (Hint: Use Exhibit 15.2 and perhaps the advanced search function.)
3  If you find multiple CPGs for your topic, do a comparison of the available CPGs to decide which one best fits your clinical population. (Hint: Use the comparison function on the NGC site to accomplish this.)
4  Now, download the AGREE collaboration instrument.
5  Next, critically appraise and score the domains of the CPG you selected.
6  Briefly describe your appraisal of your chosen guideline. Would you recommend its implementation at your practice site? If not, why not?

## REFERENCES

AGREE Collaboration. (2001). Appraisal of guidelines for research and evaluation (AGREE) instrument. Retrieved February 1, 2008 from http://www.agreecollaboration.org

Atkins, D., Best, D., Briss, P.A., Eccles, M., Falck-Ytter, Y., Flottorp, S., et al. (2004a). Grading quality of evidence and strength of recommendations. *British Medical Journal, 328*(7457), 1490; retrieved December 16, 2008, from http://bmj.bmjjournals.com/cgi/reprint/328/7454/1490

Atkins, D., Briss, P. A., Eccles, M., Flottorp, S., Guyatt, G. H., Harbour, R. T., et al. (2005). GRADE Working Group: Systems for grading the quality of evidence and the strength of recommendations II: Pilot study of a new system. *BMC Health Service Research, 5*(1), 25.

Atkins, D., Eccles, M., Flottorp, S., Guyatt, G. H., Henry, D., Hill, S., et al. (2004b). GRADE Working Group: Systems for grading the quality of evidence and the strength of recommendations I: Critical appraisal of existing approaches. The GRADE Working Group. *BMC Health Service Research, 4*(1), 38.

Berg, A. O. (1998). Dimensions of evidence. *Journal of the American Board of Family Practice, 11,* 216–223.

Berg, A. O., Atkins, D. J., & Tierney, W. (1997). Clinical practice guidelines in practice and education. *Journal of General Internal Medicine, 12* (Suppl. 2), S25–S33.

Castro, J., Wolf, F., Karras, B., Tolentino, H., Marcelo, A., & Maramba, I. (2003). Critically appraised topics (CAT) peer-to-peer network. Annual Symposium proceedings [electronic resource] / AMIA Symposium 2003, p.806.

Cook, D. J., Greengold, N. L., Ellrodt, G., & Weingarten, S. R. (1997). The relation between systematic reviews and practice guidelines. *Annals of Internal Medicine, 127,* 210–216.

Cote, P., & Hayden, J. (2001). Clinical practice guidelines: The dangerous pitfalls of avoiding methodological rigor. *Journal of the Canadian Chiropractic Association, 45*(3), 154–155.

*Daubert v. Merrell Dow Pharmaceuticals, Inc., 509,* U.S. 579 (1993).

*Denton Regional Medical Center v. Lacroix* (1997), 947 SW 2D941 (Tex. Appeal).

Dong, P., Wong, L., Ng, S., Loh, M., & Mondry, A. (2004). Quantitative evaluation of recall and precision of CAT Crawler, a search engine specialized on retrieval of Critically Appraised Topics. *BMC Medical Informatics and Decision Making, 4*(21), 1–7.

Gibbons, R., Smith, Jr., S. C., & Antman, E. (2003a). American College of Cardiology/ American Heart Association clinical practice guidelines, part 1: Where do they come from? Circulation, *107,* 2979–2986.

Gibbons, R., Smith, Jr., S. C., & Antman, E. (2003b). American College of Cardiology/American Heart Association clinical practice guidelines, part II: Evolutionary changes in a continuous quality improvement project. *Circulation, 107,* 3101.

Gray, J. A. (2005). Evidence-based and value-base healthcare. *Evidence-based Healthcare and Public Health, 9,* 317–318.

Guyatt, G., Gutterman, D., Baumann, M. H., Addrizzo-Harris, D., Hylek, E. M., Phillips, B., et al. (2006). Grading strength of recommendations and quality of evidence in clinical guidelines: Report from an American College of Chest Physicians Task Force. *CHEST, 129*(1), 174–181.

Harris, R. P., Helfand, M., Woolf, S. H., Lohr, K. N., Mulrow, C. D., Teutsch, S. M., et al. (2001). Current methods of the U.S. Preventive Services Task Force: A review of the process. *American Journal of Preventative Medicine, 20*(Suppl. 3), 21–35.

Haynes, R. B. (1993). Some problems in applying evidence in clinical practice. *Annals of the New York Academy of Sciences, 703,* 210–224.

*Helling v. Carey* (1974). 83 Washington State. 2d 514, 519 P. 2d 981.

Hyams, A., Brandenburg, J., Lopsitz, S., Shapiro, D., & Brennan, T. (1995) Practice guidelines in malpractice litigation: A two way street. *Annals of Internal Medicine, 122, 150–433.*

Hyams, A. L., Shapiro, D. W., & Brennan, T. A. (1996). Medical practice guidelines in malpractice litigation: An early retrospective. *Journal of Health Politics, Policy and Law, 21*(2), 289–313.

Institute of Medicine (IOM). (1990). *Clinical Practice Guidelines: Directions for a new program.* Ed. M. J. Field and K.N Lohr. Washington, DC: National Academies Press.

Institute of Medicine (IOM). (1999). *To Err Is Human: Building a Safer Health System.* Ed. L. Kohn, J. M Corrigan, & M.S. Donaldson. Washington, DC: National Academies Press.

Institute of Medicine (IOM). (2001). *Crossing the Quality Chasm: A New Health System for the 21st Century.* Washington, DC: National Academies Press.

Institute of Medicine (IOM), Committee on Reviewing Evidence to Identify Highly Effective Clinical Services Board on Health Care Services. (2008). In J. Eden, B. Wheatley, B. McNeil, & H. Sox (Eds.), *Knowing what works in health care: A Roadmap for the Nation.* Washington, DC: National Academies Press.

Jadad, A. R., Moher, M., Browman, G. P., Booker, L., Sigouin, C., Fuentes, M., et al. (2000). Systematic reviews and meta-analyses on treatment of asthma: Critical evaluation. *British Medical Journal, 320*(7234), 537–540.

Lohr, K. N. (1995). Guidelines for clinical practice: What they are and why they count. *Journal of Law and Medical Ethics, 23*(1), 49–51.

Lohr, K.N., & Field, M. J. (1992). A provisional instrument for assessing clinical practice guidelines. In M. J. Field & K. N. Lohr (Eds.), *Guidelines for clinical practice: From development to use.* Washington DC: National Academies Press.

*Lowry v. Henry Mayo Newhall Memorial Hospital* (1986), 229 Cal. Reports RPTR 620.

Roscoff, A. (2001). Evidence-based medicine and the law: The courts confront clinical practice guidelines. *Journal of Health Politics, Policy and Law, 26*(2), 327–368.

Rycroft-Malone, J. (2003). Consider the evidence. *Nursing Standard, 17*(45), 21.

Sackett, D. L., Rosenberg, W. M., Gray, J., Haynes, R. B., & Richardson, W.S. (1996). Evidence based medicine: What it is and what it isn't. *BMJ, 312,* 71–72.

Shekelle, P. G., Ortiz, E., Rhodes, S., Morton, S. C., Eccles, M. P., Grimshaw, J. M., et al. (2001). Validity of the Agency for Healthcare Research and Quality clinical practice guidelines: How quickly do guidelines become outdated? *Journal of the American Medical Association, 286*(12), 1461–1467.

Solomon, R. P. (2002). Clinical guidelines in the United States: Perspective on law and litigation. In J. Tingle & C. Foster (Eds.), *Clinical Guidelines: Law, Policy, and Practice.* London: Cavendish.

Stevens, K. R. (2004a). *ACE Star Model of EBP: The Cycle of Knowledge Transformation.* Retrieved December 12, 2008, from http://www.acestar.uthscsa.edu/Learn_model.htm

Stevens, K. R. (2004b). *ACE Star Model of EBP: Knowledge Transformation.* San Antonio: Academic Center for Evidence-Based Practice, University of Texas Health Science Center at San Antonio. Retrieved December 12, 2008, from http://www.acestar.uthscsa.edu

Straus, E. P., Richardson, W. S., Glasziou, P., & Haynes, R. B. (2005). *Evidence-based medicine: How to practice and teach EBM* (3rd ed.). Edinburgh: Elsevier.

Thomas, L., Cullum, M., McColl, E., Rousseau, N., Soutter, J., & Steen, N. (2000). Guidelines in professions allied to medicine. *Cochrane Database of Systematic Reviews,* No. CD000349.

Treadwell, J. R., Tregear, S. J., Reston, J. T., & Turkelson, C. M. (2006). A system for rating the stability and strength of medical evidence. *BMC Medical Research Methodology, 6,* 52, [doi:10.1186/1471–2288–6-52]. Retrieved February 1, 2008, from http://www.biomedcentral.com/1471–2288/6/52

West, S., King, V., Carey, T., Lohr, K., McCoy, N., Sutton, S., et al. (2002). Systems to rate the strength of scientific evidence. Evidence Report/Technology Assessment No. 47. (Prepared by the Research Triangle Institute-University of North Carolina Evidence-Based Practice Center under Contract No. 290–97–0011). AHRQ Publication No 02-E016. Rockville, MD: Agency for Healthcare Research and Quality.

# 16 Program Evaluation

MARITA G. TITLER

The use of program evaluation has grown rapidly to meet the obligation to provide effective services, make subsequent decisions about continuing specific programs, and improve future programming (Posavac & Carey, 2007; Shadish, Jr., Cook, & Leviton, 1995). Program evaluation has its roots in sociology, education, public health, and other related fields (Shadish, Jr., Cook, & Leviton, 1995; Sufflebeam & Shinkfield, 2007). As a type of research, program evaluation helps society and those responsible for various social and service programs to understand the context of the program (e.g., schools, primary care) and whether the program meets goals and objectives. At first glance, program evaluation appears simple. However, entire books, collegiate courses, and doctoral programs focus on program evaluation theories, methods, and models (Sufflebeam & Shinkfield, 2007). Although it is beyond the scope of this chapter to provide a comprehensive understanding of program evaluation, the reader can gain basic knowledge about the process and stimulate his or her interest in learning more, especially about the principles and steps of program evaluation and their application to health care. The reader is referred to several excellent resources on this topic in this regard (American Evaluation Association, 2008a; Centers for Disease Control Evaluation Working Group, 2008; Holden & Zimmerman, 2008; Posavac & Carey, 2007; Shadish, Jr., Cook, & Leviton, 1995; Spaulding,

2008; Sufflebeam & Shinkfield, 2007; W. K. Kellogg Foundation, 2008; Western Michigan University Evaluation Center, 2008).

Application of program evaluation to health care is essential as economic resources for new clinical programs shrink and the viability and impact of existing programs are questioned. Examples of areas in health care subject to program evaluation include case management, health education, faculty practice, hospital-based nursing orientation, school-based health centers, tobacco cessation programs, pregnancy prevention, hospital-based pain management programs, and hospital-based fall prevention programs (Barkauskas et al., 2004; Becker et al., 2007; Chan, Mackenzie, Tin-Fu, & Ka-yi Leung, 2000; Cramer, Mueller, & Harrop, 2003; Dykeman, MacIntosh, Seaman, & Davidson, 2003; Hackbarth & Gall, 2005; Hulton, 2007; Jacobson Vann, 2006; Logan, Boutotte, Wilce, & Etkind, 2003; Menix, 2007; Meyer & Meyer, 2000). These studies have used various frameworks and methods, but common across them were two goals: to analyze new or existing programs within a specific social context (e.g., school setting, hospital, community) to produce information for evaluating the programs' effectiveness and to use this information to make decisions about program refinement, revisions, and/or continuation.

## OVERVIEW AND PRINCIPLES OF PROGRAM EVALUATION

Program evaluation is defined as the systematic collection, analysis, and reporting of descriptive and judgmental information about the merit and worth of a program's goals, design, process, and outcomes to address improvement and accountability and to increase understanding of the phenomenon (Posavac & Carey, 2007; Sufflebeam & Shinkfield, 2007). A distinguishing feature of program evaluation is that it examines programs—a set of specific activities designed for an intended purpose and that has quantifiable goals and objectives. Because programs come in a variety of shapes and sizes, the models and methods for evaluating them are also varied (Sufflebeam & Shinkfield, 2007).

A number of different models of program evaluation are available and are briefly summarized in Table 16.1 (Posavac & Carey, 2007; Sufflebeam & Shinkfield, 2007).

There is no clear consensus or agreement about use of any one model in program evaluation. An overriding principle in selecting a model is to understand completely the program that is being evaluated, the context

Table 16.1

## OVERVIEW OF SELECTED MODELS FOR PROGRAM EVALUATION

| MODEL | DESCRIPTION | CONSIDERATIONS |
|---|---|---|
| Objective-based | Uses objectives written by the creators of the program and the evaluator. The objectives depict the overarching purpose of the evaluation and guide the type of information to be used in the evaluation. This approach includes an emphasis on and an evaluation based on the stated program goals and objectives. Evaluation data collection activities stem from the objectives. | Most prevalent model used for program evaluation. Some evaluators become so focused on the objectives that that they neglect to examine why programs succeed or fail, to consider any additional positive effects or undesired side effects of the program, or to ask whether the program objectives were the best ones for the people served. |
| Goal-free evaluation | Assumption is that evaluators work more effectively if they do not know the goals of a program. Considerable effort is spent studying the program as administered, the staff, the clients, the setting, and records to identify all positive and negative impacts of the program. The program staff and funders decide whether evaluation findings demonstrate that the program meets the needs of the clients. | This approach is expensive, and the rather open-ended nature may be threatening to staff. Projects that receive funding are required to show specific outcomes based on objectives, and, if the outcomes are not included in the evaluation, the appropriate data may not be collected. |
| Expert-oriented model | The focus is on the evaluator as a content expert carefully examines a program to render a judgment about its quality. The evaluators judge a program or service on the basis of an established set of criteria as well as their own expertise in the area. Some decisions are based on objective quantified information as well as on qualitative impressions. This approach is often used when the entity being evaluated is large, complex, and unique. | Agencies that grant accreditation to institutions, programs, or services send program evaluators to the sites to conduct an expert-oriented evaluation. Examples include health care accrediting bodies and accrediting agencies for specific health care programs such as organ transplant programs. Issues include specificity of criteria, interpretation of criteria by various experts, and level of content expertise of the evaluator. |

*(Continued)*

Table 16.1

**OVERVIEW OF SELECTED MODELS FOR PROGRAM EVALUATION** (CONTINUED)

| MODEL | DESCRIPTION | CONSIDERATIONS |
| --- | --- | --- |
| Naturalistic model | A naturalist evaluation is used to develop a deep and thorough understanding of a program. The evaluator becomes the data gather, using a variety of observation and qualitative techniques. By personally observing all phases of the program and holding detailed conversations with stakeholders, the evaluator attempts to gain a rich understanding of the program, its clients, and the social environment and setting. | Because of the detail included, reports often become quite lengthy. The advantage is that personal observations are often necessary to understand the meaning of numerical information about the program. |
| Participative-oriented model | Evaluators seek to involve program participants in the evaluation of the program. Evaluators invite stakeholders to participate actively in the evaluation and gain skills from the experience. Participants may develop instruments, analyze data, and report findings. | This requires close contact with community stakeholders. Some argue that this approach can compromise the validity of the evaluation. The potential benefits are that the stakeholders may be more likely to enact recommendations and that the process for improvement may take less time. |
| Improvement-focused model | Evaluators adopt an explicit assumption that program improvement is the focus of the evaluation. Evaluators help program staff discover discrepancies between program objectives and the needs of the target population, between program implementation and program plans, and between expectations of the target population and the services actually delivered. Objective information is needed, but this information should be interpreted using qualitative information, as well. Evaluators look for strengths of the program (merit and worth) and ways that the program may fall short of its goals and thus require improvement. | This approach tends to lead to an integrated understanding of the program and its effects. Some experts believe that an improvement-focused approach best meets the criteria necessary for effective evaluation. To carry out this evaluation off without threatening the staff is challenging. |

*(Continued)*

Table 16.1

| OVERVIEW OF SELECTED MODELS FOR PROGRAM EVALUATION (CONTINUED) | | |
| --- | --- | --- |
| MODEL | DESCRIPTION | CONSIDERATIONS |
| Success case model | Detailed information is sought from those who benefit most from the program. | Applied naively, this approach could lead to program managers tailoring programs to those most likely to succeed, rather than those most in need of the program. |
| Theory-driven model | Evaluations are based on a careful description of the service to be offered in the program (individuals in need), and the way the program is expected to change the participants and the outcomes to be achieved are specified. Analysis consists of discovering the relationships among (1) the services and characteristics of the participants, (2) the services and immediate changes, and (3) immediate changes and outcome variables. | Complex correlation techniques are used to analyze data and relationships. Qualitative understanding of the program may be ignored in place of quantitative approaches. This may require resources and expertise that are not available or funded. |

and history of the program, the intended purpose of undertaking a program evaluation, and the time, expertise, and resources required for conducting a program evaluation (Billings, 2000; Hackbarth & Gall, 2005; Posavac & Carey, 2007; Shadish, Jr., Cook, & Leviton, 1995; Spaulding, 2008; Sufflebeam & Shinkfield, 2007). Selection of an evaluation model should consider the needs of stakeholders who will use the evaluation results; evaluators should look for a program that will help organize the evaluation and yield the most useful information for various stakeholders (Hackbarth & Gall, 2005).

Of particular interest in health care is the Centers for Disease Control (CDC) model of program evaluation that was set forth to ensure that amid the complex transitions in health care, program directors, funders, and leaders remain accountable and committed to achieving measurable health outcomes (Billings, 2000; CDC Evaluation Working Group, 2008; Logan, Boutotte, Wilce, & Etkind, 2003). This framework, illustrated in Figure 16.1, is a practical, nonprescriptive tool, designed to summarize

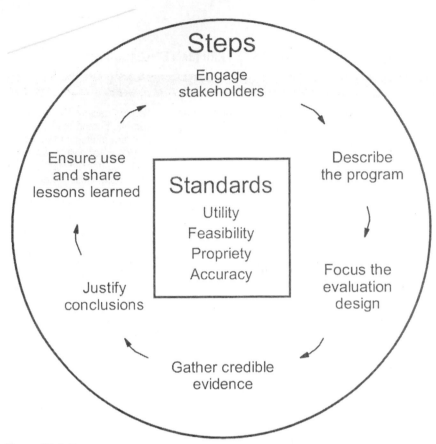

**Figure 16.1** Recommended framework for program evaluation.
From "Framework for Program Evaluation," by Centers for Disease Control, 1999. *MMWR, 48*
(RR-11). Retrieved from http://www.cdc.gov/eval/framework.htm#graphic

and organize the essential elements of program evaluation. The framework includes recommended steps in evaluation and standards for effective evaluation. The framework is a starting point for tailoring a program
evaluation, particularly for a public health effort at a particular time.

## Standards of Program Evaluation

Program evaluations are expected to meet specific standards based on
four fundamental concepts: utility, feasibility, propriety, and accuracy.
These concepts and related standards are central to the CDC model and
are from the Joint Committee on Standards for Educational Evaluation
(Sufflebeam & Shinkfield, 2007).

In brief, *utility* refers to the usefulness of an evaluation for those persons or groups involved with or responsible for implementing the program. Evaluators should ascertain the users' information needs and report the findings to them clearly, concisely, and on time. The general underlying principle of utility is that program evaluations should effectively address the information needs of clients and other audiences with a right to know and inform program improvement processes. If there is no prospect that the findings of a contemplated evaluation will be used, the evaluation should not be done.

Program evaluation should employ procedures that are *feasible*, parsimonious, and operable in the program's environment without disrupting or impairing the program. Feasibility also addresses the control of political forces that may impede or corrupt the evaluation. Feasibility standards require evaluations to be realistic, prudent, diplomatic, politically viable, frugal, and cost effective.

Evaluations should meet conditions of *propriety*. They should be grounded in clear, written agreements that define the obligations of the evaluator and the client with regard to supporting and executing the evaluation and protecting the rights and dignity of all involved. In general, the propriety standards require that evaluations be conducted legally, ethically, and with due regard for the welfare of those involved in the evaluation and those affected by the results.

*Accuracy* includes standards that require evaluators to describe the program as it was planned and executed, the background of the program, and the setting and to report valid and reliable findings. This fundamental concept and related standard requires that evaluators obtain sound information, analyze it correctly, report justifiable conclusions, and note any pertinent caveats (Sufflebeam & Shinkfield, 2007).

## Guiding Principles

In addition to these fundamental concepts and related standards of evaluation, the American Evaluation Association has set forth Guiding Principles for Evaluators intended to guide the professional practice of evaluators and to inform evaluation clients and the general public about the principles they can expect to be upheld by professional evaluators (American Evaluation Association, 2008b). These principles focus on the following areas and are fully detailed at the Association's Web site:

1   *Systematic inquiry:* Evaluators conduct systematic, data-based inquiries about whatever is being evaluated.

2   *Competence:* Evaluators provide competent performance to stakeholders.

3   *Integrity and honesty:* Evaluators ensure the honesty and integrity of the entire evaluation process.

4   *Respect for people:* Evaluators respect the security, dignity and self-worth of the respondents, program participants, clients, and other stakeholders with whom they interact.

5   *Responsibilities for general and public welfare:* Evaluators articulate and take into account the diversity of interests and values that may be related to the general and public welfare.

## FORMATIVE AND SUMMATIVE EVALUATION

*Formative and summative evaluations* are common components of program evaluation. Experts have noted that the role of formative evaluation is to assist in developing and implementing programs, whereas summative evaluation is used to judge the value of the program. It is not the nature of the collected data that determines whether an evaluation is formative or summative but the purpose for which the data are used (Sufflebeam & Shinkfield, 2007). Data for summative and formative evaluation can be *qualitative* and/or *quantitative* in nature; the former is a nonnumerical (e.g., narrative, observation) approach (quality), whereas the latter is a numerical or statistical approach (quantity).

## Formative Evaluation

Formative evaluations are used to assess, monitor, and report on the development and progress of implementing a program (Stetler et al., 2006; Sufflebeam & Shinkfield, 2007; Wyatt, Krauskopf, & Davidson, 2008). This type of evaluation offers guidance to those who are responsible for ensuring and improving the program's quality and is directed at improving operations. A well-planned and executed formative evaluation helps ensure that the purpose of the program is well defined, its goals are realistic, and its variables of interest are measurable. In addition, formative evaluation focuses on the proper training of staff that will be involved in the program implementation. During this evaluation phase, data are collected that serve to monitor the project's activities. The evaluator should interact closely with program staff, and the evaluation plan needs to be flexible and responsive to the development and implementation of the program.

As an example of formative evaluation, we will perform such an evaluation of a hypothetical pulmonary rehabilitation program. As part of the initial implementation of a pulmonary rehabilitation program, it is important that a final decision be made during the program's planning phase about the overall purpose of the program and its component parts (see Table 16.2).

The knowledge and skills of the personnel regarding the components and purpose of the program need to be assessed. For example, a pulmonary clinical nurse specialist can provide oversight for program development and implementation, including working with physical therapists, respiratory therapists, and physicians in making decisions regarding program personnel qualifications, program location, referral base for patients, the time frame for program implementation, and the projected outcomes that are used to assess the program's effectiveness.

### Key Aspects of Formative Evaluations

Delineate phases of the program and time frame for each phase.

Assess staff perceptions of program implementation to help determine how well the program runs.

Examine referral of patients into the program and whether patient enrollment is upheld.

Obtain feedback about the program from patients.

Continually feed information back to program staff and clients of the program as appropriate for the purpose of improving program planning and implementation.

## Summative Evaluation

A summative evaluation, unlike a formative evaluation, focuses on measuring the general effectiveness or success of the program by examining its outcomes. A summative evaluation includes information about whether the clinical program reached its intended goals and upheld its purpose and whether the intervention produced unanticipated

Table 16.2

### EXAMPLE OF FORMATIVE EVALUATION IN PULMONARY REHABILITATION PROGRAM

| | |
|---|---|
| Planning phase | ■ *Purpose of the Program:* To improve activity level, to reduce symptomatology, and to decrease health care resource use among patients with chronic obstructive pulmonary disease (COPD). |
| | ■ *Components of the Clinical Program:* To implement a pulmonary rehabilitation program in which physicians, clinical nurses, physical therapists, and occupational therapists collaborate to facilitate increasing activity tolerance among COPD patients through an outpatient rehabilitation program. The patients are required to learn and perform program exercises on an outpatient basis; perform these activities at home on their own or with the assistance of a friend or spouse; receive patient education about oxygen use, medication use, and management of symptoms; monitor their oxygen use; rate their ability to perform self-care behaviors; monitor their medication use; and rate their functional status on a continuing basis. |
| | ■ *Program Protocol:* Delineate the requirements of patients and the duties of staff to implement successfully the pulmonary rehabilitation program. This protocol should also include the plan for staff training and data collection and quality improvement methods. This protocol must also be clear to the staff involved in implementing the program. The patients must be clear on what is required for their participation in the rehabilitation program. |
| Imple-mentation phase | ■ *Evaluate Staff Training Program:* Examine how staff are trained to follow the program protocol, how to answer patient questions, and ways to ensure patient adherence to the program. Staff need to be trained in the correct methods of increasing activity tolerance among COPD patients, in educating patients on how to monitor their medication use and oxygen use, and in rating levels of functional status and ability to manage self-care behaviors. |
| | ■ *Process Variables:* Assess how well the program protocol is being implemented. Measure timeline and frequencies for patient recruitment into the program, determine whether number of staff involved in the program is sufficient, run focus groups or use interviews or diary data with patients and staff to determine any problems with the program implementation, and determine the barriers to efficient running of the program. Most important, determine the level of adherence of patients to their exercise requirements, their self-monitoring requirements, and their self-rating requirements, and determine the level of adherence among staff to guidelines presented to them in the program protocol. By using direct observation techniques, the evaluator can determine how well staff and patients are interacting during the outpatient phase of the program, how well the staff are collaborating to increase activity tolerance among the participating patients, and track other process variables of interest. |

outcomes; it can also compare the effectiveness of the program with that of other, similar interventions (Posavac & Carey, 2007). This type of evaluation is conducted once the changes suggested by a formative evaluation have been made and the program is completed. Summative evaluations serve to compare the effectiveness of the different treatment programs, if more than one is implemented, or to make comparisons among the "treatment" group (e.g., those enrolled in the pulmonary rehabilitation program) and a natural comparison group (e.g., those not enrolled in rehabilitation). Comparisons can also be made over time to determine the relative influence of the program at different stages. In other words, the summative evaluation also seeks to determine the long-term and lasting effects on patients of having participated in the program (Posavac & Carey, 2007; Sufflebeam & Shinkfield, 2007).

Formative and summative evaluations can be further understood in terms of *process* and *outcome*. Process refers to *how* the program is run or *how* the program reaches its desired results. A formative evaluation is process focused and requires a detailed description of the operating structure required for a successful clinical program. Outcome refers to the success of a program and the effects that it has on cost and quality of care. Outcomes can be individualized, showing the effects of the program on each of the program's clients. The evaluator in this instance seeks to determine the impact of the program on the personal lives of those involved. Outcomes can also be program based, examining the success of the program on an organizational level and determining its overall impact. These program-based outcomes are often examined in terms of their fiscal impact or success through a comparison between the clinical program and other similar programs.

## USE OF QUALITATIVE AND QUANTITATIVE DATA

*Qualitative* and *quantitative* data are both useful for program evaluations. Qualitative data, with their rich and narrative quality, provide an understanding of the impact of the program for individuals enrolled in the program. The descriptive nature of qualitative data allows one to understand the operating structure of a program and the individualized outcomes of a successful program. On the other hand, quantitative data, with their strictly numerical nature, provide statistical significance levels

and power and allow a mathematical understanding of the factors involved in a program. In addition, quantitative data provide frequency
counts and means or averages for the variables of interest. The statistical nature of quantitative data allows others to understand the overall
programmatic outcomes and makes possible direct comparisons among
clients and between program groups (if there is more than one). Most
often, evaluators and clinicians have tended to use only one of these
approaches, neglecting the beneficial provisions of the other. The two
forms of data are not necessarily at odds but instead should be used in
combination, since each supplements the weaknesses inherent in the
other. For qualitative data, direct observation and description are emphasized, as these lead to a form of discovery or an understanding of
how program factors relate on an individual or client level. Qualitative
methods also provide some insight into the context in which the program is delivered. Quantitative data tend to rely upon standardized instrumentation and variable control and provide numerical figures that
depict level of program success.

Triangulation is one way that both qualitative and quantitative data
can be incorporated into a program evaluation. Denzin (1978) has described four forms of triangulation:

1   Evaluator triangulation is the use of several program staff mem-
    bers who have direct client interaction in order to reduce any
    bias that may be introduced by using a single staff member for
    the interactions.
2   Perspective or theory triangulation is the use of various perspec-
    tives to interpret the evaluator's results.
3   Method triangulation is the use of different methods on the part
    of the evaluator to evaluate the program.
4   Data triangulation is the collection of various types of data that
    seek to answer the same questions.

Data triangulation is the type most often used in program evaluations. In order to determine effectively the success of a clinical program,
evaluators must measure and utilize several forms of data. For instance,
the evaluator can gather information from patient medical records, self-
reports made by staff and patients or a spouse, and direct observations.
By combining various types of data that seek to answer the same questions, the evaluator allows the strength in one source of data to support
the weakness in another data source (Denzin, 1978).

## STEPS IN PROGRAM EVALUATION

### Overview

Program evaluation should not focus solely on *proving* whether a program or initiative works, rather than on *improving* the program. Historically, the emphasis on the positivist scientific approach and on proving that programs work has created an imbalance in human service evaluation work—with a heavy emphasis on proving that programs work through the use of quantitative, impact designs and not enough attention to more naturalistic, qualitative designs aimed at improving programs (W. K. Kellogg Foundation, 2008). Program evaluation should consider a more pluralistic approach that includes a variety of perspectives such as whether the program works, how can it be improved, why it works or does not work, what context factors may impact the implementation and effectiveness of the program, and what are the strengths and areas for program improvement.

### Internal and External Evaluators

There are two primary ways that evaluators can relate to organizations seeking program evaluations. First, the evaluator can work for the organization and do a variety of evaluations in that setting. Second, evaluators can work for a research firm, university, or a government agency and be contracted to evaluate a specific program. The affiliation of an evaluator has implications for program evaluations; relevant considerations include the evaluator's competence and personal qualities and purpose of the evaluation (Posavac & Carey, 2007).

Factors related to competence include knowledge about the program, technical expertise, and expertise related to the type of program being evaluated. Internal evaluators have an advantage regarding knowledge of the program and have better access to program directors and administrators. A person who is physically present is likely to see the program in action, know the staff, and learn about the program from others in the organization. The more the evaluator knows about the actual program, the easier it is to ask relevant questions about the planning and interpretation of evaluation findings. The technical expertise of an evaluator is important. An external evaluator can often draw upon the resources of a greater number of individuals with expertise in various methods, such as qualitative methods, sampling techniques, and statistics, whereas an internal evaluator may have access to fewer individuals and less expertise in certain methods. Additionally, an internal evaluator may be expected to perform evaluations in a variety of different areas of an organization but may have limited content expertise or experience with some of the services being evaluated. This can limit the evaluator's insight into crucial issues in some programs. By selecting an external evaluator with content expertise or experience in the type of program being evaluated (e.g., perioperative services, case management), organizations may avoid potential errors related to inexperience.

Personal qualities such as trustworthiness, objectivity, sensitivity, and commitment to program improvement are important for program evaluation. These personal qualities may vary depending on whether the evaluator is internal or external to the organization. For example, an internal evaluator might be expected to have a higher degree of commitment to improving the program and may be trusted by program staff and administrators. In contrast, an external evaluator may be perceived as more objective and may find it easier to elicit important information. Some internal evaluators may have institutional credibility and be known as trustworthy, which influences the ability of the evaluator to carry out an evaluation. Developing a reputation for tackling sensitive issues is easier when evaluators emphasize that most program limitations are due to system issues rather than personal inadequacies among program staff. Regardless of whether the evaluator is internal or external to the organization, personal qualities of the evaluator are important considerations in program evaluations.

The purpose of the evaluation may provide some guidance to those who must decide whether to use an internal or an external evaluator. Although both internal and external evaluators can perform all types of evaluation, internal evaluators may have an advantage in performing formative evaluations because of existing positive relationships with managers and staff. These relationships can contribute to nondefensive communications between evaluator and staff, which are essential if recommendations to improve programs are to be set forth. In contrast, if a summative evaluation is the main purpose and the need to decide whether to continue, expand, or discontinue an existing program is the reason for the evaluation, an external evaluator may be more appropriate (Posavac & Carey, 2007).

## Initial Communication

When the evaluation is being conducted in an applied setting involving potentially sensitive issues (e.g., health care, public health programs), it is imperative that communication between the evaluator and program staff be clear, with agreements and expectations made explicit. Evaluators need to recognize that program administrators are managing competing demands; putting agreements in writing serves to remind all parties about the plans and serves as a record in the event that disagreements arise. Seeing developing evaluation plans described in writing can suggest implications that neither evaluators nor administrators have previously considered.

## PLANNING AND CONDUCTING THE EVALUATION: ESSENTIAL STEPS

Ideally, program evaluation should begin when programs are planned and implemented. Formative evaluation, described earlier in this chapter, is a technique often used during program planning and implementation. However, some programs may already be under way, and they may never have undergone a formal evaluation process. Evaluation of such programs requires that the evaluator understand the program and how it is being implemented as part of the evaluation process. For purposes of presenting the steps of program evaluation, the author is assuming that the program being discussed is currently under way. The CDC framework for evaluation (see Figure 16.1) will be used as the guide in describing the program evaluation steps (CDC Evaluation Working Group, 2008).

### Step 1: Engaging Stakeholders

The evaluation cycle begins by engaging stakeholders—the persons or organizations that have an investment in what will be learned from an evaluation and what will be done with the knowledge. Stakeholders includes program staff, those who derive some of their revenue or income from the program (e.g., program administrators), sponsors of the program (e.g., CEO of an organization, foundations, government agencies), and clients or potential participants in the program. Understanding the needs of intended program recipients is necessary because it is for their welfare that the program has been developed. This may require undertaking a needs assessment and gathering information on the demographics and health status indicators of the target populations. These data may reside in existing data sources (e.g., health statistics from local or state health departments) or may be collected from key informants through surveys, focus groups, or observations (Hackbarth & Gall, 2005; Laryea, Sen, Gien, Kozma, & Palacio, 1999). Stakeholders must be engaged in the inquiry to ensure that their perspectives are understood. When stakeholders are not engaged, an evaluation may fail to address important elements of a program's objectives, operations, and outcomes (Hackbarth & Gall, 2005; Posavac & Carey, 2007).

## Step 2: Describing the Program

Program descriptions convey the mission and objectives of the program being evaluated. Descriptions should be sufficiently detailed to ensure understanding of (1) program goals and strategies, (2) the program's capacity to effect change, (3) its stage of development, and (4) how it fits into the larger organization and community. Program descriptions set the frame of reference for all subsequent decisions in an evaluation. The description enables the evaluator to compare the program with similar programs and facilitates attempts to connect program components to their effects. Moreover, different stakeholders may have different ideas regarding the program's goals and purposes. Working with stakeholders to formulate a clear and logical program description will bring benefits before data are available to evaluate the program's effectiveness. Aspects to include in a program description are need (nature and magnitude of the problem or opportunity addressed by the program; target populations; changing needs), expected effects (what the program must accomplish to be considered successful; immediate and long-term effects; potential unintended consequences), activities (what activities the program undertakes to effect change, how these activities are related, who does them), resources (time, talent, technology, equipment, information, money, and other assets available to conduct program activities; congruence between desired activities and resources), stage of development (newly implemented or mature); and context (setting and environmental influences within which the program operates). An understanding of environmental influences such as the program's history, the politics involved, and the social and economic conditions within which the program operates is required to design a context-sensitive evaluation and to aid in interpreting findings accurately (Barkauskas et al., 2004; Jacobson Vann, 2006; Menix, 2007).

Questions to facilitate program descriptions include who wants the evaluation; what the focus of the evaluation should be; why an evaluation is wanted; when the evaluation is wanted; and what resources are available to support the evaluation. Addressing these questions will assist in helping individuals understand the goals of the program evaluation, arrive at an overall consensus on the purpose of evaluations, and determine the time and resources available to carry out the evaluation. These questions also assist in uncovering the assumptions and conceptual basis of the program. For example, diabetes care programs may be based on the chronic-care model, a disease-management model, or a health-belief model, and it is important that the evaluator understand the program's conceptual basis in order to understand essential information to include in the program evaluation (Berg & Wadhwa, 2007).

Development of a logic model is part of the work of describing the program. A logic model sequences the events for bringing about change by synthesizing the main program elements into a picture of how the program is supposed to work. Often, this model is displayed in a flow chart, map, or table to portray the sequence of steps that will lead to the desired results. One of the virtues of a logic model is its ability to summarize the program's overall mechanism of change by linking processes (e.g., exercise) to eventual effects (e.g., improved quality of life, decreased coronary risk). The logic model can also display the infrastructure needed to support program operations. Elements that are connected within a logic model generally include inputs (e.g., trained staff, exercise equipment, space), activities (e.g., supervised exercise three times per week, education about exercise at home), outputs (e.g., increased distance walked), and results, whether immediate (e.g., decreased dyspnea with activities of daily living), intermediate (e.g., ability to participate in desired activities of life, improved social interactions), or long term (e.g., improved quality of life). Creating a logic model allows stakeholders to clarify the program's strategies and reveals assumptions about the conditions necessary for the program to be effective. The accuracy of a program description can be confirmed by (1) consulting with diverse stakeholders, and (2) comparing reported program descriptions with direct observation of the program activities (CDC Evaluation Working Group, 2008; Dykeman, MacIntosh, Seaman, & Davidson, 2003; Ganley & Ward, 2001; Hulton, 2007).

## Step 3: Focusing the Evaluation Plan

On the basis of the information gained in steps 1 and 2, the evaluator needs to set forth a focused evaluation plan (see Table 16.3). A thorough plan anticipates the program's intended uses and creates an evaluation

Table 16.3

## EXAMPLES OF STEPS 3, 4, AND 5 FOR FORMATIVE AND SUMMATIVE EVALUATIONS

| COMPONENTS | FORMATIVE EVALUATION | SUMMATIVE EVALUATION |
|---|---|---|
| Selecting and Defining Variables of Interest | Focus on process variables that determine how well the program is running.<br>Are patients being recruited?<br>■ Has staff been properly trained in the program protocol?<br>■ Are staff members following program protocol?<br>■ Are patients adhering to program requirements? | Focus on outcome variables that determine the effectiveness of the program.<br>■ Were patients and staff satisfied with the program?<br>■ Did patient health improve significantly?<br>■ Were medical resources reduced as a result of the program?<br>■ Are patients continuing the program on their own once the program is completed? |
| Measuring Variables of Interest | Focus on ways to measure how well the program is being run. Use:<br>■ Focus groups to discuss problem areas and ways to improve the program.<br>■ Direct observation to measure how the staff are following protocol.<br>■ Staff diary data to measure problems that occur on a daily basis.<br>■ Interviews of patients to determine how well they are adhering to the program requirements. | Focus on ways to measure the impact the program has had. Use:<br>■ Self-reports of patients and staff to report on the progress of the patient in terms of health status, functioning, symptomatology.<br>■ Collateral reports from spouses of patients to get a second rating on the patient's improvements.<br>■ Biomedical data to determine changes in biological parameters of functioning.<br>■ Chart abstractions to measure health care resource use. |

*(Continued)*

Table 16.3

### EXAMPLES OF STEPS 3, 4, AND 5 FOR FORMATIVE AND SUMMATIVE EVALUATIONS (CONTINUED)

| COMPONENTS | FORMATIVE EVALUATION | SUMMATIVE EVALUATION |
|---|---|---|
| Selecting a Program Evaluation Design | Use descriptive designs or narrative accounts.<br>■ Allow for a narrative account of how well the program is being run.<br>■ Provide feedback from patients and staff on areas in need of improvement.<br>■ Document patient adherence levels to the program requirements.<br>■ Track process variables over the implementation of the program. | Use experiment, quasi-experimental, or sequential designs (when possible).<br>■ Allow for a comparison among groups of patients that were assigned to groups that received the program or did not receive the program.<br>■ Use random assignment to program groups whenever possible.<br>■ Use over-time examinations, if resources permit.<br>■ Allow for determination of impact that the program has had on patients' lives. |
| Collecting Data | Use uniform collection procedures that do not disrupt the program implementation.<br>■ Collected data must be coded according to a uniform system that translates narrative data into meaningful groupings. For example, focus group comments can be grouped into comments about staff-related problems, patient-related problems, recruitment difficulties, adherence difficulties, and so on.<br>■ Program evaluators should not bias data collection strategies by holding preconceptions about how well the program is being run. | Use systematic procedures for vollecting data across groups (if more than one) and across time.<br>■ Collected data must be coded with a uniform system that translates the data into numerical values so that data analysis can be conducted. For example, responses to a question about health status that includes responses such as *poor, fair, good,* and *excellent* need to be coded as 0, 1, 2, or 3.<br>■ Across-time data collection must follow the same procedures. For example, all patients receive self-reports either in the mail or from the program site. The procedures must not vary |

*(Continued)*

Table 16.3

**EXAMPLES OF STEPS 3, 4, AND 5 FOR FORMATIVE AND SUMMATIVE EVALUATIONS** (CONTINUED)

| COMPONENTS | FORMATIVE EVALUATION | SUMMATIVE EVALUATION |
|---|---|---|
| Evaluating Data Analysis | Use both qualitative and quantitative approaches.<br>■ Qualitative approaches provide a narrative description of the process variables and allow for descriptive understanding of how well the program is running.<br>■ Quantitative approaches provide frequency counts and means or averages for some of the variables of interest. For example, frequencies for patient recruitment can be computed for time periods in order to determine when lags in recruitment occurred and give insights into possible reasons for the lag.<br>■ Allows evaluators to make recommendations based on data. | Use both qualitative and quantitative approaches.<br>■ Qualitative approaches provide a narrative description of the impact that the program has had on individual patients. Quotes from patients to exemplify the personal impact can be used.<br>■ Quantitative approaches provide a statistical comparison between groups (if more than one) or across time. Can determine whether the program was effective in increasing patient health status, increasing staff and patient satisfaction, and reducing health care resources utilized.<br>■ Quantitative approaches can also be used to make comparisons with other similar clinical programs.<br>■ Enables evaluators to make recommendations based on data. |

From "Framework for Program Evaluation," by Centers for Disease Control, 1999. *MMWR*, *48*(RR-11). Retrieved from http://www.cdc.gov/eval/framework.htm#graphic

strategy with the greatest chance of being useful, feasible, ethical, and accurate. Although the components of the plan may differ somewhat depending on the information and understanding of the program gained in steps one and two, essential elements of the evaluation plan are discussed here.

## Purpose

Articulating an evaluation's purpose (i.e., intent) prevents premature decision making regarding how the evaluation should be conducted. Characteristics of the program, particularly its stage of development and context, influence the evaluation's purpose. The purpose may include gaining insight into program operations that affect program outcomes so that that knowledge can be put to use in designing future program modifications; describing program processes and outcomes for the purpose of improving the quality, effectiveness, or efficiency of the program; and assessing the program's effects by examining the relationships between program activities and observed consequences. It is essential that an evaluation purpose be set forth and agreed upon, as this will guide the types and sources of information to be collected and analyzed.

## Selecting and Defining Variables of Interest

Defining carefully and accurately the *independent* (process and context) and *dependent* (outcome) variables to be measured is an essential part of focusing the evaluation plan. This step is likely the most daunting, as well as the most important. Selection and definition of the variables must be precise enough so as not to be cumbersome for evaluation staff or for data analysis, yet must retain variables that are both meaningful and measurable. During formative evaluations, *process* variables are of primary interest, whereas during summative evaluations both *process* and *outcome* variables are of interest. Again, to return to the pulmonary rehabilitation example discussed previously, a process variable of importance would be whether or not patients were learning how to exercise on their own while at home. An outcome variable in this example would be defined as the level at which patients were still exercising 6 months to 1 year following the completion of the formal program.

**Independent or Process Variables.** An important independent or process variable is the level of patient adherence to any treatments or self-care regimens prescribed by the program. More than 25 years of research indicates that, on average, 40% of patients fail to adhere to the recommendations prescribed to them to treat their acute or chronic conditions (DiMatteo & DiNicola, 1982). A program's effectiveness cannot be determined unless it is known how well patients adhere to the requirements of the program, which should be a focus of formative evaluations. Patient nonadherence has been found to be a causal factor in the time and money wasted in medical visits (Haynes, Taylor, & Sackett, 1979) and must not be overlooked in determining how well a clinical program is being implemented; how well a program is implemented is intimately linked to the level of patient adherence to the requirements of the program. For instance, if a program introduces barriers to adherence (e.g., by requiring time-intensive self-care routines, by introducing complex treatments with numerous factors to remember, by making it difficult to get questions answered, or by having uninformed or untrained staff), patient adherence will be diminished. A complement to patient adherence is the issue of how well the nursing staff maintains or adheres to the program's protocol. The integrity of an intervention or program is not upheld unless the staff assigned to carry it out are diligent in following procedures and protocol (Kirchhoff & Dille, 1994). In addition to assessing patient adherence, program evaluators need to ascertain the level at which staff members are adhering to the program.

The process variables include how well patients are recruited into the program, how well trained and informed the staff are about the program's purpose and importance, the barriers (if any) to the implementation of the program, the level at which the program site is conducive to conducting a well-run program, and the perceptions held by staff and patients of the usefulness of the program. These factors generally are easier to correct than are issues of patient and staff adherence. For this reason, evaluators need to spend a considerable amount of time assessing and adjusting patient and staff adherence to program procedure and protocol.

Every project is located within a community or a larger organization. This context has some influence on how the program works and on its effectiveness. Questions about which contextual factors have the greatest impact on program success and which context factors may help or hinder the optimization of the program's goals and objectives are likely to arise in program evaluations. Variables such as leadership style, cultural competence, organizational culture, and collaboration are all examples of contextual factors that the evaluator should consider in selecting independent variables. Gathering such information through either quantitative or qualitative techniques will help the evaluator understand why some component of the program worked or did not work (Greenhalgh, Robert, Bate, Macfarlane, & Kyriakidou, 2005; Stetler, McQueen, Demakis, & Mittman, 2008). Other contextual areas that may be worth examining are the federal and state climates, particularly how these climates may be impacting the program, how they may have changed over time, and the impact of these changes on program processes and effectiveness (Randell & Delekto, 1999). For example, if payment for pulmonary rehabilitation is not available through third-party payors, including Medicare, the impact of this contextual factor should be addressed in the evaluation.

**Dependent or Outcome Variables.** Examples of dependent or outcome variables (Fitzgerald & Illback, 1993) that are measured by social scientists and health care services evaluators in determining the effectiveness of health care programs include:

- Patient health status and daily functioning
- Patient satisfaction with providers and medical care received
- Health care provider satisfaction
- Medical cost containment

Evaluators and nurses alike should consider each of these variables as outcomes of a clinical program. The evaluator who conducts a program evaluation and who attempts to determine the effectiveness or success of a program should pay particular attention to these four outcomes.

The first important outcome variable defines and measures whether the program has facilitated the patient to improve his or her health and/ or functional status. The outcome of importance is whether the program has improved the quality of the patient's life and whether health goals have been achieved. If the program does not increase these outcome variables and the protocol or intervention has been followed (i.e., patient and staff have adhered to the program), then the program's effectiveness is questionable. Although expectations for health improvements may not be a focus of the program, client health status is an important outcome variable that needs to be examined. For this reason, measurements of patient health status taken multiple times and in multiple ways through triangulation techniques over the course of the program and even after the program is completed must be a focus of evaluations.

An important outcome of the health care delivery and program evaluation is patient satisfaction. Research suggests that an intervention that decreases a patient's satisfaction with his or her health care may lead to poorer health (Kaplan, Greenfield, & Ware, Jr., 1989), poorer adherence to treatments (Ong, DeHaes, Hoos, & Lammes, 1995), poorer attendance at follow-up appointments (DiMatteo, Hays, & Prince, 1986), and greater interest in obtaining health care elsewhere (Ross & Duff, 1982) than is the case among patients whose satisfaction has increased. Evaluators need to take into account changes in patient satisfaction with the program, in particular, and with their health care, in general, because any decrease in satisfaction can point to problems in the program's purpose, scope, and execution.

Another outcome that is often overlooked is that of nursing staff satisfaction. Slevin, Somerville, and McKenna (1996) measured staff satisfaction during the evaluation of a quality improvement initiative and found that satisfaction among the nurses was related to better interpersonal care of patients. Level of satisfaction can pertain directly to the process and implementation of the intervention or can be more generally defined and include professional satisfaction. Any program that introduces frustrations for the nursing staff will likely not be conducted in the fashion that was intended, will serve to diminish the quality of care delivered, and perhaps will influence the two outcomes already discussed, patient satisfaction and health status. The staff that must implement the intervention on a daily basis and that must interact and negotiate with patients must be satisfied with the new program. Thus, evaluation of programs also must address the impact that the program has on the staff involved, and not simply the impact that it has on the patients (Slevin, Somerville, & McKenna, 1996).

Finally, of considerable importance to program evaluation is the outcome variable of cost containment and/or reduction. An effective program is one that improves the quality and delivery of care, while maintaining and perhaps even reducing medical costs to both the organization and the patient. This evaluation outcome, however, is generally long term in nature and requires multiple follow-ups, which can pose a considerable burden for programs with highly limited resources. The data that may be available to assist in this aspect of outcome evaluation include information about any patient hospitalizations and related lengths of stay, emergency room visits, regular doctor office visits, supplies and equipment costs, and personnel time. Program evaluators can work collaboratively with financial management personnel to acquire this necessary information.

## Measuring Variables

The next step is to select the way in which each variable of interest will be measured. In making this decision, it is important to consider, first, the many ways in which variables can be assessed and measured (e.g., self-reports, biomedical instrumentation, direct observation, or chart abstraction) and, second, the source from which the data will be collected (e.g., patient, staff, or medical records). Measurement is an important element of program evaluation, for without rigorous, reliable, and valid information, the data obtained and subsequent recommendations are questionable.

Program evaluators need to consider, if possible, the use of highly valid and reliable research instruments, rather than the development of new instruments to measure the variables of interest. Many forms of instrumentation exist, and many have been used in previous evaluations of new clinical programs.

---

**Benefits of Using Published Instruments to Gather Self-Report Information**

- Gathered information has a greater chance of being reliable and valid. That is, the instrument measures what it intends to measure and has internal consistency.
- The program evaluator has a normative group by which to compare ranges, means, and standard deviations on the instrument to the sample being evaluated.
- The instrument is composed of items or questions that are understandable by the majority of respondents.
- The instrument has a response format that both fits with the stem of the question and is responded to with relative ease.

---

Several reference books are available that have compiled a multitude of research instruments and normative data for measures (Frank-Stromberg & Olsen, 2004; Robinson, Shaver, & Wrightsman, 1991; Stewart & Shamdasani, 1990).

Fitzgerald and Illback (1993) delineate the various methods of obtaining information and corresponding data sources to consider in program evaluation. *Self-reports* from patients and staff are likely the most widely used technique for acquiring information about the process and effects of an intervention. These measures are completed by participants and staff involved in clinical programs, and they can often be completed at the individual's leisure. These measures can either be user friendly, allowing the individual to complete the questionnaire by circling his or her response to the various items, or research friendly, requiring the individual to transfer his or her responses onto a computer-scannable form. The main advantages of self-reports are their ease of use, their cost efficiency, their limited coding requirements, and the lack of need for highly trained staff to implement their use. The main disadvantage is the prevalent belief that self-report instruments elicit self-presentation tendencies (i.e., the tendency of individuals to present themselves in a socially desirable manner or in a positive light). This view is often unfounded, as many measurement experts now hold the view that most of the people, most of the time, are accurate in their self-reported responses (Stewart & Ware, Jr., 1992; Ware, Jr., Davies-Avery, & Donald, 1978).

In addition to self-report inventories completed by the participant, *collateral reports* can be obtained. These reports rely upon the same instruments as those used for self-reports, with slight modifications in wording regarding the tense. These measures can provide additional information about the patient and can even serve to provide a check on the patient's responses. Collateral reports are completed by an individual very close (usually a spouse) to the study participant. These types of reports have not been used to a great extent in nursing research, though they have been used extensively in psychological research. These collateral measures have been found to be highly correlated with the self-report data and can serve as either a validity check on the self-report data or an additional source of variant information to be used in the program evaluation. For instance, if the collateral reports are consistently lower than self-reports in measures for health status, then the evaluator may feel compelled to question the level of honesty of the responses.

Use of *structured* and *unstructured interviews* is another method for acquiring information. The practice of interviewing participants either in face-to-face interactions or over the telephone provides benefits beyond those of self-report questionnaires but also introduces a few drawbacks. The benefits of interviews include the ability to clarify any confusing questions or items for participants, to increase participant rates in the program, to obtain more complete information (individuals are often more likely to leave questions blank on questionnaires), and to obtain narrative accounts that are not restricted by standardized questions and response formats. The main drawback to interviews, however, is the need for highly trained interviewers who are taught not to lead individuals into answers and who are not biased (preferably interviewers should be blinded to the purpose of the program). Another drawback includes the reduced ability to acquire vast amounts of information, which self-report questionnaires more easily achieve.

*Direct observation* is an alternative method of measurement that does not rely upon the reports of the participants in the project. Observations, like interviews, require highly trained observers. In order to effectively obtain data, observers must record very specific and narrow pieces of information and may need to reduce the amount of time a particular action is observed. For instance, a patient may be observed through the use of time sampling techniques in which only the first five minutes or last five minutes of every hour are observed and recorded. In addition, direct observations can provide information only about observable behaviors and does not allow insight into the perceptions or attitudes of the participants.

A variation on interviews and direct observations is the use of *focus groups* (Becker et al., 2007; Laryea et al., 1999; Packer, Race, & Hotch, 1994; Wyatt, Krauskopf, & Davidson, 2008). The information obtained from focus groups is qualitative and helps evaluators performing formative and summative evaluations to assess areas that need to be further refined, changed altogether, or even eliminated. Focus groups were first utilized by market researchers and have been a favored method by which to obtain information about consumer preferences (Stewart & Shamdasani, 1990). The use of focus groups, however, is becoming more widespread among program evaluators seeking to understand patient preferences and expectations. For example, a focus group can be used to gather pertinent information from a group of patients who receive the clinical program or to obtain feedback about how the program is proceeding. Focus groups can also be used to learn how patients talk about the program or its directive and to ascertain patients' perceptions about the program and its effectiveness and utility (Morgan, 1988; Stewart & Shamdasani, 1990).

Stewart and Shamdasani (1990) discuss the role of focus groups in program evaluation and define the focus group technique as the collective interview of usually 8 to 12 individuals who are brought together to discuss a particular topic for an hour or two. The group is generally directed by a trained moderator who keeps the discussion focused on the topic of interest, enhances group interaction, and probes for necessary details. Morgan (1988) points out that information acquired from group discussions is often more readily accessible than it would be for individual interviews, as individual members are cued or primed to give information that they would not give in an interview. The topic of interest can vary depending on whether this technique is used during formative or summative evaluation of the program's success.

*Biomedical data* include laboratory tests, blood pressure, heart and respiratory rates, and other types of data that require the use of a bioinstrument for collection (e.g., use of blood pressure monitor, heart rate monitor, or stress tests). Because of the expense of medical tests, their use as the sole means of data collection in program evaluation may not be practical. If the program requires use of biomedical data collection as part of its protocol, however, the evaluator might be able to acquire this information. The type of biomedical information collected for program evaluations must provide information relevant to the program and its evaluation and must hold meaning outside basic medical parameters. In other words, biomedical information is useless unless it can be translated into information that is directly meaningful in the determination of a program's effectiveness (e.g., if the program's goal is to reduce hypertension, then the bioinstrumentation must demonstrate that blood pressure has been lowered among the program's participants).

*Medical record reviews* or *chart abstractions* are another source of data to consider when conducting a program evaluation. Use of medical records as a data source requires development of a standardized evaluation form and coding scheme to use in abstracting data. These types of reviews need highly trained chart abstractors who are clear about the information to be gathered and the need to be systematic in the review process. Chart reviews often allow for the gathering of information that cannot be found by any other fashion. The main drawback is that patient charts are not always totally complete and readable and often contain inaccurate patient health histories. The main advantage of this method is that the evaluator is relying upon an already developed set of data; no new data need to be collected, and retrospective data can be collected and used as part of the evaluation.

*Diary data* are another source of data that can be utilized to measure the variables of interest. Diary data can be completed by either the health care provider or the patient and provide information that is immediate and time relevant. Data can be collected once a day (a nightly count of food consumed for that day), several times a day (when every prescription medication is taken), or even randomly (when a beeper goes off and the patient is required to write down the relevant information). The main disadvantage of using diary data is that patients and staff may not always take the necessary time to complete the forms completely or accurately. Diary data, however, are a true advance in data collection when used in triangulation with the other forms of data discussed.

---

**Ways to Measure Variables**

*Self-reports* obtained from patients or staff

*Collateral reports* obtained from family members

*Structured or unstructured interviews* conducted by a trained interviewer

*Direct observation* of the program implementation mechanisms

*Focus groups* on benefits of and problems with the clinical program

*Biomedical information* to substantiate progress of patient

*Medical record* or chart abstractions

*Diary data* obtained from patients or staff

---

## Selecting the Design

The next step is to select the method that will provide the information necessary to determine a program's effectiveness. Numerous evaluation methods are available that serve as both practical and efficient means to determine the effectiveness of clinical programs. In order for program evaluations to determine whether or not the outcomes of interest have improved, the program evaluation must be conducted with precision and stringency. Following is a list of evaluation methods or designs that an evaluator can consider in choosing a technique for program evaluation. Each design, briefly reviewed here, is different in terms of the amount of the time and financial expense required to implement it, the type of analysis plan necessary, the level of control it offers the evaluator over the variables of interest, and the level of associated statistical power (Rossi & Freeman, 1989).

True *randomized controlled experiments* (RCTs) involve a comparison between one or more experimental groups that receive an intervention and a control group that does not receive the intervention. Participants in the experimental group(s) participate in the clinical program that is intended to affect a measurable outcome, while those in the control group serve as a comparison (Chan et al., 2000). The key component to true experiments is the random assignment of subjects to either the experimental or the control group. This assignment theoretically eliminates any individual differences among the groups prior to the implementation of the program. For this reason, in experimental designs the outcomes can be attributed to the program and not to differences among the participants of the program. Observed group differences in the selected program outcomes determine the level of program success or failure. In other words, for the program to be deemed a success, it must have a significant, beneficial effect on the experimental group in comparison to its effect on individuals in the comparison group. If the clinical program is conducted in an experimental manner, program evaluators can decide to use this design in the evaluation by assigning either all of the participants to be evaluated or by randomly selecting an equal number of participants from each group (experimental and control) for the evaluation.

According to program evaluation experts, this type of design is difficult to do in a dynamic, real-world setting where programs reside. Furthermore, this design requires withholding ongoing feedback regarding information related to program improvement during the experiment (Sufflebeam & Shinkfield, 2007). Opportunities to meet the requirements of randomized experiments in program evaluation, particularly in service fields such as health care and social service, are quite limited. This type of design is costly and may not be feasible, and the information it provides may not be useful in addressing the purpose of the program evaluation. The expectation of federal agencies and government mandates that program evaluations employ RCTs has had a crippling and wasteful influence on the practice of program evaluations (Sufflebeam & Shinkfield, 2007).

Both quantitative and qualitative approaches to data collection are appropriate in experimental designs. Before comparing group data, however, the evaluator should perform a formative evaluation that focuses on how well the experiment is being conducted and whether random assignment to the groups is being upheld. The summative evaluation will allow for comparisons between the groups in an attempt to illustrate the program's causal effect on outcomes. Qualitative data are useful in experimental designs because they can make it clear whether the program is being carried out as intended and can clarify differences of perceptions among members of the experimental and the control groups. By providing a narrative description of the impact of the program on the individuals, the qualitative data provide further support for the evaluator's conclusions about the program's effectiveness; by offering a narrative of the way in which the program or intervention is being carried out, they give the evaluator in this type of design information that elucidates the quantitative findings.

*Quasi-experiments* involve the same intervention and comparison component as true experiments, except that quasi-experiments differ in one critical way: Random assignment of subjects or participants to a "treatment" group is not feasible. For instance, a clinical program may have the goal of understanding the effect of gender differences on some health-related area. Since we cannot randomly assign individuals to be in either the male or the female group, this design inherently involves a quasi-experiment. The evaluation process for quasi-experiments is similar to that for true experiments. The main difference, however, occurs during the summative evaluation. Since random assignment to treatment groups cannot be done, it is not possible to be certain that changes in outcome variables are the result of the intervention or clinical program. Differences among the individuals in the assigned groups prior to group assignment cannot be ruled out as the cause for observed changes in the outcome variable(s) of interest.

One drawback to both experiments and quasi-experiments is the need for a control or natural comparison group. This need for an additional group can pose a limitation for sites where patient participation is limited, recruitment of patients takes a great deal of time, or there is no natural comparison group available. In addition, some have argued the ethical implications of providing some patients with care or experimental care and not providing equivalent care to other patients. For these reasons, a *cross-sequential design* might be the most practical. In the cross-sequential design, the program evaluator observes or assesses several different groups of patients over several time periods, but each group is observed initially in the same period, for example, 6 weeks after admission to the program (Rosenthal & Rosnow, 1991). This type of design allows the time of measurement and the patient group to serve as the basis for comparison, eliminating the need for a control group. In essence, a cross-sequential design simultaneously compares several different groups of patients on a set of variables observed during one time period. The evaluator is able to control for possible variations in how the program is conducted. If patients observed during the beginning of the program have different outcomes from those recruited later in the program, the evaluator can attempt to determine if these differences are due to individual differences among the patients or to differences in program implementation.

Finally, *descriptive designs* are also useful to employ in program evaluations. These designs serve to track and describe key outcome variables over time and examine trends in data. Descriptive designs can be employed that utilize a cross-sectional examination of reports of patients and staff or a longitudinal examination of trends in relationships among variables of interest and provide narrative descriptions of the component parts of the program as viewed by patients and staff. These designs are particularly relevant for formative evaluations, since this phase of evaluation is focused upon the process of planning and implementing the program as well as on *how* the program is being executed. Descriptions of the program can help to illuminate problems in program execution, especially in adherence among the patients and the staff. For example, by examining the changes in functional status in a group of pulmonary rehabilitation patients over a one-year period (by including measurements before the program, during the program, and after the program), the evaluator can determine to some degree the level of success of the program. If all of the patients are observed to have increases in their reports of functional status, and this is corroborated by biomedical tests, staff reports, and diary data, then the program will likely be deemed effective.

## Sample Size in Program Evaluations

When selecting a design for program evaluation, the evaluator must consider the sample size required for an effective evaluation. Sample size depends on several factors. Among these are the expected effect size of the intervention (i.e., whether the intervention will produce a small amount or a large amount of change), the type of design used, and the analysis plan. For a further explanation of sample size and its related statistical power to detect significant effects, please refer to Chapter 13, on data analysis.

## Step 4: Gathering Credible Evidence: Data Collection

The next step in evaluation is to establish a systematic procedure for data collection. In order for the data not to become contaminated (by bias or error), trained data collectors must be utilized. The same procedures must be used for every participant in the program in order for the results of the evaluation to be trustworthy. Procedures for collecting the data to be used in the program evaluation should be the same for all individuals in the program, whether the data are collected from patients or from staff.

## Data Collection Quality

Choosing an approach to data collection and its usefulness has always posed a problem in the evaluation of new clinical programs. Once the evaluator has decided upon data source, type, measurement, and collection strategy, the integrity of the data must be ensured at all levels. In all forms of data, similar problems become evident, in that each form requires precise units of measurement. Data collection procedures and data analysis are highly sensitive to variations, and one goal of the evaluator is to ensure the uniformity across the program. All collection procedures must be systematic, and potential bias on the part of the evaluator and the staff involved in the program must be eliminated.

## Data Coding

One of the most tedious components of the evaluation process is the coding and entering of all relevant data (Coffey & Atkinson, 1996; Keppel & Zedeck, 1989; Lipsey, 1994). The protocol for coding data needs to be well developed early in program planning and, whenever possible, to follow a standardized and published method. Since many of the data collected during an evaluation may be narrative, the coding scheme for analyzing the accounts must be succinct, time efficient, and meaningful. The accounts are usually sorted through and divided into a manageable number of conceptual or programmatic categories. Often, not all of these categories will be utilized in the evaluation of the program, but, nonetheless, a systematic coding scheme needs to be followed. Additionally, all self-report data, biomedical data, and chart data need to be coded into numerical values that can be used in the computations for the final evaluations. Again, these coding procedures need to be uniform across all participants (patients and staff reports) and across all forms of data. For instance, the anchor on all items or questions should consistently be 0 or 1 and should not vary throughout the coding scheme (if the question has the first response as "poor," the code should be "0"; if the question has the first response as "none of the time," the code should be "0"; if the question has the first response as "never," the code should be "0," and so forth).

The evaluator must also remember to keep track of the direction in which questions are worded or data from charts and bioinstruments are abstracted so that these can be correctly recoded. Multiple questions that measure the same variable should be analyzed only when they are all coded in the same direction. Since many questions are asked in a negative manner to reduce response biases, these questions need to be recoded to reflect the direction of the other questions in the same scale. Recoding should follow the direction of the positively stated questions and should reflect a higher score of the variable being measured (e.g., a high score on a health status scale should reflect better health).

## Step 5: Justifying Conclusions: Data Analysis, Interpretation, and Recommendations

Techniques for analyzing, synthesizing, and interpreting findings should be agreed on before data collection begins and should thus guide this phase of program evaluation. Once all data are coded properly and entered into a database, the evaluator can take on the task of data analysis. The reader is referred to Chapter 13 for a thorough discussion of how to conduct a proper analysis. Analysis and synthesis of an evaluation's findings may detect patterns in evidence, either by isolating important findings (analysis) or by combining sources of information to reach a larger understanding (synthesis). Mixed-method evaluations require the separate analysis of each evidence element and a synthesis of all sources to allow for an examination of patterns of agreement, convergence, or complexity.

The program evaluator must be cautious in interpreting the results of an evaluation once it has been completed. Interpretation is the act of figuring out what the findings mean and is part of the overall effort to understand the evidence gathered in an evaluation. The uncovering of facts regarding a program's performance is not a sufficient basis on which to draw evaluative conclusions. Evaluation evidence must be interpreted to determine the practical significance of what has been learned. Interpretations draw on information and perspectives that stakeholders bring to the evaluation inquiry.

The results of data analysis can sometimes be confusing but are often unassuming. The determination, based on quantitative data analysis, that a program has had small effects is predominant in most evaluations;

however, that an effect is small does not mean that it is unimportant. Every evaluator should understand the size of effects for each of the various statistics and the relative importance given to each size. The effect size refers to the magnitude of the relationship between two variables; the smaller the related coefficient, the smaller the effect. The evaluator must keep in mind that the effect size coefficient is meaningful only in a statistical sense and does not mean that the effect has on the lives of individuals is small (Cohen, 1988; Rosenthal & Rosnow, 1991).

To interpret qualitative data, the evaluator should employ standard qualitative analysis techniques, using quotations and stories to illustrate themes and concepts. Qualitative information is important to include; it illustrates the basis for recommendations derived from the data, particularly for components that address program implementation.

Judgments about the program are made on the basis of data analysis and interpretation. Statements about the program are set forth and focus on the merit, worth, or significance of the program and are based on the agreed-upon values or standards set by the stakeholders in the planning stages of program evaluation. They are formed by comparing the findings and interpretations regarding the program against one or more of the selected standards. Because multiple standards can be applied to a given program, judgment statements may be somewhat incongruent. However, one of the unique features of program evaluation is that the evaluator makes judgment statements based upon standards set a priori and reflecting the perspectives of various stakeholder groups. For example, a 10% increase in pulmonary rehabilitation enrollment over a year may be viewed as positive by the program manager, whereas potential participants in the program may view this figure differently and argue that a critical threshold for access to this service has not been reached. Conflicting statements regarding a program's quality, value, or importance often indicate that stakeholders are using different standards for judgment. In the context of an evaluation, such disagreement can be a catalyst for clarifying relevant values and the worth of the program (CDC Evaluation Working Group, 2008).

## Recommendations

Recommendations are proposed actions for consideration that grow out of the evaluation. Forming recommendations is a distinct element of program evaluation that requires information beyond what is necessary to form judgments regarding program performance (CDC Evaluation

Working Group, 2008). Knowing that a program is able to reduce the risk of disease does not translate necessarily into a recommendation to continue the effort, particularly when competing priorities or other effective alternatives exist. Thus, recommendations for continuing, expanding, redesigning, or terminating a program are separate from judgments regarding a program's effectiveness. Making recommendations requires information concerning the context, particularly the organizational context, in which programmatic decisions will be made. Recommendations that lack sufficient evidence or those that are not aligned with stakeholders' values can undermine an evaluation's credibility. By contrast, an evaluation can be strengthened by recommendations that anticipate the political sensitivities of intended users and that highlight areas that users can control or influence. Sharing draft recommendations, soliciting reactions from multiple stakeholders, and presenting options instead of directive advice increase the likelihood that recommendations will be relevant and well received.

Conclusions and recommendations are strengthened by (a) summarizing the plausible mechanisms of change; (b) delineating the temporal sequence between activities and effects; (c) searching for alternative explanations and showing why they are unsupported by the evidence; and (d) showing that the effects can be repeated (CDC Evaluation Working Group, 2008). When different but equally well-supported conclusions exist, each can be presented with a summary of its strengths and weaknesses.

## Step 6: Ensure Use and Share Lessons Learned: The Written Report and Follow-Up

Lessons learned in the course of an evaluation do not automatically translate into informed decision making and appropriate action. Deliberate effort is needed to ensure that the evaluation processes and findings are used and disseminated appropriately (CDC Evaluation Working Group, 2008).

### Writing an Evaluation Plan and Report

Writing an *evaluation report* and disseminating the report to key stakeholders and administrators are the essential final steps in program evaluation (see also Chapter 22, on reporting results through publication).

**10 Components of a Program Evaluation Report**

1 The purpose of the report
2 The nature of the clinical program and its component parts
3 The setting of the program (e.g., inpatient or ambulatory care or home settings)
4 The time frame for the program
5 The program staff resources used
6 The way that data obtained during the formative evaluation were used to alter the program and improve its implementation process
7 The evaluation methods used, including the evaluation of the program process and outcome variables
8 Results of the data analysis
9 Recommendations for program revisions, refinement, and continuation
10 Summary of the program's overall effectiveness in achieving its designed purpose

A full report describing each of the 10 points listed with documents in support of these points is helpful to the individuals directly responsible for the clinical program. A short *executive summary* is useful for administrators and those individuals responsible for making decisions about whether to continue the clinical program, expand it, or downsize its scope. It is also critical in this executive summary to document clearly the association between the program and the outcomes of interest and to demonstrate clearly the benefits of the program, the cost saved, and the number of patients served.

The executive summary is usually written after the evaluator has completed the final summative report that is designed to be a more comprehensive report of the program evaluation. The executive summary needs to be as succinct and as clear as possible about the outcomes of the program. In addition, it is often best to illustrate the results with diagrams and charts. The evaluator needs to make the recommendations for the program clear and action oriented so that the executive committee or those directly responsible for the program are clear about the program's purpose and results and about the best actions to take regarding the program's future. Writing the final summative report and the subsequent executive summary on a new clinical program may seem like a daunting task, but this serves as a template for annual program reviews.

## Follow-Up

Follow-up refers to the support provided to users to enable them to disseminate and enact the program evaluation findings as appropriate (CDC Evaluation Working Group, 2008). Active follow-up might be necessary to remind intended users of the planned use of the report. Follow-up might also be required to ensure that lessons learned are not lost or ignored in the process of making complex or politically sensitive decisions. To guard against such oversight, someone involved in the evaluation should serve as an advocate for the evaluation's findings during the decision-making phase. This type of advocacy increases appreciation of what was discovered and what actions are consistent with the findings.

Facilitating use of evaluation findings also carries with it the responsibility for preventing misuse. Evaluation results are always bound by the context in which the evaluation was conducted. However, some results may be interpreted or taken out of context and used for purposes other than those agreed on. For example, individuals who seek to undermine a program might misuse results by overemphasizing negative findings without giving regard to the program's positive attributes. Active follow-up can help prevent these and other forms of misuse by ensuring that evidence is not misinterpreted and is not applied to questions other than those that were the central focus of the evaluation (CDC Evaluation Working Group, 2008).

## SUMMARY

The process of planning, conducting, and analyzing a well-devised and comprehensive clinical program evaluation is time consuming, creative, and challenging. The effort put forth in an evaluation can be rewarded with fiscal reinforcement, community recognition, and a sound future for the program. Programs that are found to be effective in terms of increasing patient and staff satisfaction, increasing patient health status, and saving medical dollars are likely the ones that will receive continued or increased funding. The main purpose of the program evaluator is to examine and protect the program's integrity at all levels, for, if integrity is not maintained, the outcomes of the program are questionable.

## SUGGESTED ACTIVITIES

1  You have been asked by the Chief Nursing Officer to evaluate the cardiovascular case management program at your community hospital. Describe how you will proceed in developing an evaluation plan for this program. Include a purpose statement for the evaluation, a list of the key stakeholders you will need to communicate with, and the program evaluation methods you will use to gather information to include in the evaluation.

2  Compare and contrast the use of an internal evaluator and an external evaluator for program evaluation. For example, what are the advantages and disadvantages of having an individual employed by the institution conduct the evaluation and of contracting with an external program evaluator?

## REFERENCES

American Evaluation Association. (2008a). Retrieved November 2008 from http://www. eval.org/

American Evaluation Association. (2008b). *Guiding principles for evaluators.* Retrieved November 2008 from http://www.eval.org/Publications/GuidingPrinciplesPrintable. asp

Barkauskas, V. H., Pohl, J., Breer, L., Tanner, C., Bostrom, A. C., Benkert, R., et al. (2004). Academic nurse-managed centers: Approaches to evaluation. *Outcomes Management, 8*(1), 57–66.

Becker, K. L., Dang, D., Jordan, E., Kub, J., Welch, A., Smith, C. A., et al. (2007). An evaluation framework for faculty practice. *Nursing Outlook, 55*(1), 44–54.

Berg, G. D., & Wadhwa, S. (2007). Health services outcomes for a diabetes disease management program for the elderly. *Disease Management, 10*(4), 226–234.

Billings, J. R. (2000). Community development: A critical review of approaches to evaluation. *Journal of Advanced Nursing, 31*(2), 472–480.

Centers for Disease Control Evaluation Working Group. (2008). November 2008, from http://www.cdc.gov/eval/

Chan, S., Mackenzie, A., Tin-Fu, D., & Ka-yi Leung, J. (2000). An evaluation of the implementation of case management in the community psychiatric nursing service. *Journal of Advanced Nursing, 31*(1), 144–156.

Coffey, A., & Atkinson, P. (1996). *Making sense of qualitative data: Complementing research strategies.* Thousand Oaks, CA: Sage.

Cohen, J. (1988). *Statistical power analysis for the behavioral sciences* (2nd ed.). Hillsdale, NJ: Erlbaum.

Cramer, M. E., Mueller, K. J., & Harrop, D. (2003). Comprehensive evaluation of a community coalition: A case study of environmental tobacco smoke reduction. *Public Health Nursing, 20*(6), 464–477.

Denzin, N. K. (1978). *The research act.* New York: McGraw-Hill.

DiMatteo, M. R., & DiNicola, D. D. (1982). *Achieving patient compliance: The psychology of the medical practitioner's role.* New York: Pergamon Press.

DiMatteo, M. R., Hays, R. D., & Prince, L. M. (1986). Relationship of physicians' nonverbal communication skill to patient satisfaction, appointment noncompliance, and physician workload. *Health Psychology, 5,* 581–594.

Dykeman, M., MacIntosh, J., Seaman, P., & Davidson, P. (2003). Development of a program logic model to measure the processes and outcomes of a nurse-managed community health clinic. *Journal of Professional Nursing, 19*(3), 197–203.

Fitzgerald, E., & Illback, R. J. (1993). Program planning and evaluation: Principles and procedures for nurse managers. *Orthopaedic Nursing, 12*(5), 39–45.

Frank-Stromberg, M., & Olsen, S. J. (2004). *Instruments for clinical health care research.* Boston: Jones & Bartlett.

Ganley, H. E., & Ward, M. (2001). Program logic: A planning and evaluation method. *Journal of Nursing Administration, 31*(1), 4, 39.

Greenhalgh, T., Robert, G., Bate, P., Macfarlane, F., & Kyriakidou, O. (2005). *Diffusion of innovations in health service organisations: A systematic literature review.* Malden, MA: Blackwell.

Hackbarth, D., & Gall, G. B. (2005). Evaluation of school-based health center programs and services: The whys and hows of demonstrating program effectiveness. *Nursing Clinics of North America, 40,* 711–724.

Haynes, R. B., Taylor, D. W., & Sackett, D. L. (1979). *Compliance in health care.* Baltimore: Johns Hopkins University Press.

Holden, D. J., & Zimmerman, M. A. (2008). *A practical guide to program evaluation planning: Theory and case examples.* Thousand Oaks, CA: Sage.

Hulton, L. J. (2007). An evaluation of a school-based teenage pregnancy prevention program using a logic model framework. *Journal of School Nursing, 23*(2), 104–110.

Jacobson Vann, J. C. (2006). Measuring community-based case management performance: Strategies for evaluation. *Lippincott's Case Management, 11*(3), 147–157.

Kaplan, S. H., Greenfield, S., & Ware, Jr., J. E. (1989). Assessing the effects of physician-patient interactions on the outcomes of chronic disease. *Medical Care, 27,* S110–S127.

Keppel, G., & Zedeck, S. (1989). *Data analysis for research designs.* New York: W. H. Freeman.

Kirchhoff, K. T., & Dille, C. A. (1994). Issues in intervention research: Maintaining integrity. *Applied Nursing Research, 7,* 32–38.

Laryea, M., Sen, P., Gien, L., Kozma, A., & Palacio, T. (1999). Using focus groups to evaluate an education program. *International Journal of Psychiatric Nursing Research, 4*(3), 482–488.

Lipsey, M. W. (1994). Identifying potentially interesting variables and analysis opportunities. In H. Cooper & L. V. Hedges (Eds.), *The handbook of research synthesis* (pp. 111–123). New York: Russell Sage Foundation.

Logan, S., Boutotte, J., Wilce, M., & Etkind, S. (2003). Using the CDC framework for program evaluation in public health to assess tuberculosis contact investigation programs. *International Journal of Tuberculosis and Lung Disease, 7*(12), S375–S383.

Menix, K. D. (2007). Evaluation of learning and program effectiveness. *Journal of Continuing Education in Nursing, 38*(5), 201–231.

Meyer, R. M., & Meyer, M. C. (2000). Utilization-focused evaluation: Evaluating the effectiveness of a hospital nursing orientation program. *Journal for Nurses in Staff Development, 16*(5), 202–208.

Morgan, D. L. (1988). *Focus groups as qualitative research.* Sage University Paper Series on Qualitative Research Methods, Vol. 16. Beverly Hills, CA: Sage.

Ong, L. M. L., DeHaes, J. C. J. M., Hoos, A. M., & Lammes, F. B. (1995). Doctor-patient communication: A review of the literature. *Social Science & Medicine, 40,* 903–918.

Packer, T., Race, K. E. H., & Hotch, D. F. (1994). Focus groups: A tool for consumer-based program evaluation in rehabilitation agency settings. *Journal of Rehabilitation, 60,* 30–33.

Posavac, E. J., & Carey, R. G. (2007). *Program evaluation: Methods and case studies* (7th ed.). Upper Saddle River, NJ: Pearson Education.

Randell, C. L., & Delekto, M. (1999). Telehealth technology evaluations process. *Journal of Healthcare Information Management, 13*(4), 101–110.

Robinson, J. P., Shaver, P. R., & Wrightsman, L. S. (1991). *Measures of personality and social psychological attitudes.* San Diego: Academic Press.

Rosenthal, R., & Rosnow, R. L. (1991). *Essentials of behavioral research: Methods and data analysis.* New York: McGraw-Hill.

Ross, C. E., & Duff, R. S. (1982). Returning to the doctor: The effects of client characteristics, type of practice, and experience with care. *Journal of Health and Social Behavior, 23,* 119–131.

Rossi, P., & Freeman, H. (1989). *Evaluation: A systematic approach* (4th ed.). Newbury Park, CA: Sage.

Shadish, Jr., W. R., Cook, T. D., & Leviton, L. C. (1995). *Foundations of program evaluation: Theories of practice.* Thousand Oaks, CA: Sage.

Slevin, E., Somerville, H., & McKenna, H. (1996). The implementation and evaluation of a quality improvement initiative at Oaklands. *Journal of Nursing Management, 4,* 27–34.

Spaulding, D. T. (2008). *Program evaluation in practice: Core concepts and examples for discussion and analysis.* San Francisco: Jossey-Bass.

Stetler, C. B., Legro, M. W., Wallace, C. M., Bowman, C., Guihan, M., Hagedorn, H., et al. (2006). The role of formative evaluation in implementation research and the QUERI experience. *Journal of General Internal Medicine, 21,* S1–8.

Stetler, C. B., McQueen, L., Demakis, J., & Mittman, B. S. (2008). An organizational framework and strategic implementation for system-level change to enhance research-based practice: QUERI services. *Implementation Science, 3,* 30.

Stewart, A. L., & Ware, Jr., J. E. (1992). *Measuring functioning and well-being.* Durham, NC, and London: Duke University Press.

Stewart, D. W., & Shamdasani, P.M. (1990). *Focus groups: Theory and practice.* Applied Social Research Methods Series, Vol. 20. Newbury Park, CA: Sage.

Sufflebeam, D. L., & Shinkfield, A. J. (2007). *Evaluation theory, models and applications.* San Francisco: Jossey Bass.

W. K. Kellogg Foundation. (2008). Retrieved November 2008 from http://www.wkkf. org/

Ware, Jr., J. E., Davies-Avery, A., & Donald, C. A. (1978). *Conceptualization and measurement of health for adults in the health insurance study. Vol. V, General Health Perceptions.* Santa Monica, CA: RAND Corporation.

Western Michigan University Evaluation Center. (2008). Retrieved November 2008 from http://www.wmich.edu/evalctr/

Wyatt, T. H., Krauskopf, P. B., & Davidson, R. (2008). Using focus groups for program planning and evaluation. *Journal of School Nursing, 24*(2), 71–77.

# 17 Implementing Evidence-Based Practice

SUSAN ADAMS AND MARITA G. TITLER

The use of evidence-based practice (EBP) has become the expected standard in health care; yet in spite of decades of high-quality health care research and a growing evidence base, its impact at the point of care remains inconsistent. It has long been recognized that the availability of high-quality research does not ensure that findings will be used to improve patient outcomes (Clancy, Slutsky, & Patton, 2004; Institute of Medicine, 2001; McGlynn et al., 2003). In fact, recent findings in both the United States and the Netherlands indicate that 30% to 40% of patients do not receive evidence-based care, and 20% to 25% of patients receive unneeded or potentially harmful care (Graham et al., 2006).

In an effort to improve patient care, government bodies and individual organizations have focused time, attention, and resources on compiling and evaluating research findings, as shown by the increase in published systematic reviews (Institute of Medicine, 2008). The findings from these reviews on topics relevant to preventive, acute, and chronic health care have been used to develop behavioral interventions, evidence-based health care programs, and evidence-based guidelines and protocols. However, despite these efforts, use of evidence-based practices at the point of care remains inconsistent (Clancy et al., 2004; Grimshaw et al., 2004; Institute of Medicine, 2007b; Srinivasan & Fisher, 2000; Taylor, Auble, Calhoun, & Mosesso, 1999; Wang, Berglund, & Kessler, 2000).

There is a need for focused research to identify effective strategies to increase the use of evidence-based programs, guidelines, and protocols (Institute of Medicine, 2007a; Leape, 2005; Rubenstein & Pugh, 2006; Sung et al., 2003) and to answer questions such as these: What strategies are effective in increasing the use of EBP? Are these strategies effective in all settings (e.g., acute care, long-term care, school health, primary care)? Are they effective with all end users (e.g., nurses, physicians, pharmacists, and housekeeping staff)? And are they effective with different evidence-based health care practices (prescribing drugs, hand washing, fall prevention)? In summary, we need to know what strategies to use in what setting and with whom for varying topics when implementing evidence-based practices in an organization.

This chapter describes the field of implementation science, a relatively new area of study that is addressing these questions through research. Included are emerging definitions, an overview of promising models, the current state of the science, and information on developing a program of research. The chapter concludes with suggestions for future research needed to move the field forward.

## DEFINITION OF TERMS

*Implementation,* simply stated, is putting into effect the decision to adopt a change in practice (e.g., a research finding or an evidence-based health care practice). *Implementation research* is the investigation of strategies to increase the rate and extent of adoption and sustainability of EBP by individuals and organizations to improve clinical and operational decision making (Eccles & Mittman, 2006; Titler, Everett, & Adams, 2007). It includes research to (1) understand context variables that influence adoption of EBPs, and (2) test the effectiveness of interventions to promote and sustain use of evidence-based health care practices. *Implementation science* denotes both the systematic investigation of methods, interventions, and variables that influence adoption of evidence-based health care practices and the organized body of knowledge gained through such research (Eccles & Mittman, 2006; Rubenstein & Pugh, 2006; Sussman, Valente, Rohrbach, Skara, & Pentz, 2006; Titler & Everett, 2001; Titler et al., 2007).

Because implementation research is a young science, there are no standardized definitions of commonly used terms (Graham et al., 2006). This is evidenced by differing definitions and the interchanging of terms that, in fact, may represent different concepts to different people. Adding to the confusion, terminology may vary depending on the country in which the research was conducted. A recent study done by Graham et al. (2006) reported identifying 29 terms in nine countries that refer to some aspect of translating research findings into practice. For example, researchers in Canada may use the terms *research utilization, knowledge-to-action, knowledge transfer,* or *knowledge translation* interchangeably, while researchers in the United States, the United Kingdom, and Europe may be more likely to use the terms *implementation* or *research translation* to express similar concepts (Graham & Logan, 2004; Graham et al., 2006; Titler & Everett, 2001). Table 17.1 provides examples of currently used definitions of common terms describing concepts related to implementation science. While these definitions provide an explanation of terms used in articles about implementation science, terms such as *implementation, dissemination, research translation,* and *knowledge transfer* may be used interchangeably, and the reader must determine the exact meaning from the content of the article.

The interchange of terms leads to confusion about how implementation research fits into the broader picture of conduct and use of research. One way to understand this relationship is to compare implementation research and the commonly used scientific terms for the steps of scientific discovery: basic research, methods development, efficacy trials, effectiveness trials, and dissemination trials (Sussman et al., 2006). For example, the term *translation* denotes the idea of moving something from one form to another. The National Institutes of Health (NIH) uses this term to describe the process of moving basic research knowledge that may be directly or indirectly relevant to health behavior changes into a form that eventually has impact on patient outcomes (Sussman et al., 2006). NIH has increased emphasis on translation research and has divided the concept into Type I and Type II. Type I translation research focuses on the first three steps of research, that is, basic, or "bench" research, and the movement of that research forward through methods development and efficacy trials. Type II describes the movement through the last two steps of the research process: effectiveness trials and dissemination trials. Implementation research is a subset of Type II translation research as denoted by NIH and focuses on the last step of the research process: actual use of the information to change practice. Building a common taxonomy of terms in implementation science is of primary importance to this field and must involve input from a variety of stakeholders and researchers from various disciplines (e.g., health care,

Table 17.1

## DEFINITIONS ASSOCIATED WITH EVIDENCE-BASED PRACTICE

| | DEFINITION | SOURCE |
|---|---|---|
| Diffusion | "The process by which an innovation is communicated through certain channels over time among members of a social system" | Rogers, E. (2003). *Diffusion of innovations* (5th ed). New York: Simon & Schuster, p. 5 |
| Dissemination | "The targeted distribution of information and intervention materials to a specific public health or clinical practice audience. The intent is to spread knowledge and the associated evidence-based intervention." | NIH, retrieved September 22, 2007, from http://grants.nih.gov/grants/guide/pa-files/PAR-07-086.html |
| Dissemination Research | "The study of the processes and variables that determine and/or influence the adoption of knowledge, interventions or practice by various stakeholders" Research about "how, when, by whom, and under what circumstances research evidence spreads throughout the agencies, organizations, and front line workers providing public health and clinical services." | Dobbins, M., Ciliska, D., Cockerill, R., Barnsley, J., & DiCenso, A. (2002). A framework for the dissemination and utilization of research for health-care policy and practice. *Online Journal of Knowledge Synthesis for Nursing, 9*(7), p. 2 NIH retrieved 4/46/09 from http://grants.nih.gov/grants/guide/pa-files/PAR-07-086.html |
| Evidence | "Knowledge that has been derived from a variety of sources and that has been tested and found to be credible" | Jones, M., & Higgs, J. (2000). Will evidence-based practice take the reasoning out of practice? In J. Higgs & M. Jones (Eds.), *Clinical reasoning in the health professions.* Boston. Butterworth Heinemann, p. 311 |
| Implementation | "The use of strategies to adopt and integrate evidence-based health interventions and change practice patterns within specific settings." | NIH, retrieved April 26, 2009, from http://grants.nih.gov/grants/guide/pa-files/PAR-07-086.html |

*(Continued)*

Table

## DEFINITIONS ASSOCIATED WITH EVIDENCE-BASED PRACTICE (CONTINUED)

| | DEFINITION | SOURCE |
|---|---|---|
| Implementation Research | "The scientific study of methods to promote the systematic uptake of clinical research findings and other evidence-based practices into routine practice" in order to improve the quality and effectiveness of health care | Graham, I. D., Logan, J., Harrison, M. B., Straus, S. E., Tetroe, J., Caswell, W., et al. (2006). Lost in knowledge translation: Time for a map? *Journal of Continuing Education in the Health Professions, 26*(1), 13–24 |
| Implementation Science | "The investigation of methods, interventions, and variables that influence adoption of evidence-based healthcare practices by individuals and organizations to improve clinical and operational decision making and includes testing the effectiveness of interventions to promote and sustain use of evidence-based healthcare practices"<br>"All aspects of research relevant to the scientific study of methods to promote the uptake of research findings into routine health care in both clinical and policy contexts." | Titler, M. G., Everett, L. Q., & Adams, S. (2007). Implications for implementation science. *Nursing Research, 56*(4 Suppl.), S53–S59, p. S53<br>Graham, I. D., Logan, J., Harrison, M. B., Straus, S. E., Tetroe, J., Caswell, W., et al. (2006). Lost in knowledge translation: Time for a map? *Journal of Continuing Education in the Health Professions, 26*(1), 13–24. |
| Knowledge to Action | A broad concept that encompasses both the transfer of knowledge and the *use* of knowledge by practitioners, policymakers, patients and the public, including use of knowledge in practice and/or the decision making process. The term is often used interchangeably with knowledge transfer or knowledge translation. | Graham, I. D., Logan, J., Harrison, M. B., Straus, S. E., Tetroe, J., Caswell, W., et al. (2006). Lost in knowledge translation: Time for a map? *Journal of Continuing Education in the Health Professions, 26*(1), 13–24. |
| Knowledge Transfer | "Knowledge transfer is used to mean the process of getting knowledge used by stakeholders." | Graham, I. D., Logan, J., Harrison, M. B., Straus, S. E., Tetroe, J., Caswell, W., et al. (2006). Lost in knowledge translation: Time for a map? *Journal of Continuing Education in the Health Professions, 26*(1), 13–24. |

*(Continued)*

# Table 17.1

## ITH EVIDENCE-BASED PRACTICE (CONTINUED)

| | | SOURCE |
|---|---|---|
| | ...iew of 'knowledge ...ni-directional flow of knowledge from researchers to users." | Canadian Institutes of Health Research,, retrieved April 26, 2009, from http://www.cihr-irsc.gc.ca/e/26574.html |
| Knowledge Trans-lation | "Knowledge translation is the exchange, synthesis and ethically-sound application of knowledge - within a complex system of interactions among researchers and users"- | Canadian Institutes of Health Research,, Retrieved April 26, 2009, from http://www.cihr-irsc.gc.ca/e/26574.html |
| Research Utili-zation | A process directed toward transfer of specific research into practice through the systematic use of a series of activities | Horsley, J., Crane, A., Crabtree, M., & Wood, D. (1983). Using research to improve nursing practice: A guide. Philadelphia: W. B. Saunders |
| Translation Research | Testing the effectiveness of interventions on the rate and extent of adoption of evidence-based practices by nurses, physicians, and other health care providers | Titler, M., & Everett, L. (2001). Translating research into practice. Critical Care Nursing Clinics of North America, 12(4), 587–604 |
| | Translation research broadly studies and examines factors that facilitate efficacious and effective translation of research into everyday health policies and programs; evaluates the effectiveness of the administrative, management, policy, healthcare and health practice decisions and/or use of research knowledge; and describes the experience and roles of the stakeholders, practitioners, and participants. | National Institutes of Health, retrieved September 22, 2007, from http://grants.nih.gov/grants/guide/rfa-files/RFA-CD-07-005.html |

From *Understand the Context for Translation of Evidence-Based Practice Into School Nursing,* by S. Adams, 2007. Unpublished dissertation. University of Iowa College of Nursing. Reprinted with permission.

organizational science, psychology, and health services research) (Institute of Medicine, 2007b).

## IMPLEMENTATION MODELS

Several models are available to guide the overall process of evidence-based practice (Rosswurm & Larrabee, 1999; Stetler, 2001; Titler et al., 2001). Most of these models include implementation as a concept, but the focus of EBP models is primarily on identifying clinical problems, collecting and analyzing evidence, making the decision to use the evidence to change practice, and evaluating the change after implementation. Little detail and little guidance are provided regarding the actual process of implementation. Users of these models are told to "implement," a directive that fails to take into account the complexity of the process of implementation. Implementing and sustaining change is a complex and multifaceted process, requiring attention to both individual and organizational factors (Titler, 2008).

Many experts believe that using a model specifically focused on implementation provides a framework for identifying factors that may be pertinent in different settings or circumstances, and allows for testing and comparing tailored strategies for individual settings. The hope is this will allow for some generalization of results (Grimshaw, Eccles, Walker, & Thomas, 2002; ICEBeRG, 2006). While no single model may apply to all situations, a model must be sufficiently specific to guide both implementation research and implementation at the point of care but general enough to cross various populations.

Several attempts have been made to search for and organize the multitude of theories, models, and frameworks that are used to promote changes in practice or behavior. Just as the terms for implementation science are often used interchangeably, although technically they are not the same, the terms *conceptual frameworks/models* and *theoretical framework/models* are often used interchangeably, although they differ in their level of abstraction (ICEBeRG, 2006; Kitson et al., 2008; Meleis, 2005). In this discussion, the term *model* will be used as a general term, unless the model is specifically identified as a theory or conceptual framework by its creator. A model, then, for our purposes, is a set of general concepts and propositions that are integrated into a meaningful configuration to represent how a particular theorist views the phenomena of interest, in this case the transfer of evidence into practice (Fawcett, 2005).

Although an extensive review of all models suggested for possible use in implementation science is beyond the scope of this chapter, several promising models are discussed in some detail. For a summary of additional models, the review by Grol and colleagues (2007) is recommended. Included in their recent review of models relevant to quality improvement and implementation of change in health care are cognitive, educational, motivational, social interactive, social learning, social network, social influence theories, as well as models related to team effectiveness, professional development, and leadership. Additional work by the Improved Clinical Effectiveness Through Behavioural Research Group (ICEBeRG) has resulted in the development of an implementation database consisting of planned action models, frameworks and theories that explicitly describe both the concepts and the action steps to be considered or taken. This database was developed from a search of social science, education, and health literature that focused on practitioner or organizational change (http://www.iceberg-grebeci.ohri.ca/research/kt_theories_db.html).

## Diffusion of Innovations

Probably the most well known and frequently used theory for guiding change in practice is the Diffusion of Innovations Theory by Everett Rogers. Rogers (2003) proposed that the rate of adoption of an innovation is influenced by the nature of the innovation, the manner in which the innovation is communicated, and the characteristics of the users and the social system into which the innovation is introduced. Rogers's theory has undergone empirical testing in a variety of different disciplines (Barta, 1995; Charles, 2000; Feldman & McDonald, 2004; Greenhalgh, Robert, Macfarlane, Bate, & Kyriakidou, 2004; Lia-Hoagberg, Schaffer, & Strohschein, 1999; Michel & Sneed, 1995; Rogers, 2003; Rutledge, Greene, Mooney, Nail, & Ropka, 1996; Wiecha et al., 2004).

According to Rogers, an innovation can be used to describe any idea or practice that is perceived as new by an individual or organization; evidence-based health care practices are considered an innovation according to this theory. Rogers acknowledges the complex, nonlinear interrelationships among organizational and individual factors as people move through five stages when adopting an innovation: knowledge/awareness, persuasion, decision, implementation, and evaluation (2003).

## Translation Research Mod

The Translation Research M
is built on Rogers's Diffusio
develop and test strategies
health care (see Figure 17.1
adoption can be influenced
fect each area identified by
(e.g., the use of EBP guid(
channels (e.g., use of opin
social system (e.g., modify
ship support) and individ
focus groups).

The Translation Research Model has been u·c·
in a series of multisite experimental studies funded by the Agency ··
Healthcare Research and Quality (PI Titler, RO1 HS10482, and PI
Titler AHRQ RO2) and the National Cancer Institute (PI Herr R01-
CA115363–01). Strong points of this model are its simplicity and its
focus on specific implementation strategies that have been tested for
effectiveness, that is, the "how" of implementation which is often overlooked in other models.

## The PARiHS Framework

The PARiHS framework (Promoting Action on Research Implementation in Health Services) is another promising model proposed to help
practitioners understand and guide the implementation process. Developed in 1998 as a result of work with clinicians to improve practice,
the framework has undergone concept analysis and has been used as a
guide for structuring research and implementation projects at the point
of care (Ellis, Howard, Larson, & Robertson, 2005; Wallin, Rudberg, &
Gunningberg, 2005; Wallin, Ewald, Wikblad, Scott-Findlay, & Arnetz,
2006). This framework proposes that implementation is a function of the
relationship among the nature and strength of the evidence, the contextual factors of the setting, and the method of facilitation used to introduce the change. Kitson and colleagues suggested that the model may
be best used as part of a two-stage process: first, the practitioner uses the
model to perform a preliminary evaluation measure of the elements of
the evidence and the context and, second, the practitioner uses the data
from the analysis to determine the best method to facilitate change. A

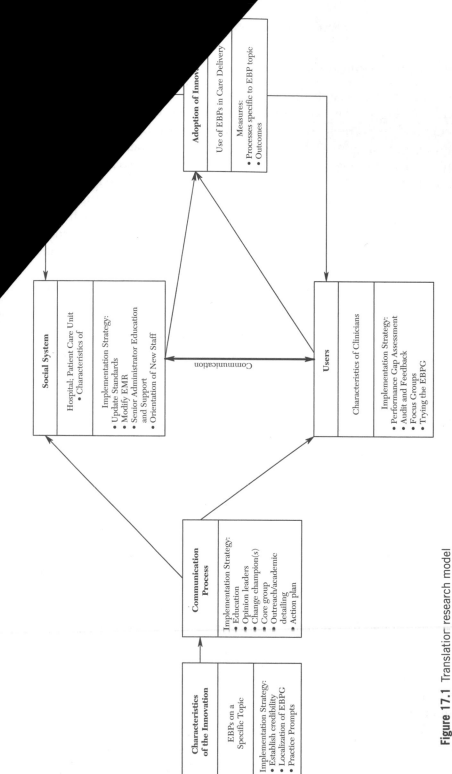

**Figure 17.1** Translation research model
From "Translating Research into Practice: Considerations for Critical Care Investigators," by M. G. Titler & L. Q. Everett, 2001. *Critical Care Nursing Clinics of North America, 13*(4), 587–604.

strong point of this model is its ability to adapt the facilitation process to the level of evidence and the level of context support available, making it adaptable to various situations. For example, if one or two of the components are weak (e.g., poor organizational support), this may be overcome by increased or targeted facilitation. Although the model is promising, it offers few specifics to guide the actual facilitation process. According to Kitson, the PARiSH framework is still under development and has not been tested as a conceptual framework, and its usefulness has not been quantified (Kitson et al., 2008).

## The Knowledge Transfer Framework

The Knowledge Transfer Framework (KTF) (see Figure 17.2) was developed by the Agency for Healthcare Research and Quality (AHRQ) to speed the transfer of results from AHRQ's safety research portfolio into health care practice (Nieva et al., 2005). This framework uses the term *knowledge transfer* to denote a three-stage process that includes (1) knowledge creation and distillation; (2) diffusion and dissemination; and (3) end-user adoption, implementation, and institutionalization.

Although originally designed for the translation of safety research into health care practice, the creators of the framework suggest that it may be relevant to other research initiatives whose focus is the uptake of evidence into practice settings. The framework is broad in scope, but the final stage is pertinent to our discussion of implementation. The suggested strategies are similar to those proposed by both Rogers and Titler; however, there are a few key differences, most notably the use of partnerships and the inclusion of the end users throughout the entire research process. Because implementation of evidence-based health care practices in actual practice settings involves complex and unpredictable interactions, external partnerships may be useful in providing the network of support needed to assess and evaluate these complex relationships and to facilitate the transfer of evidence into practice.

## Conceptual Model of Diffusion in Service Organizations

Although it does not provide specific strategies for the implementation process, the *conceptual model of diffusion in service organizations* by Greenhalgh and colleagues (2005) provides a framework for identifying variables that should be considered when implementing change in organizations. Based on a systematic review of literature on diffusion

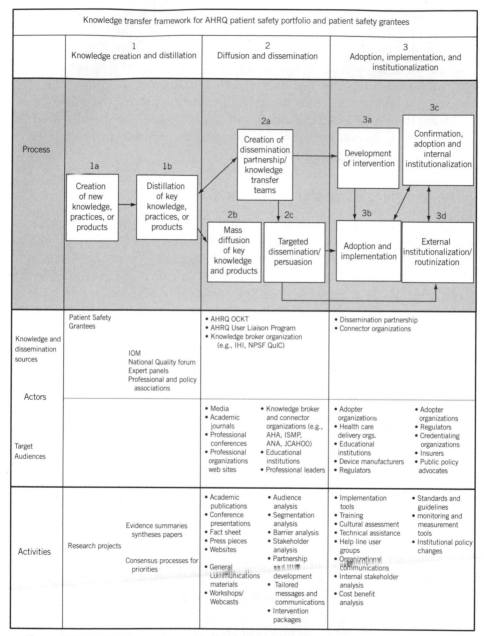

**Figure 17.2** AHRQ Knowledge Transfer Framework (KTF).
From "From Science to Service: A Framework for the Transfer of Patient Safety Research Into Practice," by V. F. Nieva, R. Murphy, N. Ridley, N. Donaldson, J. Combes, P. Mitchell, et al., 2005. In K. Henriksen, J. Battles, E. Marks, & D. I. Lewin (Eds.), *Advances in patient safety: From research to implementation: Vol. 2, Concepts and methodology* (pp. 441–453, AHRQ Publication No. 05-0021-2). Rockville, MD: Agency for Healthcare Research and Quality.

and sustainability of innovations in organizations, the model is intended primarily as a memory aid for those considering different aspects of a complex situation and their interaction. As such, it does not provide specific strategies to achieve implementation but rather provides general points to remember. For example, the model suggests that when looking at the characteristics of the adopter the practitioner should consider the adopter's needs, motivation, values and goals, skills, learning styles, and social networks (Greenhalgh, Robert, Bate, Macfarlane, & Kyriakidou, 2005). The conceptual model of diffusion in service organizations provides an understanding of the variables that should be considered when conducting implementation research or implementing a change in practice.

## STATE OF THE SCIENCE

When implementing EBP, as previously stated, it is helpful to use a model to provide structure and guidance in targeting interventions to increase the rate of adoption. For this discussion we will use the Translation Model (see Figure 17.1) as a guide for providing an overview of implementation strategies. To be effective, it is recommended that the practitioner use multifaceted strategies to affect the various areas identified in the model, that is, the characteristics of the innovation (in this case an evidence-based health care practice), the communication channels, the social system, and the individual users (Feldman, Murtaugh, Pezzin, McDonald, & Peng, 2005; Greenhalgh et al., 2004; Nieva et al., 2005; Rogers, 2003; Rubenstein & Pugh, 2006).

### Innovation

The nature or characteristics of the EBP influences the rate of adoption; however, the attributes of an evidence-based health care practice as perceived by the users and stakeholders are not stable but change depending on the interaction between the users and the context of practice (Dopson, FitzGerald, Ferlie, Gabbay, & Locock, 2002; Greenhalgh et al., 2005). For example, an identical guideline for improving pain management may be viewed as pertinent and not complex by users in one setting (e.g., labor and delivery) but as less of a priority and as difficult to implement by staff in another unit (e.g., gero-psychiatry). While a positive perception of the evidence-based practice alone is not sufficient to ensure adoption, it is important that the information be perceived as pertinent and presented in a way that is credible and easy to understand (Greenhalgh et al., 2004; Greenhalgh et al., 2005; Kitson, Harvey, & McCormack, 1998; Rogers, 2003; Rycroft-Malone et al., 2004; Titler, 2008). Some characteristics of the innovation known to influence the rate of adoption are the complexity or simplicity of the evidence-based health care practice, the credibility and pertinence of the evidence-based health care practice to the user, and the ease or difficulty of assimilating the change into existing behavior (Rogers, 2003; Titler & Everett, 2001). However, while these characteristics are important, the decision to use and sustain an EBP is complex. This is evident in the continued failure to achieve a consistent high rate of adherence to handwashing recommendations in spite of the relative simplicity of the process and the knowledge of its pertinence to optimal patient outcomes.

EBP guidelines are one tested method of presenting information (Grimshaw et al., 2004; Guihan, Bosshart, & Nelson, 2004). EBP guidelines are designed to assimilate large, complex amounts of research information into a useable format (Grimshaw et al., 2004; Lia-Hoagberg et al., 1999). Appropriately designed guidelines are adaptable and easy to assimilate into the local setting (See Appendix B for an example). Empirically tested methods of adapting guidelines and protocols to the local practice setting include practice prompts, quick reference guides, decision-making algorithms, and computer-based decision support systems (Eccles & Grimshaw, 2004; Feldman et al., 2005; Grimshaw et al., 2006; Wensing, Wollersheim, & Grol, 2006).

## Communication

The method and the channels used to communicate with potential users about an innovation influence the speed and extent of adoption of the innovation (Rogers, 2003; Titler & Everett, 2001). Communication channels include both formal methods of communication that are established in the hierarchical system and informal communication networks that occur spontaneously throughout the system. Communication networks are interconnected individuals who are linked by patterned flows of information (Rogers, 2003).

Mass-media communication methods are effective in raising awareness at the population or community level, for example, of public health issues such as the need for immunizations and screenings and include the use of television, radio, newspapers, pamphlets, posters, and leaflets

(Grilli, Ramsay, & Minozzi, 2002; Lam et al., 2003; Randolph & Viswanath, 2004; Rogers, 2003; Silver, Rubini, Black, & Hodgson, 2003). Many acute-care EBP implementation projects also use awareness campaigns in the early stages that may include similar strategies (e.g., bulletin boards, flyers, posters, and newsletters). While research has been done on the effectiveness of mass-media campaigns at the population level to guide message content and delivery to the general public (Grilli et al., 2002; Randolph & Viswanath, 2004), less evidence is available to guide the message content or delivery methods needed to affect the rate of adoption of EBP among health care workers (Titler, 2008).

Interpersonal communication is more effective than mass-media communication in persuading people to change practice (Rogers, 2003). Communication strategies tested in health care systems that use interpersonal communication channels include education (Davis, Thomson, Oxman, & Haynes, 1995; Grimshaw et al., 2001; Forsetlund et al., 2009), opinion leaders (Doumit, Cattellari, Grimshaw, & O'Brien, 2007; Locock, Dopson, Chambers, & Gabbay, 2001), change champions (Guihan et al., 2004), facilitators (Kitson et al., 1998; Stetler et al., 2006), audit and feedback (Grimshaw et al., 2004; Hysong, Best, & Pugh, 2006; Jamtvedt, Young, Kristoffersen, O'Brien, & Oxman, 2006), and outreach consultation and education by experts (Bero et al., 1998; Davis et al., 1995; Feldman & McDonald, 2004; Hysong et al., 2006; Titler, 2008).

The literature indicates that education using didactic teaching strategies such as the traditional dispersion of educational material and formal conference presentations may increase awareness but has little impact on changing practice. Interactive teaching methods, especially when combined with other methods, have proven more effective (Bero et al., 1998; Grimshaw et al., 2001; Forsetlund et al., 2009). Educational strategies that lead to improvement in EBP adherence include educational meetings with an interactive component, small-group educational meetings (which are more effective than large-group meetings), and educational meetings that include an opportunity to practice skills (Forsetlund et al., 2009).

Opinion leaders are informal leaders from the local peer group who are viewed as respected sources of information and judgment regarding the appropriateness of the innovation (Rogers, 2003). They are trusted to evaluate new information and to determine the appropriateness of the innovation for the setting. Opinion leaders have been effective in promoting the adoption of EBP (Doumit et al., 2007), especially in combination with other strategies such as outreach and performance feedback (Dopson et al., 2002; Doumit et al., 2007; Forsetlund et al., 2009; Locock et al., 2001; Soumerai et al., 1998). While the effects of opinion leaders in natural settings have been well documented, selecting and engaging opinion leaders for specific projects is complex (Greenhalgh et al., 2004; Grimshaw, Eccles et al., 2006; Titler, 2008). For changes in practice that involve multiple disciplines, opinion leaders should be selected from each of the various disciplines involved. These opinion leaders must be respected members of their group, competent, knowledgeable, and enthusiastic about the innovation, and able to understand how the new practice fits with the group norms (Collins, Hawks, & Davis, 2000). Opinion leaders can be self-selected (e.g., volunteer to be a leader for a particular EBP), identified by program implementers as known leaders, selected as a result of their position (e.g., local advanced practice nurse), or nominated by staff members to lead the project (Titler, 2002).

Change champions are expert practitioners from the local peer group who promote the use of the innovation (Rogers, 2003). Change champions are nurses who provide information and encouragement, are persistent, and have positive working relationships with their colleagues (Titler, 2008). The use of change champions has proven effective in many settings (Estabrooks, O'Leary, Ricker, & Humphrey, 2003; Rycroft-Malone et al., 2004; Titler, 2002). Research suggests that nurses prefer interpersonal communication with peers rather than other sources of information, so the presence of a change champion is crucial in facilitating the adoption of the innovation (Adams & Barron, 2009; Estabrooks, O'Leary, et al., 2003; Estabrooks, Chong, Brigidear, & Profetto-McGrath, 2005).

Using a core group or team that has the same goal of promoting evidence-based practice, along with the change champion, increases the likelihood of obtaining the critical mass of users necessary to promote and sustain the adoption of the practice change (Dopson et al., 2002; Nelson et al., 2002; Rogers, 2003; Titler, 2006, 2008). Members of the core group should represent the various shifts and days of the weeks and should assume responsibility for providing information, daily reinforcement of the change, and positive feedback to several of their peers. Conferencing with the core group, opinion leaders, and change champions during implementation of the innovation is recommended to provide additional support and guidance (Horbar et al., 2004; Titler, 2008; Titler & Everett, 2001).

Educational outreach, also called academic detailing, is one-on-one communication between an external topic expert and health care practitioners in their practice setting to provide information on the practice change. The expert should be knowledgeable about the research base for the evidence-based practice change and able to respond to questions and concerns that arise during implementation. Feedback on performance and/or education may be provided at that time. When used alone or in combination with other strategies, outreach has proven effective in adoption of EBP (Feldman & McDonald, 2004; Hendryx et al., 1998; Horbar et al., 2004; O'Brien et al., 2007).

A related concept is the facilitator role identified as an essential component in the PARiHS model of translation of EBP (Harvey et al., 2002). The facilitator role may range from task-focused activities (e.g., outreach, academic detailing) to holistic interactions designed to enable individuals, teams, and organizations to change practice (Harvey et al., 2002; Kitson et al., 1998; Stetler et al., 2006). The facilitator may be internal to the organization or external to the organization, and facilitation may encompass more than one individual (both internal and external), in contrast to outreach, which is typically external to the organization (Greenhalgh et al., 2005; Stetler et al., 2006; Titler, 2008).

## Users of the Innovation

Several studies have analyzed attitudes and characteristics that influence adoption of EBP by individual users (Estabrooks, Floyd, Scott-Findlay, O'Leary, & Gushta, 2003; Milner, Estabrooks, & Myrick, 2006; Rogers, 2003). Characteristics such as favorable attitude toward research and previous involvement in research studies are consistently associated with use of research findings in practice (Estabrooks, Floyd, et al., 2003). Additional characteristics such as educational level, professional role (e.g., management versus staff nurse), autonomy, conference attendance, cooperativeness and self-efficacy, job satisfaction, professional association membership, and time spent reading professional journals may influence one's readiness to adopt EBP, but the findings are not consistent across various studies (Estabrooks, 1999; Hutchinson & Johnston, 2004; McKenna, Ashton, & Keeney, 2004; Milner et al., 2006).

Implementation strategies targeted to the individual user include audit and feedback and performance gap assessment (PGA). PGA and audit and feedback have consistently shown positive effects on changing practice behavior of providers (Berwick, 2003; Bradley, Holmboe, et al., 2004; Horbar et al., 2004; Hysong et al., 2006; Jamtvedt et al., 2006; McCartney, Macdowall, & Thorogood, 1997). PGA is the provision of *baseline* performance data specific to the EBPs being implemented (e.g., pain assessment, fall rates) to practitioners at the beginning of the implementation process (Jamtvedt et al., 2006), accompanied by a discussion about the gap between current practices and the desired evidence-based practices. For example, investigators who were testing the effectiveness of a translating-research-into-practice intervention for acute pain management in older adults met with physicians and nurses at each experimental site at the beginning of the implementation process to review indicators of acute pain management (e.g., avoid meperidine prescription) specific to their setting and to discuss gaps between current practices and recommended evidence-based practices in areas such as frequency of pain assessment, dosing of opiods, and around-the-clock administration of analgesics (Titler et al., 2009). Audit and feedback follows PGA and consists of ongoing audit of performance indicators specific to the EBP being implemented (e.g., pain assessment, fall rates), followed by presentation and discussion of the data with staff members. For example, investigators testing the TRIP intervention followed the PGA strategy, with ongoing audit and feedback of pain data collected by concurrent medical record abstraction of older adult patients admitted during the implementation phase and presentation of data in graph form to nurses and physicians every 6 weeks for 10 months (six reports). Although these strategies show a consistently positive effect on adoption of EBPs, the effect size varies between studies. Greater effectiveness is associated with additional factors such as low baseline compliance and increased intensity of the feedback (Bero et al., 1998; Davis et al., 1995; Grimshaw et al., 2001; Grimshaw et al., 2004; Hysong et al., 2006; Jamtvedt et al., 2006). Organizations with a successful record of EBP guideline adherence provide nonpunitive, individualized feedback in a timely manner throughout the implementation process (Hysong et al., 2006). Timely feedback is feedback that is provided monthly or more frequently; those organizations that provide feedback at longer intervals or inconsistently have lower adherence to guidelines (Hysong et al., 2006). Providing individual feedback, as opposed to unit or facility level feedback, is also associated with better adherence to EBP guidelines. Offering positive feedback, in addition to pointing out areas where the practitioner can improve performance, provides better results than providing feedback only when staff members fall short of optimal performance (Hysong et al., 2006).

## Social System

The social system or context of care delivery influences adoption of an innovation (Fraser, 2004a, 2004b; Institute of Medicine, 2001; Rogers, 2003; Vaughn, McCoy, & BootsMiller, 2002). To date, much of implementation research has focused on acute and primary care. However, health care is delivered in a wide variety of health care delivery systems, including occupational settings, school settings, long-term care and assisted-living facilities, and homes and community settings through public health and home health care agencies. These settings have obvious differences because of their unique natures, but, even within similar settings, each organization has its own character and feel. This is a result of the interaction of individuals through communication channels and social networks within the organizational structure and hierarchy, as well as interaction with the larger community as a whole. It is important to remember that the resulting social system is unique to each setting and is complex and dynamic (Garside, 1998; Greenhalgh et al., 2005; Scott, Mannion, Davies, & Marshall, 2003a, 2003b).

When choosing strategies to increase adoption of EBP, it is necessary to focus on both the organizational structures and the individual adopters within the social system. For example, requiring a change in pain assessment frequency by individual caregivers but not providing the accompanying organizational changes (appropriate forms, changes in the electronic charting system, inclusion of the new standards in performance evaluations) is shortsighted and reduces the likelihood the change will be sustained in practice. Organizational procedures and policies should support the use of EBPs and should contain language explicitly requiring their use in all policies and protocols instituted in the organization (Titler & Everett, 2001). The expectation that practice will be based on evidence and participation in research activities should be a written part of job evaluations, as well.

There are several structural characteristics that are consistently associated with increased use of EBP, such as size, slack resources, and urbanicity. Organizations that are larger in size and divided into differentiated and specialized semiautonomous units are associated with innovativeness. Slack resources (i.e., uncommitted resources) are associated with larger organizations and may be partially responsible for the impact of organization size on adoption rates. Larger organizations may have more resources available, both financial and human, to support EBP in practice. Urbanicity provides organizations with access to more interpersonal and mass media channels, access to resources and education opportunities, exposure to new ideas, and contact with other innovative organizations (Greenhalgh et al., 2005; Rogers, 2003; Titler, 2008).

There is no question that leadership at all levels in the organization is critical to adoption of EBP. The leader defines and communicates the organization's goals and vision (Bradley, Holmboe, et al., 2004; Bradley, Schlesinger, Webster, Baker, & Inouye, 2004; Institute of Medicine, 2001). Most early studies focused on measurable characteristics such as educational background and tenure of individuals holding key leadership positions (Greenhalgh et al., 2005). The wider contribution of leadership is harder to explicitly measure but includes efforts in areas such as promoting a climate that facilitates adoption, which can include communication style, providing a nonpunitive environment for risk taking, providing resources for EBP projects, providing time for research activities, and promoting a learning environment (Greenhalgh et al., 2005; Stetler, 2003; Titler, 2002, 2008). Other influences of leadership include setting role expectations that include the use research in practice, providing role clarity, and supporting democratic and inclusive decision-making processes (Bradley, Webster, et al., 2004; Institute of Medicine, 2001; McCormack et al., 2002; Meijers et al., 2006; Rutledge & Donaldson, 1995). However, little research has been done on specific leadership strategies at the unit manager level that may impact the adoption of EBP.

Additional strategies are (1) the use of multidisciplinary teams, especially in the care of chronic illnesses, and (2) the revising of professional roles (Wensing et al., 2006). Both strategies have been effective in improving patient outcomes through better adherence to recommended EBP guidelines and also have resulted in reduced health care costs (Wensing et al., 2006). The use of multidisciplinary teams seeks to improve communication and cooperation between professional groups (e.g., physicians and nurses) and also to streamline services (Zwarenstein & Reeves, 2006). However, all teams are not created equal, and measuring characteristics of teams that improve patient outcomes is difficult. Some characteristics of high-functioning teams that show positive impact on patient care include team composition, stability, collaboration, time allotted for the various tasks, explicit, appropriate task and role definitions, and having a team leader (Schouten et al., 2008). A related strategy, revision of professional roles (e.g., reassigning prevention interventions to non-physician staff, such as nurses), has also resulted in improved patient outcomes through better adherence to EBP guidelines (Zwarenstein & Reeves, 2006).

Documentation systems for effective data recording aid in the implementation and sustainability of guidelines and protocols by providing appropriate forms for outcome measurement and information for quality-improvement programs (Garside, 1998; Greenhalgh et al., 2004; Titler, 2008; Wensing et al., 2006). In addition, access to computer technology can improve professional performance and client outcomes in two ways. First, use of data recording, patient record keeping, computer prompts, and reminders increase adherence to EBP (Rappolt, Pearce, McEwen, & Polatajko, 2005; Wensing & Grol, 1994; Wensing et al., 2006). Second, information systems, including computer technology, allow for better knowledge acquisition and management (Bradley, Holmboe, et al., 2004; Titler, 2008; Wensing et al., 2006). The Institute of Medicine's 2001 report, *Crossing the Quality Chasm: A New Health System for the 21st Century,* stresses the importance of computerized information technology systems, but in order to take advantage of these systems, health care workers need not only access but the skills to use them (Institute of Medicine, 2001). Organizations that provide needed resources and access to support for EBP, such as technology and sufficient training to allow staff to become proficient, libraries, research findings, computer databases, journals, time and financial support for continuing education, and time for research participation and implementation, are more likely to implement and sustain EBP in practice (Bryar et al., 2003; Dopson, Locock, Chambers, & Gabbay, 2001; Estabrooks, 2003; Estabrooks, O'Leary, et al., 2003; Meijers et al., 2006; Pravikoff, Tanner, & Pierce, 2005; Titler, 2008).

## DESIGNING IMPLEMENTATION STUDIES

The Institute of Medicine Forum on the Science of Quality Improvement and Implementation Research has sponsored several workshops on implementation science in which researchers have addressed various perspectives in conducting studies in this field (http://www.nap.edu). Methods used in implementation studies range from qualitative, phenomenological studies to randomized controlled trials. Links between generalizable scientific evidence for a given health care topic and specific contexts create opportunities for experiential learning in implementation science (Institute of Medicine, 2007a). Given this perspective, qualitative methods may be used to better understand why specific implementation strategies work in some settings and not in others. For example, an investigator might ask why CMS-regulated evidence-based practices for heart failure patients are adhered to in some hospitals and not others. A study designed to understand these differences might use qualitative approaches such as interviews with front-line staff, observation of clinical care delivery, and practitioner focus groups (Tripp-Reimer & Doebbeling, 2004). This qualitative study would generate hypotheses for future investigations. Such studies provide a sound basis for empirical studies on the effectiveness of implementation interventions.

Rigorous evaluations of implementation interventions provide a solid base of research that can be built upon. Much can be learned from empirical evaluation of naturally occurring adoption efforts such as the implementation of rapid-response teams in acute-care settings. Implementation studies that investigate natural experiments provide several benefits, including testing the relationships among various individual and system factors and the level of practice adoption. Understanding these factors and their relationships is important as one designs studies to test the effectiveness of implementation interventions.

At the IOM workshops, Grimshaw discussed the disagreement in the field of implementation science regarding the use of randomized controlled trials (RCTs) to evaluate the effectiveness of implementation interventions (Institute of Medicine, 2007a, 2007b). There is some antipathy to the use of RCTs in complex social contexts such as the process of implementation of EBPs, although others believe RCTs to be an extremely valuable method of evaluating these interventions. Randomized trials of implementation interventions tend to be pragmatic and focus on effectiveness in order to elucidate whether an intervention will be effective in a real-world setting. Such RCTs, unlike RCTs that focus on efficacy (e.g., drug trials), have broad inclusion criteria and are designed to improve our understanding of both the influence of context on the effectiveness of the intervention and why changes occurred. One method of achieving this understanding is to use observational approaches in conjunction with data from the RCT to test multilevel hypotheses about which interventions work and which do not. RCTs build on the knowledge generated by observational studies and case studies (Institute of Medicine, 2007a). The best method to evaluate a given intervention depends upon the research question(s), hypotheses, and the specifics of the implementation intervention. One should always attempt to choose a mixture of the best possible methods, given the individual circumstances.

Building this body of research knowledge will require development in many areas. Theoretical developments are needed to provide frameworks and predictive theories that will lead to generalizable research such as studies on how to change individual and organizational behavior. Methodological developments are also required, as are exploratory studies aimed at improving our understanding of the experiential and organizational learning that accompanies implementation. Rigorous evaluations are needed to evaluate the effectiveness and efficiency of implementation interventions, and partnerships are needed to encourage communication among researchers, theorists, and implementers and to help researchers understand what types of knowledge are needed and how that knowledge can best be developed (Dawson, 2004; Titler, 2004a, 2004b; Tripp-Reimer & Doebbeling, 2004).

## FUTURE DIRECTIONS

While the evidence-base for implementation strategies is growing, there is much work to be done. In 2003, the U.S. Invitational Conference "Advancing Quality Care Through Translation Research" convened, funded in part by the Agency for Healthcare Research and Quality (1 R13 HS014141–01). The objective was to set forth a future research agenda for translation (or implementation) science. Seventy-seven participants representing 25 states and all geographic regions of the United States were selected to attend on the basis of their knowledge and skills in research, education, practice, and public policy; the goal was to advance a translation science agenda.

Conference participants recommended giving high priority to testing multifaceted, interdisciplinary implementation interventions in a variety of settings, and to designing multisite studies that increase understanding about what interventions work in similar types of settings (e.g., acute care) with different contextual factors. Priority was also given to comparing the effectiveness of implementation interventions in different types of clinical settings (e.g., acute versus home health) to foster understanding of the components of the intervention that need modification depending on type of setting. These implementation priorities are congruent with recommendations of others (Dopson et al., 2002; Greenhalgh et al., 2004; Grimshaw et al., 2004; Kirchhoff, 2004).

A unique finding of the U.S. Invitational Conference was the call to prioritize research on (1) methods for engaging stakeholders to increase their support; and (2) implementation of clinical topics for nursing practice based on existing guidelines and synthesis reports.

The conference attendees identified these recommended research priorities for implementation science:

- Test implementation strategies across different types and contexts of care delivery to determine which strategies are most effective for which type of health care setting and context.
- Test interdisciplinary approaches (e.g., physicians, nurses, physical therapists) to implementation.
- Test combined or multiple implementation strategies such as education plus use of opinion leaders plus audit and feedback.
- Test various dissemination methods and implementation strategies such as electronic information technology, communication strategies, and facilitator roles.
- Determine best methods for engaging stakeholders to promote the use of evidence in practice.
- Focus on measurement and methodological issues encountered in translation science regarding process measures, outcome measures, intervention/TRIP dose, core dependent measures (e.g., process versus outcome measures), organizational context, nested designs, and qualitative methods.
- Investigate leadership and organizational context variables and measures that promote EBPs.
- Develop and test measures of organizational readiness for EBP.
- Determine ways to create practice cultures that facilitate change.
- Test organizational-level interventions that promote EBPs.

## SUMMARY

The use of EBP remains sporadic in spite of a growing evidence base and the increasing availability of systematic reviews and predeveloped EBP guidelines. Implementation science provides a research focus for identifying effective strategies to increase the use of evidence-based programs, guidelines, and protocols in different settings and among different end users. Because this is a young science, standardized definitions have not been established. Commonly used terms were identified in this chapter, along with promising models to guide implementation at the point of care. The current evidence base for implementation strategies is growing, and, while additional research is needed, there is sufficient evidence to warrant use of evidence-based strategies when implementing a change in practice.

## SUGGESTED ACTIVITIES

1   You are the nurse manager of an adult surgical inpatient unit (30 beds) at a 500-bed community hospital. Staff are changing practice for assessment of bowel mobility following abdominal surgery. The practice change includes "giving up" listening for bowel sounds. Describe an implementation plan with specific implementation strategies for making this change in practice.

2   You are the school nurse supervising other school nurses in a rural consolidated school district. This school district includes three high schools, five elementary schools, and four middle schools. There are nine school nurses: two covering the high schools, two covering the middles schools, and 5 covering the elementary schools.

   a   Select a topic of interest to school nurses to promote the health of the population of students with a rationale for why this topic was selected.

   b   Identify evidence sources for each topic.

   c   Describe implementation strategies for the selected topics.

## REFERENCES

Adams, S. (2007). Understanding the context for translation of evidence-based practice into school nursing. Unpublished dissertation. University of Iowa College of Nursing, Iowa City.

Adams, S., & Barron, S. (2009). Use of evidence-based practice in school nursing: Prevalence, associated variables and perceived needs. *Worldviews on Evidence-Based Nursing, 5*(4), 1–11.

Barta, K. M. (1995). Information-seeking, research utilization, and barriers to research utilization of pediatric nurse educators. *Journal of Professional Nursing: Official Journal of the American Association of Colleges of Nursing, 11*(1), 49–57.

Bero, L. A., Grilli, R., Grimshaw, J. M., Harvey, E., Oxman, A. D., & Thomson, M. A. (1998). Closing the gap between research and practice: An overview of systematic reviews of interventions to promote the implementation of research findings. The Cochrane effective practice and organization of care review group. *British Medical Journal (Clinical Research Edition), 317*(7156), 465–468.

Berwick, D. M. (2003). Disseminating innovations in health care. *Journal of the American Medical Association, 289*(15), 1969–1975.

Bradley, E. H., Holmboe, E. S., Mattera, J. A., Roumanis, S. A., Radford, M. J., & Krumholz, H. M. (2004). Data feedback efforts in quality improvement: Lessons learned from U.S. hospitals. *Quality & Safety in Health Care, 13*(1), 26–31.

Bradley, E. H., Schlesinger, M., Webster, T. R., Baker, D., & Inouye, S. K. (2004). Translating research into clinical practice: Making change happen. *Journal of the American Geriatrics Society, 52*(11), 1875–1882.

Bradley, E. H., Webster, T. R., Baker, D., Schlesinger, M., Inouye, S. K., Barth, M. C., et al. (2004). Translating research into practice: Speeding the adoption of innovative health care programs. *Issue Brief (Commonwealth Fund), (724),* 1–12.

Bryar, R. M., Closs, S. J., Baum, G., Cooke, J., Griffiths, J., Hostick, T., et al. (2003). The Yorkshire BARRIERS project: Diagnostic analysis of barriers to research utilisation. *International Journal of Nursing Studies, 40*(1), 73–84.

Charles, R. (2000). The challenge of disseminating innovations to direct care providers in health care organizations. *Nursing Clinics of North America, 35*(2), 461–470.

Clancy, C. M., Slutsky, J. R., & Patton, L. T. (2004). Evidence-based health care 2004: AHRQ moves research to translation and implementation. *Health Services Research, 39*(5), xv–xxiii.

Collins, B. A., Hawks, J. W., & Davis, R. (2000). From theory to practice: Identifying authentic opinion leaders to improve care. *Managed Care, 9*(7), 56–62.

Davis, D. A., Thomson, M. A., Oxman, A.D., & Haynes, R. B. (1995). Changing physician performance. A systematic review of the effect of continuing medical education strategies. *Journal of the American Medical Association, 274*(9), 700–705.

Dawson, J. D. (2004). Quantitative analytical methods in translation research. *Worldviews on Evidence-Based Nursing 1*(Suppl. 1), S60–S64.

Dopson, S., FitzGerald, L., Ferlie, E., Gabbay, J., & Locock, L. (2002). No magic targets! Changing clinical practice to become more evidence based. *Health Care Management Review, 27*(3), 35–47.

Dopson, S., Locock, L., Chambers, D., & Gabbay, J. (2001). Implementation of evidence-based medicine: Evaluation of the promoting action on clinical effectiveness programme. *Journal of Health Services Research & Policy, 6*(1), 23–31.

Doumit, G., Gattellari, M., Grimshaw, J., & O'Brien, M. A. (2007). Local opinion leaders: Effects on professional practice and health care outcomes. *Cochrane Database of Systematic Reviews, 1,* CD000125.

Eccles, M. P., & Grimshaw, J. M. (2004). Selecting, presenting and delivering clinical guidelines: Are there any "magic bullets"? *Medical Journal of Australia, 180* (6 Suppl.), S52–S54.

Eccles, M. P., & Mittman, B. S. (2006). Welcome to implementation science. *Implementation Science, 1*(1). Retrieved April 22, 2009, from http://www.implementation science.com/

Ellis, I., Howard, P., Larson, A., & Robertson, J. (2005). From workshop to work practice: An exploration of context and facilitation in the development of evidence-based practice. *Worldviews on Evidence-Based Nursing 2*(2), 84–93.

Estabrooks, C. A. (1999). Modeling the individual determinants of research utilization. *Western Journal of Nursing Research, 21*(6), 758–772.

Estabrooks, C. A. (2003). Translating research into practice: Implications for organizations and administrators. *The Canadian Journal of Nursing Research = Revue Canadienne De Recherche En Sciences Infirmieres, 35*(3), 53–68.

Estabrooks, C. A., Chong, H., Brigidear, K., & Profetto-McGrath, J. (2005). Profiling Canadian nurses' preferred knowledge sources for clinical practice. *Canadian Journal of Nursing Research = Revue Canadienne de Recherche en Sciences Infirmières, 37*(2), 118–140.

Estabrooks, C. A., Floyd, J. A., Scott-Findlay, S., O'Leary, K. A., & Gushta, M. (2003). Individual determinants of research utilization: A systematic review. *Journal of Advanced Nursing, 43*(5), 506–520.

Estabrooks, C. A., O'Leary, K. A., Ricker, K. L., & Humphrey, C. K. (2003). The Internet and access to evidence: How are nurses positioned? *Journal of Advanced Nursing, 42*(1), 73–81.

Fawcett, J. (2005). *Contemporary nursing knowledge: Analysis and evaluation of nursing models and theories* (2nd ed.). Philadelphia: F. A. Davis.

Feldman, P. H., & McDonald, M. V. (2004). Conducting translation research in the home care setting: Lessons from a just-in-time reminder study. *Worldviews on Evidence-Based Nursing 1*(1), 49–59.

Feldman, P. H., Murtaugh, C. M., Pezzin, L. E., McDonald, M. V., & Peng, T. R. (2005). Just-in-time evidence-based e-mail "reminders" in home health care: Impact on patient outcomes. *Health Services Research, 40*(3), 865–885.

Forsetlund, L., Bjørndal, A., Rashidian, A., Jamtvedt, G., O'Brien, M. A, Wolf, F., et al. (2009). Continuing education meetings and workshops: Effects on professional practice and health care outcomes. *Cochrane Database of Systematic Reviews, 2,* CD003030.

Fraser, I. (2004a). Organizational research with impact: Working backwards. *Worldviews on Evidence-Based Nursing, 1*(Suppl. 1), S52–59.

Fraser, I. (2004b). Translation research: Where do we go from here? *Worldviews on Evidence-Based Nursing, 1*(Supp. 1), S78–S83.

Garside, P. (1998). Organisational context for quality: Lessons from the fields of organisational development and change management. *Quality in Health Care, 7*(Suppl.), S8–S15.

Graham, I. D., & Logan, J. (2004). Innovations in knowledge transfer and continuity of care. *Canadian Journal of Nursing Research = Revue Canadienne de Recherche en Sciences Infirmières, 36*(2), 89–103.

Graham, I. D., Logan, J., Harrison, M. B., Straus, S. E., Tetroe, J., Caswell, W., et al. (2006). Lost in knowledge translation: Time for a map? *Journal of Continuing Education in the Health Professions, 26*(1), 13–24.

Greenhalgh, T., Robert, G., Bate, P., Macfarlane, F., & Kyriakidou, O. (2005). *Diffusion of innovations in health service organisations: A systematic literature review.* Malden, MA: Blackwell.

Greenhalgh, T., Robert, G., Macfarlane, F., Bate, P., & Kyriakidou, O. (2004). Diffusion of innovations in service organizations: Systematic review and recommendations. *Milbank Quarterly, 82*(4), 581–629.

Grilli, R., Ramsay, C., & Minozzi, S. (2002). Mass media interventions: Effects on health services utilisation. *Cochrane Database of Systematic Reviews, 1,* CD000389.

Grimshaw, J. M., Eccles, M., Thomas, R., MacLennan, G., Ramsay, C., Fraser, C., et al. (2006). Toward evidence-based quality improvement. evidence (and its limitations) of the effectiveness of guideline dissemination and implementation strategies 1966–1998. *Journal of General Internal Medicine: Official Journal of the Society for Research and Education in Primary Care Internal Medicine, 21*(Suppl. 2), S14–S20.

Grimshaw, J. M., Eccles, M. P., Greener, J., Maclennan, G., Ibbotson, T., Kahan, J. P., et al. (2006). Is the involvement of opinion leaders in the implementation of research findings a feasible strategy? *Implementation Science, 1*(3). Retrieved April 22, 2009, from http://www.implementationscience.com/

Grimshaw, J. M., Eccles, M. P., Walker, A. E., & Thomas, R. E. (2002). Changing physicians' behavior: What works and thoughts on getting more things to work. *Journal of Continuing Education in the Health Professions, 22*(4), 237–243.

Grimshaw, J. M., Shirran, L., Thomas, R., Mowatt, G., Fraser, C., Bero, L., et al. (2001). Changing provider behavior: An overview of systematic reviews of interventions. *Medical Care, 39*(8, Suppl. 2), II2–II45.

Grimshaw, J. M., Thomas, R. E., MacLennan, G., Fraser, C., Ramsay, C. R., Vale, L., et al. (2004). Effectiveness and efficiency of guideline dissemination and implementation strategies. *Health Technology Assessment (Winchester, England), 8*(6), iii–iv, 1–72.

Grol, R. P., Bosch, M. C., Hulscher, M. E., Eccles, M. P., & Wensing, M. (2007). Planning and studying improvement in patient care: The use of theoretical perspectives. *Milbank Quarterly, 85*(1), 93–138.

Guihan, M., Bosshart, H. T., & Nelson, A. (2004). Lessons learned in implementing SCI clinical practice guidelines. *SCI Nursing: A Publication of the American Association of Spinal Cord Injury Nurses, 21*(3), 136–142.

Harvey, G., Loftus-Hills, A., Rycroft-Malone, J., Titchen, A., Kitson, A., McCormack, B., et al. (2002). Getting evidence into practice: The role and function of facilitation. *Journal of Advanced Nursing, 37*(6), 577–588.

Hendryx, M. S., Fieselmann, J. F., Bock, M. J., Wakefield, D. S., Helms, C. M., & Bentler, S. E. (1998). Outreach education to improve quality of rural ICU care. Results of a randomized trial. *American Journal of Respiratory and Critical Care Medicine, 158*(2), 418–423.

Horbar, J. D., Carpenter, J. H., Buzas, J., Soll, R. F., Suresh, G., Bracken, M. B., et al. (2004). Collaborative quality improvement to promote evidence based surfactant for preterm infants: A cluster randomised trial. *British Medical Journal (Clinical Research Edition), 329*(7473), 1004.

Hutchinson, A. M., & Johnston, L. (2004). Bridging the divide: A survey of nurses' opinions regarding barriers to, and facilitators of, research utilization in the practice setting. *Journal of Clinical Nursing, 13*(3), 304–315.

Hysong, S. J., Best, R. G., & Pugh, J. A. (2006). Audit and feedback and clinical practice guideline adherence: Making feedback actionable. *Implementation Science, 1*(9). Retrieved April 22, 2009, from http://www.implementationscience.com/

ICEBeRG (Interventions the Improved Clinical Effectiveness Through Behavioural Research Group). (2006). Designing theoretically informed implementation. *Implementation Science, 1*(4). Retrieved April 22, 2009, from http://www.implementation science.com/

Institute of Medicine. (2001). *Crossing the quality chasm: A new health system for the 21st century.* Washington, DC: National Academies Press.

Institute of Medicine. (2007a). *Advancing quality improvement research: Challenges and opportunities.* Workshop Summary. Washington, DC: National Academies Press.

Institute of Medicine. (2007b). *The state of quality improvement and implementation research: Expert reviews.* Workshop Summary. Washington, DC: National Academies Press.

Institute of Medicine. (2008). *Knowing what works in health care: A roadmap for the nation.* Committee on Reviewing Evidence to Identify Highly Effective Clinical Services. Washington, DC: National Academies Press.

Jamtvedt, G., Young, J. M., Kristoffersen, D. T., O'Brien, M. A., & Oxman, A. D. (2006). Audit and feedback: Effects on professional practice and health care outcomes. *Cochrane Database of Systematic Reviews, 2*, CD000259.

Kirchhoff, K. T. (2004). State of the science of translational research: From demonstration projects to intervention testing. *Worldviews on Evidence-Based Nursing* *1*(Suppl. 1), S6–S12.

Kitson, A., Harvey, G., & McCormack, B. (1998). Enabling the implementation of evidence-based practice: A conceptual framework. *Quality in Health Care,7*(3), 149–158.

Kitson, A., Rycroft-Malone, J., Harvey, G., McCormack, B., Seers, K., & Titchen, A. (2008). Evaluating the successful implementation of evidence into practice using the PARiHS framework: Theoretical and practical challenges. *Implementation Science, 3*(1). Retrieved April 22, 2009, from http://www.implementationscience.com/

Lam, T. K., McPhee, S. J., Mock, J., Wong, C., Doan, H. T., Nguyen, T., et al. (2003). Encouraging Vietnamese-American women to obtain Pap tests through lay health worker outreach and media education. *Journal of General Internal Medicine: Official Journal of the Society for Research and Education in Primary Care Internal Medicine, 18*(7), 516–524.

Leape, L. L. (2005). *Advances in patient safety: From research to implementation* (3rd ed.). Rockville, MD: Agency for Healthcare Research and Quality.

Lia-Hoagberg, B., Schaffer, M., & Strohschein, S. (1999). Public health nursing practice guidelines: An evaluation of dissemination and use. *Public Health Nursing (Boston, Mass.), 16*(6), 397–404.

Locock, L., Dopson, S., Chambers, D., & Gabbay, J. (2001). Understanding the role of opinion leaders in improving clinical effectiveness. *Social Science & Medicine, 53*(6), 745–757.

McCartney, P., Macdowall, W., & Thorogood, M. (1997). A randomised controlled trial of feedback to general practitioners of their prophylactic aspirin prescribing. *British Medical Journal (Clinical Research Edition), 315*(7099), 35–36.

McCormack, B., Kitson, A., Harvey, G., Rycroft-Malone, J., Titchen, A., & Seers, K. (2002). Getting evidence into practice: The meaning of "context." *Journal of Advanced Nursing, 38*(1), 94–104.

McGlynn, E. A., Asch, S. M., Adams, J., Keesey, J., Hicks, J., DeCristofaro, A., et al. (2003). The quality of health care delivered to adults in the United States. *New England Journal of Medicine, 348*(26), 2635–2645.

McKenna, H., Ashton, S., & Keeney, S. (2004). Barriers to evidence-based practice in primary care: A review of the literature. *International Journal of Nursing Studies, 41*(4), 369–378.

Meijers, J. M., Janssen, M. A., Cummings, G. G., Wallin, L., Estabrooks, C. A., & Halfens, R. (2006). Assessing the relationships between contextual factors and research utilization in nursing: Systematic literature review. *Journal of Advanced Nursing, 55*(5), 622–635.

Meleis, A. (2005). *Theoretical nursing* (3rd ed.). Philadelphia: Lippincott, Williams & Wilkins.

Michel, Y., & Sneed, N. V. (1995). Dissemination and use of research findings in nursing practice. *Journal of Professional Nursing: Official Journal of the American Association of Colleges of Nursing, 11*(5), 306–311.

Milner, M., Estabrooks, C. A., & Myrick, F. (2006). Research utilization and clinical nurse educators: A systematic review. *Journal of Evaluation in Clinical Practice, 12*(6), 639–655.

Nelson, E. C., Batalden, P. B., Huber, T. P., Mohr, J. J., Godfrey, M. M., Headrick, L. A., et al. (2002). Microsystems in health care: Part 1. learning from high-performing front-line clinical units. *Joint Commission Journal on Quality Improvement, 28*(9), 472–493.

Nieva, V., Murphy, R., Ridley, N., Donaldson, N., Combes, J., Mitchell, P., et al. (2005). From science to service: A framework for the transfer of patient safety research into practice. In K. Henriksen, J. Battles, E. Marks, & D. I. Lewin (Eds.), *Advances in patient safety: From research to implementation: Vol. 2, Concepts and methodology* (pp. 441–453, AHRQ Publication No. 05-0021-2). Rockville, MD: Agency for Healthcare Research and Quality.

O'Brien, M. A., Rogers, S., Jamtvedt, G., Oxman, A. D., Odgaard-Jensen, J., Kristoffersen, D. T., et al. (2007). Educational outreach visits: effects on professional practice and health care outcomes. *Cochrane Database of Systematic Reviews, 4,* CD000409.

Pravikoff, D. S., Tanner, A. B., & Pierce, S. T. (2005). Readiness of U.S. nurses for evidence-based practice. *American Journal of Nursing, 105*(9), 40–51.

Randolph, W., & Viswanath, K. (2004). Lessons learned from public health mass media campaigns: Marketing health in a crowded media world. *Annual Review of Public Health, 25,* 419–437.

Rappolt, S., Pearce, K., McEwen, S., & Polatajko, H. J. (2005). Exploring organizational characteristics associated with practice changes following a mentored online educational module. *Journal of Continuing Education in the Health Professions, 25*(2), 116–124.

Rogers, E. (Ed.). (2003). *Diffusion of innovations* (5th ed.). New York: Simon & Schuster.

Rosswurm, M. A., & Larrabee, J. H. (1999). A model for change to evidence-based practice. *Image—the Journal of Nursing Scholarship, 31*(4), 317–322.

Rubenstein, L. V., & Pugh, J. (2006). Strategies for promoting organizational and practice change by advancing implementation research. *Journal of General Internal Medicine: Official Journal of the Society for Research and Education in Primary Care Internal Medicine, 21*(Suppl. 2), S58–S64.

Rutledge, D. N., & Donaldson, N. E. (1995). Building organizational capacity to engage in research utilization. *Journal of Nursing Administration, 25*(10), 12–16.

Rutledge, D. N., Greene, P., Mooney, K., Nail, L. M., & Ropka, M. (1996). Use of research-based practices by oncology staff nurses. *Oncology Nursing Forum, 23*(8), 1235–1244.

Rycroft-Malone, J., Harvey, G., Seers, K., Kitson, A., McCormack, B., & Titchen, A. (2004). An exploration of the factors that influence the implementation of evidence into practice. *Journal of Clinical Nursing, 13*(8), 913–924.

Schouten, L. M., Hulscher, M. E., Akkermans, R., van Everdingen, J. J., Grol, R. P., & Huijsman, R. (2008). Factors that influence the stroke care team's effectiveness in reducing the length of hospital stay. *Stroke: A Journal of Cerebral Circulation, 39*(9), 2515–2521.

Scott, T., Mannion, R., Davies, H., & Marshall, M. (2003a). The quantitative measurement of organizational culture in health care: A review of the available instruments. *Health Services Research, 38*(3), 923–945.

Scott, T., Mannion, R., Davies, H. T., & Marshall, M. N. (2003b). Implementing culture change in health care: Theory and practice. *International Journal for Quality in Health Care: Journal of the International Society for Quality in Health Care,* 15(2), 111–118.

Silver, F. L., Rubini, F., Black, D., & Hodgson, C. S. (2003). Advertising strategies to increase public knowledge of the warning signs of stroke. *Stroke: A Journal of Cerebral Circulation,* 34(8), 1965–1968.

Soumerai, S. B., McLaughlin, T. J., Gurwitz, J. H., Guadagnoli, E., Hauptman, P. J., Borbas, C., et al. (1998). Effect of local medical opinion leaders on quality of care for acute myocardial infarction: A randomized controlled trial. *Journal of the American Medical Association,* 279(17), 1358–1363.

Srinivasan, R., & Fisher, R. S. (2000). Early initiation of post-PEG feeding: Do published recommendations affect clinical practice? *Digestive Diseases and Sciences,* 45(10), 2065–2068.

Stetler, C. B. (2001). Updating the Stetler model of research utilization to facilitate evidence-based practice. *Nursing Outlook,* 49(6), 272–279.

Stetler, C. B. (2003). Role of the organization in translating research into evidence-based practice. *Outcomes Management,* 7(3), 97–103; quiz 104–105.

Stetler, C. B., Legro, M. W., Rycroft-Malone, J., Bowman, C., Curran, G., Guihan, M., et al. (2006). Role of "external facilitation" in implementation of research findings: A qualitative evaluation of facilitation experiences in the Veterans Health Administration. *Implementation Science,* 1(23). Retrieved April 22, 2009, from http://www.implementationscience.com/

Sung, N. S., Crowley, W. F., Jr., Genel, M., Salber, P., Sandy, L., Sherwood, L. M., et al. (2003). Central challenges facing the national clinical research enterprise. *Journal of the American Medical Association,* 289(10), 1278–1287.

Sussman, S., Valente, T. W., Rohrbach, L. A., Skara, S., & Pentz, M. A. (2006). Translation in the health professions: Converting science into action. *Evaluation & the Health Professions,* 29(1), 7–32.

Taylor, D. M., Auble, T. E., Calhoun, W. J., & Mosesso, V. N., Jr. (1999). Current outpatient management of asthma shows poor compliance with international consensus guidelines. *Chest,* 116(6), 1638–1645.

Titler, M., Herr, K., Brooks, J., Xie, X., Ardery, G., Schilling, M., et al. (2009). Translating research into practice intervention improves management of acute pain in older hip fracture patients. *Health Services Research,* 44(1), 264–287.

Titler, M. G. (2002). *Toolkit for promoting evidence-based practice.* Iowa City: University of Iowa Hospitals and Clinics.

Titler, M. G. (2004a). Methods in translation science. *Worldviews on Evidence-Based Nursing,* 1(1), 38–48.

Titler, M. G. (2004b). Translation science: Quality, methods and issues. *Communicating Nursing Research,* 37, 15, 17–34.

Titler, M. G. (2006). Developing an evidence-based practice. In G. LoBiondo-Wood, & J. Haber (Eds.), *Nursing research: Methods and critical appraisal for evidence-based practice* (6th ed.). St. Louis, MO: Mosby.

Titler, M. G. (2008). The evidence for evidence-based practice implementation. In R. Hughes (Ed.), *Patient safety and quality—an evidence-based handbook for nurses* (1st ed.). Rockville, MD: Agency for Healthcare Research and Quality. Retrieved April 22, 2009, from http://www.ahrq.gov/qual/nurseshdbk/

Titler, M. G., & Everett, L. Q. (2001). Translating research into practice. considerations for critical care investigators. *Critical Care Nursing Clinics of North America, 13*(4), 587–604.

Titler, M. G., Everett, L. Q., & Adams, S. (2007). Implications for implementation science. *Nursing Research, 56*(4 Suppl.), S53–S59.

Titler, M. G., Kleiber, C., Steelman, V. J., Rakel, B. A., Budreau, G., Everett, L. Q., et al. (2001). The Iowa model of evidence-based practice to promote quality care. *Critical Care Nursing Clinics of North America, 13*(4), 497–509.

Tripp-Reimer, T., & Doebbeling, B. (2004). Qualitative perspectives in translational research. *Worldviews on Evidence-Based Nursing, 1,* S65–S72.

Vaughn, T. E., McCoy, K. D., BootsMiller, B. J., Woolson, R. F., Sorofman, B., Tripp-Reimer, T., et al. (2002). Organizational predictors of adherence to ambulatory care screening guidelines. *Medical Care, 40*(12), 1172–1185.

Wallin, L., Ewald, U., Wikblad, K., Scott-Findlay, S., & Arnetz, B. B. (2006). Understanding work contextual factors: A short-cut to evidence-based practice? *Worldviews on Evidence-Based Nursing, 3*(4), 153–164.

Wallin, L., Rudberg, A., & Gunningberg, L. (2005). Staff experiences in implementing guidelines for kangaroo mother care—a qualitative study. *International Journal of Nursing Studies, 42*(1), 61–73.

Wang, P. S., Berglund, P., & Kessler, R. C. (2000). Recent care of common mental disorders in the united states: Prevalence and conformance with evidence-based recommendations. *Journal of General Internal Medicine: Official Journal of the Society for Research and Education in Primary Care Internal Medicine, 15*(5), 284–292.

Wensing, M., & Grol, R. (1994). Single and combined strategies for implementing changes in primary care: A literature review. *International Journal for Quality in Health Care, 6*(2), 115–132.

Wensing, M., Wollersheim, H., & Grol, R. (2006). Organizational interventions to implement improvements in patient care: A structured review of reviews. *Implementation Science, 1,* (2). Retrieved April 22, 2009, from http://www.implementationscience.com/

Wiecha, J. L., El Ayadi, A.M., Fuemmeler, B. F., Carter, J. E., Handler, S., Johnson, S., et al. (2004). Diffusion of an integrated health education program in an urban school system: Planet health. *Journal of Pediatric Psychology, 29*(6), 467–474.

Zwarenstein, M., & Reeves, S. (2006). Knowledge translation and interprofessional collaboration: Where the rubber of evidence-based care hits the road of teamwork. *Journal of Continuing Education in the Health Professions, 26*(1), 46–54.

# Evaluating the Impact of Evidence-Based Practice and Communicating Results

# 18

# Cost as a Dimension of Evidence-Based Practice

ROBERT J. CASWELL

The guiding principle of evidence-based practice (EBP) is this: results obtained from careful investigation drive professional practice—in short, find out what works and then do it. However, the realities of the marketplace remind us that there is a difference between effectiveness and efficiency. Not every action that improves outcomes is necessarily worth doing. Without a good understanding of cost, our research is incomplete and our recommendations for practice may waste resources that could have been used more productively elsewhere—which is exactly the sort of issue evidence-based practice (EBP) is designed to address.

The range of cost-related considerations in evidence-based nursing practice is quite large. Among the many topics, here are some examples:

- *Cost measurement for purposes of payment.* One of the most straightforward tasks is the measurement of work done and the cost associated with it so that payment may be appropriately responsive. This has been a continuing controversy in nursing, which is so often "buried" in other categories of payment.
- *Cost of specific nursing interventions.* Many research studies examine the cost and benefit/effectiveness of particular clinical, educational, or other interventions undertaken by nurses.

**363**

- *Technology assessment.* Nursing is frequently a critical component of innovations in care, whether related to drugs, medical devices, or other therapies.
- *Input substitution.* A significant stream of research looks at the use of nursing to replace other inputs in producing care (e.g., advanced practice nurses in primary-care settings as a substitute for physician time). Whether the principal motivation is cost saving or quality enhancement, cost is a part of the evaluation.
- *Organizational and staffing models.* In some cases, nursing itself is the subject of study. Investigations of different staffing patterns or ways of organizing work can give very valuable information to practitioners, and cost is an essential element.

There should be no difficulty finding multiple examples of the categories listed in the literature. A few articles are suggested at the end of the chapter, but these are only a small sample of what is available. It is the intention of this chapter to equip you to read this sort of literature with understanding and a critical eye, because it is too often the case that, in the published literature, cost elements are addressed poorly.

## WHAT IS COST?

### Cost Versus Price

The words *cost* and *price* are frequently interchangeable in everyday speech, but they represent different ideas in economics. When you go into a store and ask how much something costs, you are really asking for a price. Although the words may be interchangeable, the concepts are not: *price* represents the amount that must be paid in order to gain ownership or use of something, whereas *cost* measures the resources that are used. For example, the *price* of this book is whatever was paid in order to buy it from its previous owner. The *cost* of this book is the paper and ink required to print it, the labor of those who were involved in writing, printing, transporting, and marketing it, and so on. The distinction between price and cost is particularly important in health care, where prices can be extremely complex and far removed from the apparent buyer. What is the price of a coronary artery bypass graft performed on a person insured under both Medicare and a private supplemental policy? One might reasonably ask, "The price to whom?" It is even possible for the *price* to the recipient of care to be zero—hospitals and other providers frequently treat patients as charity cases, providing care to the patients without any intention of billing them (note that this is different from a "bad debt," which is recorded when a patient is billed but does not pay). It is *not,* however, possible for the *cost* to be zero because real resources will have been consumed in providing the service.

Even though price and cost are emphatically not the same thing, they are not unrelated. The party that incurs the cost will be very interested in whether the price received is sufficient to pay for the resources used. In the example of "free" hospital care, it is unlikely that the price to all parties will be zero; for instance, the price not paid by a particular patient may cause the prices to other patients to be higher, as the provider attempts to collect enough from other payers in order to recoup the cost—the real resources consumed. Similarly, even though true cost is measured in resources, it is not unusual to encounter price (or "expenditure") used as a proxy measure. When data on cost are difficult to obtain, price is often used to represent the cost of an action from the point of view of the patient or payer (e.g., Stone & Walker, 1995, where cost is defined as "the economic impact of charges"). It is the responsibility of the researcher to identify clearly what measure is being used and the extent to which it departs from the real cost of the resources.

## Opportunity Cost

The fact that cost is conceptually a measurement of resources leads us to one of the most important ways of thinking about cost. The *opportunity cost* of any particular use of resources is the loss of the alternative uses of the same resources. The time you are using to read this chapter has an opportunity cost in that you have lost the opportunity to use that time for other, competing purposes (e.g., sleeping, watching television, walking the dog). In order to make a good decision, one should always put resources to their most valuable use.

The concept of opportunity cost is quite powerful and makes it easy to understand why persons who are paid on a piece-work basis (e.g., physicians paid on a fee-for-service basis) may choose to take short vacations or constantly look at their watches during meetings. Those of us who are paid by salary may be equally skilled, but the opportunity cost to us of spending more time at a particular activity can be quite different.

In fact, it is opportunity cost that is the fundamental reason why cost analysis must be part of EBP. Every use of resources imposes a cost in the form of the lost alternative uses of the resources. Thus, we cannot completely justify doing something as good evidence-based practice, even if it contributes positively to a patient outcome, unless we can be satisfied that the outcome is sufficiently good to be worth sacrificing the other things we could have done with the resources (e.g., the nurse's time, the equipment).

## Cost Is in the Eye of the Beholder

The examples of the opportunity cost of time for a salaried professional and for someone paid a fee for service should provide a clue that cost may not be the same when measured from different points of view. The most common cause for costs to appear different is variation in the level of inclusiveness or aggregation. For example, persons who smoke generally have higher health care costs than those who do not. It is also true that the health care costs attributable to smoking can be reduced by quitting smoking, even at relatively older ages. Therefore, it would save money for all of us as taxpayers if we could convince older persons to quit smoking and thus use fewer services paid for by Medicare, right? The answer is that it depends on your point of view. If smoking cessation leads to a longer life span, it may be that the higher health care costs resulting from needing care for more years will more than offset the savings that result from reducing the costs attributable to smoking. Thus, if your point of view is simply to reduce total expenditures in the Medicare program, it might be better to encourage smoking and hope people die sooner. If you adopt a broader concept of cost, including the lost productivity of persons who are ill, the costs to others in the society from passive smoke, fires, the psychic cost of watching family members suffer lung disease, and so on, then encouraging smoking cessation would be quite appropriate. The point is obviously that cost can be measured meaningfully only after one has decided on the boundaries that are relevant to the decision or evaluation at hand. The work of LaGodna and Hendrix (1989) illustrates this principle: the authors computed the cost of impaired nurses from the separate points of view of the nurse, the employer, and the profession. Although the estimates themselves are rough, the elements of cost that are included in each are quite distinct (e.g., lost income, hiring cost, investigation and adjudication). This is not an isolated example, because cost is *always* measured from a particular point of view. For instance, a study of *Chlamydia trachomatis* screening of army recruits found very different estimates of savings depending on whether one counted only the projected savings to the military from the screening or also the savings accruing in the private sector (Howell, McKee, Gaydos, Quinn, & Gaydos, 2000).

## CONCEPTS OF COST MEASUREMENT AND BEHAVIOR

### Direct Versus Indirect Cost

In almost every complex activity, some of the cost can be attributed easily to the output of that activity itself. When a laboratory test is done, it is clear that the chemicals used, the time of the technician, and the time of a pathologist to examine the results are all direct resource costs incurred to perform the test. It is less clear how one should consider the cost of having a laboratory manager, or of routine cleaning of the lab, or of having excess capacity available so that urgently needed tests can be done immediately. These are all examples of *indirect* cost; they are not attributable directly to any particular output of the laboratory but are nevertheless necessary for the overall activity to be done. That is, the true cost of a particular output such as a simple urinalysis would be understated if only the direct costs were considered. However, because the indirect costs are not attached to specific outputs, they must be *allocated* in some way.

Cost allocation has become a critical activity for health care organizations as they struggle to understand the true costs of their activities in order to manage those costs and to set prices that are both competitive and adequate. There are many examples of such cost allocation problems in nursing; it is easy to attribute the cost of nursing to a specific patient when identifiable procedures are being performed, but much less so for general care and especially for activities of coordination and management provided simultaneously to multiple patients. Thus, the typical practice of including nursing cost as a part of the "room rate" of the hospital blurs the distinction between these direct and indirect components of cost and effectively assumes that all patients in a particular room category receive identical nursing services, which is unlikely to be true (Welton, Fischer, DeGrace, & Zone-Smith, 2006). The usual approach to a more careful indirect cost allocation is to arrive at an *allocation basis,* which serves as a sort of proxy for the relationship between the indirect cost and the outputs (see Exhibit 18.1). For example, it is common to allocate the cost of housekeeping on the basis of the number

Exhibit 18.1

**TYPICAL ALLOCATION BASES FOR INDIRECT COST**

| WHEN ALLOCATING COST FROM THIS INDIRECT COST CENTER | IT MIGHT BE DIVIDED AMONG OTHER AREAS ON THE BASIS OF |
|---|---|
| Housekeeping Department | Relative size of each area in square feet |
| Nursing Administration | Number of patient days in each area |
| Personnel Department | Number of employees or paid hours in each area |
| Admissions Department | Number of admissions or discharges in each area |
| Clinic Management | Number of patient visits in each area |

of square feet in an area, possibly weighted by some other factor such as special procedures needed in areas requiring infectious disease control measures. A further discussion of the practical issues involved in such allocations is found at the end of the chapter.

## Explicit Versus Implicit Cost

The principle of opportunity cost described earlier—such as the cost of your time in reading this chapter—reminds us that not all costs involve a payment transaction. *Explicit* costs are those for which there is an actual expenditure, such as the salary and retirement benefit cost of hiring an employee. *Implicit* costs are those that need to be recognized in a decision, even though there is no actual payment made. Although there are many kinds of implicit costs, two are seen quite frequently: foregone earnings and depreciation. The implicit cost of foregone earnings is one with which almost everyone is familiar. It can arise, as in the example used earlier, when a person paid fee-for-service uses time for other, unpaid purposes. Perhaps less obviously, it arises whenever one makes a decision about how to finance a large purchase: if a clinic pays cash for an X-ray machine rather than borrowing the money, the explicit cost of the interest payment on a debt is avoided. However, the opportunity to *earn* interest on the cash that was used is also lost. These lost interest earnings are an implicit cost of cash financing. This same reasoning can be extended to much more complex decisions. The other best-known implicit cost is depreciation, which simply means that something may lose value over time either through actual deterioration or obsolescence. If a diagnostic device must be replaced approximately every 5 years, then it is reasonable to think that there is an implicit cost of using the device equal to approximately one-fifth of the replacement cost per year, in addition to the explicit cost of operating the device. If the owner of the device recognizes this implicit cost and sets aside the money for depreciation at this rate (even though it is not due to anyone as a payment), then at the end of the 5 years there will be a fund from which the needed replacement can be purchased.

## Cost Variability With Output

If the number of patients in a neonatal intensive care unit doubles, does the cost of providing nursing care double, more than double, or less than double? This sort of question is particularly important for planning and budgeting purposes and is the subject of a very large body of the research on cost in health care. Some costs do not change at all as the quantity of output changes, at least as long as the change isn't too large. For instance, the cost of utilities (e.g., light, heat), insurance, and nursing administration might not change at all as the number of patients in the neonatal ICU varies. These costs are described as *fixed costs*. Conversely, any costs that do change as the quantity of output changes, such as supplies or overtime hours, are *variable costs*. Using these two definitions, we can describe a simple relationship:

$$\text{Total Cost} = \text{Fixed Cost} + \text{Variable Cost}$$
$$(\text{or, symbolically, TC} = \text{FC} + \text{VC})$$

Describing a cost as fixed or variable depends on the time span that is relevant. If one is speaking of the cost in a particular patient care area during the next shift, almost all of the costs will be fixed because it is too late to make any meaningful changes in them. If the time span stretches to several months or years, then most or all of the costs become variable because we could make very radical changes in the way the work is accomplished, including the use of new technologies, hiring a different mix of staff, building a new building, and so on. In most situations, some costs are fixed and some are variable, although there is clearly a continuum depending upon how easily the cost can be changed. As mentioned earlier, the practice of incorporating nursing into the per diem room charge for hospital care effectively treats nursing as a fixed cost per patient day (though variable per patient because of differences in length of stay). This should be understood as a result of historical practices in reimbursement persisting from a time when nursing care was simpler and more uniform, rather than any actual assertion that nursing costs are in fact fixed, and may result in an undervaluing of nursing care (Welton, Unruh, & Halloran, 2006).

## Total Cost Versus Unit Cost

For some management and budgetary purposes, it is enough to know the total cost of all the activity in an organization or some relevant part. For example (though this is oversimplified), the hospitals in the Veterans Health Administration system are given an annual budget allocation and are simply expected to meet their care responsibilities within that budget. One could argue that, from the point of view of the agency granting the funds, all that matters is that the costs not exceed what was authorized in total. However, many decisions require information on the cost per unit of output. "Unit" in this case means whatever is used to measure the quantity of output. In nursing, the unit might be a specific procedure, a patient visit, or a patient day in an inpatient setting. Obviously, it is important that the units used to measure work be meaningful representations. In a setting in which all the patients are quite similar, cost per patient visit could be a reasonable measure, though it would obviously be an inappropriate measure for an emergency department that treats both trauma and minor sprains.

The most common measure of unit cost is the *average cost*, which can be calculated easily from the simple equation presented earlier for total cost ($TC = FC + VC$). If we divide both sides of the equation by Q, symbolizing the quantity of output (e.g., neonatal intensive care patient days), each of the variables becomes a measure per unit of output (i.e., cost per neonatal intensive care patient day):

$$\frac{TC}{Q} = \frac{FC}{Q} + \frac{VC}{Q} \quad \text{or,}$$

Average Total Cost = Average Fixed Cost + Average Variable Cost

We can be sure that average fixed cost ($FC/Q$) will decline as the quantity of output gets larger, because the fixed cost in the numerator will stay the same and the quantity in the denominator will grow. This pattern is what financial managers sometimes describe as "spreading the overhead." That is, the fixed cost is spread over more and more units as output grows. We can't be as sure what will happen to average variable cost, and therefore to average total cost, as output grows. For instance, in a setting with plenty of excess physical capacity (e.g., patient beds, examining rooms, equipment), it may be that the average variable cost will remain rather stable because the only thing that will change as output grows is hours of labor and the supplies used. On the other hand, in a setting that is operating close to capacity it may be very expensive to try to expand output (as the staff attempt to work around problems of inadequate equipment, long waiting times for procedures, and so on), causing average cost to rise very fast as output grows. The discovery of these relationships between cost per unit and the level of output is yet another of the heavily researched topics in health care cost.

One of the most important uses of unit cost measurements is in making predictions about the impact of change. For instance, if we have an underutilized inpatient area with extra beds available, what would be the additional cost of treating just one more patient? It could be the same as the average cost of the patients we're already treating but usually won't be. The reason is that we would not incur any more fixed cost, and the additional variable cost might depend on how many patients we already have, the capabilities of the staff, and so forth. The appropriate measure for this situation is called *marginal cost,* which refers to the change in cost per unit of change in output. We have already seen above that average total cost is simply total cost divided by the amount of output (TC/Q). Marginal cost is similar but is calculated as the *change* in total cost divided by the *change* in output:

$$\text{Marginal Cost} = \text{MC} = \frac{\Delta TC}{\Delta Q}$$

(where $\Delta$ represents a change in the variable)

Because the quantity of output can change in either direction, marginal cost either represents the additional cost per unit of increased output (e.g., the additional cost of one more patient day in cardiology) or the reduction in cost per unit of decreased output (one fewer patient day in cardiology). The managerial and policy uses of marginal cost are many, but the most common is related to estimating the response of cost to a fluctuating workload. In the short run, many costs are fixed, and the marginal cost of changes in workload may be considerably below the average cost per unit of work. From a practical point of view, this simply means that the existing staff may just "work harder" to cover a small increase in workload, so total cost does not go up by much. Note that this reasoning also applies when the workload is falling: the marginal cost saved by a downward fluctuation in workload may be small, because there is no opportunity to adjust the fixed costs. Marginal cost has also been used to analyze broader issues such as estimates of the savings from closing hospital beds or diverting patients to an alternate setting (see, e.g., Williams, 1996). Much of the research in nursing has used proxy measures that are closer to average variable cost rather than marginal cost when estimating the impact of change. For example, Pappas (2007) uses a variety of measures, including RN salary cost or salary plus supply cost, to estimate changing cost as length of stay varies. While this might be a reasonable estimate for additional cost of an additional day for a particular patient whose condition is stable, it is probably not as good a measure for the change in cost resulting from additional patients on a given day (i.e., more patient days because of more patients rather than more days with the same patient). Similar incremental cost estimation issues are addressed by Needleman and colleagues (2006) in their examination of the impact of variations in nurse staffing on the avoidance of adverse outcomes, including avoided hospital days.

## EVALUATING COST AS A DIMENSION OF OUTCOMES

In the research context, we frequently want to analyze whether a particular decision seems appropriate, given the cost that was (or will be) incurred. As noted at the beginning of the chapter, this is the essence of EBP. A variety of evaluative approaches may be used, depending upon the nature of the question being asked and the realistic opportunities for data collection (see Exhibit 18.2 for examples). The researcher should note that titles of articles in the literature are not a reliable guide to the technique being used. Although such terms as *cost-benefit* and *cost-effectiveness* have specific meanings, they are sometimes used in a rather loose and inaccurate manner; only careful reading can establish whether the claimed analytic methods are present.

### Cost Identification

At the most basic level, the evaluation of cost is simply a careful aggregation incorporating all the elements that are relevant from the viewpoint of the evaluator. The technique in this case is quite straightforward: first,

Exhibit 18.2

## CHOOSING THE CORRECT COST EVALUATION CONCEPT

CHOOSING THE CORRECT COST EVALUATION CONCEPT

| RESEARCH QUESTION | MOST APPROPRIATE COST CONCEPT[a] | PRINCIPAL ISSUES |
|---|---|---|
| What is the cost (e.g., of this action, program, intervention)? | Cost identification/ minimization analysis (estimation of total, average, and/or marginal cost) | ■ Point of view (i.e., inclusiveness) <br> ■ Indirect cost allocation |
| Is this worth doing (or, how much of this is worth doing)? | Cost-benefit analysis | ■ Valuation of nonmonetary benefits <br> ■ Discount rate |
| Which alternative way of doing this is the best? | Cost-effectiveness analysis or cost-utility analysis | ■ Subjective or objective evaluation of principal outcomes and side effects <br> ■ Discount rate |

[a]The determination of which cost concept is most appropriate can depend on many things, but the choices indicated are likely to be helpful in the majority of circumstances.

define the boundaries of the viewpoint that has been chosen (e.g., is transportation cost to the hospital that is borne by the patient's family relevant in the evaluation?); second, identify each of the components of cost (e.g., supplies, employee turnover); and third, perform the measurements and sum the costs. This frequently involves the researcher in problems of *valuation*, if some of the relevant costs are not obvious or don't have clear monetary units. Valuation addresses such concerns as the proper cost to assign to a lengthened response time of nursing resulting from some kind of reorganization of duties or the cost of using capital equipment (Hundley et al., 1995).

Many applications of the cost identification approach involve comparison of alternatives that are assumed to have identical, or at least very similar, outcomes other than cost. In these situations, cost identification is essentially cost minimization, choosing the alternative that achieves the outcome and costs the least. In this instance, cost identification/minimization is a short-cut version of cost-effectiveness analysis, which is detailed later in this chapter. Cost identification is also appropriate when it has already been determined that a course of action is desirable but the question is financial feasibility. The sorts of results reported in the literature range from crude averages (Regan, Byers, & Mayrovitz, 1995) to very detailed attempts to adjust for factors that affect cost (Mauskopf, Paul, Wichman, White, & Tilson, 1996). A typical study applying the cost mini-mization approach evaluated the use of nurse-led intermediate care units for patients who no longer needed acute hospital care (Walsh, Steiner, Pickering, & Ward-Basu, 2005). Because there was no difference of inter-est in patient outcomes between the control group and the experimental group, the evaluation could be based entirely on the difference in cost.

## Cost-Benefit Analysis

In theory, *cost-benefit analysis* (CBA) is the closest of any of the evalua-tion methods to reproducing the logic of the ordinary market decision. It asks the question "Does the benefit of this action exceed the cost?"

In the context of health care, cost-benefit analysis is used when the goal is to determine the net value of an action or the appropriate level of expenditure on a particular intervention: "How do the benefits of this program compare to its costs?" or "How do the benefits and costs of this program change as the level of program activity is changed?" Thus, at least in principle, CBA can be used to answer questions such as "Is this worth doing at all?" or "How much more of this is it worth doing?"

CBA requires that all benefit and cost values, regardless of what they represent, be expressed in monetary terms. This allows the calculation of a net value (benefit minus cost). Stating *cost* in monetary terms is usu-ally straightforward, but in the case of health programs it can sometimes be quite difficult to put the *benefits* into dollar units. For instance, if the purpose of the program is to extend life expectancy by avoiding car-diovascular disease (e.g., by preventive use of statin drugs), what is the appropriate *monetary* value of the benefit?

The basic equation of cost-benefit analysis is the calculation of a net present value (NPV):

$$NPV = \sum_{i=1}^{t} \frac{B_i - C_i}{(1 + r)^i}$$

where $i$ = a particular time period, one of $t$, the total number of time periods included in the analysis

$Bi$ = benefits in time period $i$

$Ci$ = costs in time period $i$

$r$ = the appropriate discount rate (see explanation that follows)

We speak of NPV as *net* because costs are subtracted from benefits and as a *present value* because the evaluation is made from the point of view of the current time period, even though the costs and benefits may occur in the future (in the case of something like immunizations, perhaps decades later). The summation sign ( ) indicates that we are adding up the net benefit (benefit minus cost) over all time periods included in the analysis. A positive net present value means that, over the relevant time span, the value of the benefits exceeds the value of the costs (and the reverse, of course, for a negative NPV). Although there are many possible complications, one can generalize simply by saying that anything with a positive NPV is "worth doing" and that the higher the NPV, the better the activity is. One of the most common complicating factors is a limited budget, which may mean that some projects with a positive NPV must be forgone. This returns us to the real world of EBP, in which we must not only note the existence of an improvement but be ready to use evidence to make difficult tradeoff decisions.

The *discount rate* in the cost-benefit equation is essentially an interest rate, used to incorporate the impact of time into the analysis (note that this is a special use of the word "discount," which can also have its usual meaning of a price reduction; one must rely on the context to know which is correct). For instance, a cost of $100 that will not be incurred until 5 years in the future is clearly different from a cost of $100 now, and the same is true of a $100 benefit that is delayed for 5 years rather than occurring now. Space does not permit a complete explanation of the discount calculations here, but they are straightforward and readily available in texts on economic evaluation (e.g., Drummond, Stoddart, & Torrance, 2005).

The larger challenge for CBA is often the need to measure benefits in monetary terms. For that reason, CBA is most readily applied when the benefits are naturally monetary—for instance, avoided costs of treatment. In a simple example, Catz, Zifroni, and Philo (2005) estimated the impact of using a computerized mattress system in which one of the measures of benefit was the nursing labor cost avoided by not having to reposition patients as often.

## Cost-Effectiveness Analysis

Unlike cost-benefit analysis, *cost-effectiveness analysis* (CEA) allows the measure of outcome or benefit to be left in nonmonetary units. This means that CEA is sometimes more straightforward to undertake, as there may be natural measures of effectiveness (e.g., years of life saved). It attempts to answer the question "Which of the known ways of achieving the outcome we want produces the most of that outcome per dollar spent on the program?" Clearly, CEA is not appropriate for the comparison of programs with widely variant purposes. For example, it is hard to compare meaningfully the cost-effectiveness of two programs if the outcome of one is the number of dental caries avoided by fluoridating water and the outcome of the other is lives saved by immunization. However, it would be appropriate to compare the cost of saving lives (or the number of lives saved per dollar spent) for two different methods of implementing immunization. CEA can be used when the purpose is to decide whether something is worth doing, but only if there is a standard of some kind against which the result can be tested. For example, is it worth spending X dollars per additional cancer detected in a screening program? There is no obvious analytical answer, but one could compare a new program and the cost per cancer detected in existing screening programs. For programs that have more generalizable outcomes (e.g., life years saved), it is more feasible to create some kind of standard for comparison (i.e., does the cost per life year saved in this program compare favorably to the cost per life year saved in other programs, regardless of how that is accomplished?). CEA is particularly widely used in technology assessment, determining whether it is appropriate to switch from one way of doing something to a new way (e.g., new drugs, medical devices, procedures).

Cost-effectiveness is always expressed as a ratio in which the changes in cost are customarily in the numerator and the changes in effectiveness (the outcome measure) are in the denominator. The changes in cost and effectiveness that create the ratio fall logically into four possible patterns that illustrate the use of CEA in evaluating a program for implementation:

1 *Increased effectiveness, reduced cost:* This is the happiest situation, in which the outcome is improved and cost reduced, so the program would clearly be accepted.

2 *Reduced effectiveness, increased cost:* The worst situation, which offers no reason to accept the program.

3 *Increased effectiveness, increased cost:* This is probably the most common situation, in which an improved outcome is possible only with increased cost. The decision to accept the program must consider the effectiveness of the new program against that of other alternatives in order to know whether it is sufficiently attractive.

4   *Reduced effectiveness, reduced cost:* The mirror image of the preceding situation, evaluated in almost the same manner. However, it can be more difficult in practice to justify accepting a lesser outcome, even if it can be achieved at a cost that is attractive. Practical examples abound in health care, including the evaluation of drugs for formularies, in which there may be pressure to select drugs that are both "good enough" and available at much lower cost than newer drugs.

## Cost-Utility Analysis

*Cost-utility analysis* (CUA) is actually a type of cost-effectiveness analysis in which the effectiveness measure reflects *subjective* valuation as well as objective outcome. For instance, a person facing extensive chemotherapy might not evaluate the additional life span gained as being worth as much as the same life span without the side effects of the treatment because of the impact of the side effects on the perceived quality of life. In standard cost-effectiveness analysis, side effects are important because they may diminish the objective effectiveness of the program or require additional treatment; for instance, a screening program might result in a small number of adverse reactions that require treatment and thus add to cost. Cost-utility analysis is concerned about this impact but would add any positive or negative *subjective* evaluation by those being screened (e.g., some persons might prefer not to know that they have a condition if there is no effective treatment available). CUA may also consider varying response to the seriousness or acceptability of certain symptoms (Danese, Powe, Sawin, & Ladenson, 1996). With the exception of the adjustment of effectiveness measures, CUA follows the CEA calculations. However, there is a very extensive literature on the ways to elicit utility (subjective value) judgments from individuals in order to modify the effectiveness measures appropriately. An excellent review of methods and issues in CEA and CUA can be found in Gold, Siegel, Russell, and Weinstein (1996), which has become the standard reference for these methods.

## ISSUES IN COST MEASUREMENT AND ANALYSIS

### The Impact of Time on Value

As explained earlier, the discounting process reflects both the subjective preference to have things now rather than later and the real effect of interest rates. The choice of the discount rate can have a very substantial impact on the decision, especially if costs and benefits occur in a very different pattern over time. A common pattern in some health programs is to have all costs up front but benefits delayed or spread over several years. The choice of discount rate can raise troubling intergenerational issues—for example, the higher the discount rate applied to future benefits, the more likely one is to favor programs that achieve results quickly and thus to reject programs that are primarily preventive or aimed toward the young.

## Inflation

In addition to the influence of time on values as discussed earlier, time may create a complication in the measurements because of the phenomenon of persistently rising prices. In the context of research on cost, inflation becomes important if the time periods under study extend fairly far into the future (or into the past). If so, it may be that any measures with monetary value will have to be adjusted so that comparisons are not misleading. For instance, expenditure for a typical day in the hospital has increased hugely over the period since the introduction of Medicare and Medicaid, in the mid-1960s. Some of that increase in expenditure represents a real change in utilization, but some is nothing more than the change in prices attached to equivalent units. Depending upon the purpose of the research, it may be appropriate to remove the effect of inflation by expressing all the monetary magnitudes in "constant dollars" of one particular time period. This is a complex topic beyond the space available here, but it has been treated extensively in the literature (see, e.g., Feldstein, 2005; Getzen, 1992; Newhouse, 1989).

## Geographic Variability

Research that is done in a single location does not need to consider geographic variability, but any that compares sites may need to account for variation in prices and costs due to such things as variations in costs between urban and rural location. It would not be surprising to find that caring for a patient of a particular type is more expensive in Boston than in a small town in Ohio because of differences in labor costs, rent, and so on. These variations are not different in principle from the inflationary changes discussed earlier. Adjusting for geographic variation requires index numbers that measure change related to spatial location rather than to the passage of time. This has been a major issue in public programs such as Medicare that must pay for the same services in highly diverse locations. Unfortunately, the data available for measuring regional variation are not as well developed as the data for recognizing change in prices over time in a single place and are subject to more disagreement over interpretation. The researcher is likely to have very little recourse but to use the available index values, knowing that there is controversy (see, e.g., the discussion of geographic variability in nursing wages in U.S. Government Accountability Office, 2005).

## Valuation

Valuation is required in two basic situations. The first, somewhat easier to calculate, relates to choosing the appropriate cost measurement for a durable resource such as capital. This is usually handled in part as an allocation question, discussed further later in this chapter, with the monetary cost per unit of service (e.g., an hour of magnetic resonance imaging equipment time) determined by a depreciation allowance. The more difficult situation involves the need to measure intrinsically nonmonetary things such as human life or well-being in monetary terms, a task that is not unique to health care programs. It is present in many legal situations, such as compensation for workplace injury. One important difference is that in many legal settings, the value that is relevant (at least for the purposes of the court, although the injured party might not agree) is some measure of the person's worth in the labor market, such as expected lifetime income, with appropriate adjustments for uncertainty and discounting. The problem with applying this sort of reasoning in health care programs is that it would place the highest value on saving the life or health of the wealthiest persons—so the top priority would probably be given to diseases of corporate executives, professional athletes, and media figures. Note also that the effect of any discrimination in the labor market would remain systematically in the evaluation of the health program; for example, if women are paid less than men, then the analysis would continue this bias.

Because of this problem, it is more common to use measures other than income. There are several creative alternatives. For instance, if one examines the differences in wages demanded by persons with different levels of risk in their work, one can calculate an implicit value that workers assign to the possibility of injury or death. Suppose a person who undertakes a risky occupational choice (e.g., to do welding high up in a construction site rather than on the ground) is subject to an increased risk of death of 1 in 1,000 and is paid an additional $2,000 per year as extra compensation. One can simply divide the extra compensation by the increased risk to find an implied value of life: $2000/0.001, or $2 million. It is also possible to ask the question directly, usually in the form of willingness to pay to avoid a known risk. The problem with this approach is obviously that the person may view the question as entirely hypothetical, in which case the answer may be quite different from what it would be if the person actually faced the risk. As a final example, one can calculate implicit values demonstrated by policy decisions. If we are willing to spend X dollars on a program of a particular type with a known set of outcomes, what value do we appear to be placing on life or health within that program? For example, what is implied by the willingness of consumers to pay extra for automobiles with certain safety features that reduce the risk of injury or death? Although this is not very finely tuned, it can at least give a comparative standard.

In many cases the benefit or effectiveness measures may represent outcomes that should be modified in some way to account for variation in quality of life, as suggested by cost-utility analysis. For instance, a laryngectomy may extend the life of a throat cancer patient, but the evaluation of the quality differential of that longevity might vary from patient to patient, depending on the value placed upon ease of oral communication. Similarly, many therapies have relatively severe side effects that should be taken into account in evaluating outcomes. The most important point is that a complete analysis should make some attempt to determine whether such quality adjustments are likely to have a significant impact on the evaluation (e.g., an otherwise cost-effective alternative that has significant negative side effects may be less desirable than others after adjustment for change in the quality of life).

## SOME PRACTICAL CONCERNS IN RESEARCH ON COST

### Sources of Cost Data

There are three basic approaches for obtaining cost data in health care organizations. The majority of organizational providers are participants in Medicare and Medicaid, and thus there is generally a legally mandated uniform cost reporting system in place. Second, most health care providers are also engaged in major internal cost-finding and cost accounting efforts in order to negotiate reasonable payment under managed-care contracts or to establish their own prices. Finally, the researcher can collect data unique to the task at hand. The uniform data collected for public programs have the advantages of low cost, since the data have already been assembled, are readily available as public documents, and have relatively straightforward comparability from institution to institution because of the accounting standards. However, the cost reports are designed to answer the operational needs of the payment programs and thus frequently aggregate or omit items that would be useful to the researcher asking a focused question. A variety of strategies have been proposed in the literature for augmenting public data sets to improve the applicability of the cost information. These include measures of nursing intensity (e.g., Knauf, Ballard, Mossman, & Lichtig, 2006; Welton, Zone-Smith, & Fischer, 2006) and of specific activities and outcomes (Saba & Arnold, 2004). If the organization has undertaken a comprehensive cost accounting program for its own decision making, the researcher may find that these internal reports contain much greater detail; the tradeoff is that the data may lack external comparability and are proprietary, requiring that the researcher navigate cumbersome approval processes to gain access. The researcher who engages in specialized data collection will of course need organizational approval and will maintain external comparability only if there is a protocol for this purpose within the research design.

## Price Versus Cost Revisited

One of the most common confusions in research on cost in health care is the myriad ways that financial data are described. As noted earlier, *price* and *cost* refer to different concepts in economics, and this is certainly true in health care. To add to the confusion, there are multiple versions of price data, depending upon the payer: very few pay the nominal fee-for-service charges quoted by the provider, because there is almost certain to be a contractual agreement that specifies some sort of discount from these charges or an alternate payment system altogether, such as capitation (a fixed payment per patient to the provider, regardless of the quantity or cost of services provided). It is thus essential that the researcher ensure that the data being used in fact represent cost rather than one of these price variables. If it is necessary to use some form of price or expenditure as a proxy for cost, it is very important to ensure that the price concepts being used are consistent. Otherwise, it is clearly possible that apparent cost variation in comparisons might simply reflect differences in bargainers' ability to negotiate discounts rather than true differences in cost. It is also true that some payers do not recognize certain elements as acceptable cost, and there may therefore be more than one system of accounting in place for costs. One of the most common examples of this is the cost of clinical training (e.g., of physicians and nurses) in the hospital; these costs are certainly incurred, but they are sometimes quite difficult to disentangle from the actual treatment cost of particular patients. Although it may be intuitively obvious, it is important for the researcher to understand precisely what is and is not included in the cost data being used.

## Allocating Cost to Activities

Cost allocation can have two related meanings. The first, mentioned earlier, is the assignment of indirect costs, such as nursing management, to the final units of output for which a cost estimate is desired (e.g., cost per case or per patient day). Traditionally, this has meant assigning the cost of "nonrevenue departments," for which no separate charge was made, to "revenue departments" whose output was given a price. The myriad ways of paying for care have blurred this distinction, but it is still important to know the full cost of an activity.

Indirect costs are usually allocated according to a measure of activity or workload. For instance, the cost of the human resources department might be allocated to the patient care departments on the basis of the number of employees in each department. Many standard procedures are available for these allocations, including those used by the government for determining cost in the Medicare program. The other meaning of cost allocation is the estimation of relative resource requirements for different outputs within a department. The three principal methods are the ratio-of-cost-to charges (RCC), relative value units (RVU), and activity-based costing (ABC). RCC is acknowledged to be a rough estimate based on the assumption that resource use is proportional to price. RVUs have been widely used in nursing, usually in the form of some sort of severity adjustment to the basic unit of work (see, e.g., Ballard, Gray, Knauf, & Uppal, 1993; Barhyte and Glandon, 1988; Flarey, 1990; Moss, O'Connor, & Windle, 1994; Wong, Gordon, Cassard, Weisman, & Bergner, 1993). It is usually conceded that ABC, which examines cost at a very micro level and attempts to link cost allocation to "cost drivers" for each service, gives the most accurate results (Fox, Ehreth, and Issel, 1994; Llewellyn et al., 1994; West, Balas, and West, 1996).

## SUMMARY

There is a huge research literature on the costs of health care, exploring an enormous variety of descriptive and analytical cost-related questions. However, many of the basic tasks in all these studies are the same: deciding upon a consistent point of view in measuring cost, keeping price and cost as separate concepts, and using appropriate measures of cost for the question at hand. The very fact that there are so many research options suggests the importance of sensitivity analysis, in which the assumptions or approaches are varied in order to observe the impact on the results. Sensitivity analysis can discover huge differences in cost estimates—one study reports a 60% variation depending upon the options chosen (Wilson, Prescott, & Aleksandrowicz, 1988). Such a possibility for variation creates a serious responsibility for the researcher to proceed with care and to document scrupulously the method used so that the interpretation of the findings is clear.

## SUGGESTED ACTIVITIES

1   Consider a clinical nursing setting in which you have experience. During a period of one week, what costs would you describe as fixed? Variable? How would these change if the time period were one day? One month? One year?

2   For the same or another clinical setting, how many different viewpoints can you identify from which cost could be measured? In what ways would the different viewpoints affect your decision concerning which costs are relevant? Suppose you were asked to evaluate a proposal to centralize all solid organ transplant services in the state in a single hospital in order to achieve economies of scale and ensure enough volume to build a high quality program. How might the resulting cost differ from the point of view of the hospital, the payer, the patient, and his or her family?

3   Choose an article reporting an economic evaluation (cost identification/minimization, cost-benefit, cost-effectiveness, or cost-utility analysis) relevant to nursing. Critique the article with respect to its handling of cost concepts. How were costs measured? Is the point of view clear? Does the measure correctly reflect the cost that is relevant for the evaluation? What improvements could you suggest? What concerns would you have

in using the article's results for evidence-based practice (i.e., would you feel comfortable recommending action in a practice setting on the basis of the article)?

# REFERENCES

Ballard, K. A, Gray, R. F., Knauf, R. A., & Uppal, P. (1993). Measuring variations in nursing care per DRG. *Nursing Management, 24,* 33–36, 40–41.

Barhyte, D. Y., & Glandon, G. L. (1988). Issues in nursing labor costs allocation. *Journal of Nursing Administration, 18,* 16–19.

Catz, A., Zifroni, A., & Philo, O. (2005). Economic assessment of pressure sore prevention using a computerized mattress system in patients with spinal cord injury. *Disability and Rehabilitation, 27,* 1315–1319.

Danese, M. D., Powe, N. R., Sawin, C. T., & Ladenson, P. W. (1996). Screening for mild thyroid failure at the periodic health examination: A decision and cost-effectiveness analysis. *Journal of the American Medical Association, 276,* 285–292.

Drummond, M. F., Stoddart, G. L., & Torrance, G. W. (2005). *Methods for the economic evaluation of health care programmes.* New York: Oxford University Press.

Feldstein, P. J. (2005). *Health care economics.* Clifton Park: Thomson Delmar Learning.

Flarey, D. L. (1990). A methodology for costing nursing service. *Nursing Administration Quarterly, 14,* 41–51.

Fox, S., Ehreth, J., & Issel, L. M. (1994). A cost evaluation of a hospital-based perinatal case management program. *Nursing Economics, 12,* 214–220.

Getzen, T. E. (1992). Medical care price indexes: Theory, construction and empirical analysis of the U.S. series 1927–1990. In R. M. Scheffler & L. F. Rossiter (Eds.), *Advances in health economics and health services research* (Vol. 13, pp. 83–128). Greenwich, CT: JAI Press, Inc.

Gold, M. R., Siegel, J. E., Russell, L. B., & Weinstein, M. C. (Eds.). (1996) *Cost-effectiveness in health and medicine.* New York: Oxford University Press.

Howell, M. R., McKee, K. T., Gaydos, J. C., Quinn, T. C., & Gaydos, C. A. (2000). Point-of-entry screening for *C. trachomatis* in female army recruits. Who derives the cost savings? *American Journal of Preventive Medicine, 19,* 160–166.

Hundley, V. A., Donaldson, C., Lang, G. D., Cruickshank, F. M., Glazener, C. M. A., Milne, J. M., et al. (1995). Costs of intrapartum care in a midwife-managed delivery unit and a consultant-led labour ward. *Midwifery, 11,* 103–109.

Knauf, R. A., Ballard, K., Mossman, P. N., & Lichtig, L. K. (2006). Nursing cost by DRG: Nursing intensity weights. *Policy, Politics, & Nursing Practice, 7,* 281–289.

LaGodna, G. E., & Hendrix, M. J. (1989). Impaired nurses: A cost analysis. *Journal of Nursing Administration, 19,* 13–18.

Llewellyn, J., Giese, R., Nosek, L. J., Lager, J. D., Turco, S. J., Goodell, J., et al. (1994). A multicenter study of costs and nursing impact of cartridge-needle units. *Nursing Economics, 12,* 208–214.

Mauskopf, J. A., Paul, J. E., Wichman, D. S., White, A.D., & Tilson, H. D. (1996). Economic impact of treatment of HIV-positive pregnant women and their newborns with zidovudine: Implications for HIV screening. *Journal of the American Medical Association, 276,* 132–138.

Moss, M. T., O'Connor, S. A., & Windle, P. E. (1994). A perioperative acuity measurement system. *Nursing Management, 25,* 64A–B, F, H.

Needleman, J., Buerhaus, P. I., Stewart, M., Zelevinsky, K., & Mattke, S. (2006). Nurse staffing in hospitals: Is there a business case for quality? *Health Affairs, 25,* 204–211.

Newhouse, J. P. (1989). Measuring medical prices and understanding their effects. *Journal of Health Administration Education, 7,* 19–26.

Pappas, S. H. (2007). Describing costs related to nursing. *Journal of Nursing Administration, 37,* 32–40.

Regan, M. B., Byers, P. H., & Mayrovitz, H. N. (1995). Efficacy of a comprehensive pressure ulcer prevention program in an extended care facility. *Advances in Wound Care, 8,* 49–55.

Richardson, J. (1994). Cost utility analysis: What should be measured? *Social Science and Medicine, 37,* 7–21.

Saba, V. K., & Arnold, J. M. (2004). Clinical care costing method for the Clinical Care Classification System™. *International Journal of Nursing Terminologies and Classifications, 15(3),* 69–77.

Stone, P. W., & Walker, P. H. (1995). Cost-effectiveness analysis: Birth center vs. hospital care. *Nursing Economics, 13,* 299–308.

U. S. Government Accountability Office. (2005). *Medicare physician fees: Geographic adjustment indices are valid in design, but data and methods need refinement.* Report to Congressional Committees GAO-05-119. Retrieved April 28, 2009, from http://www.gao.gov/new.items/d05119.pdf

Walsh, B., Steiner, A., Pickering, R. M., & Ward-Basu, J. (2005). Economic evaluation of nurse led intermediate care versus standard care for post-acute medical patients: Cost minimisation analysis of data from a randomised controlled trial. *British Medical Journal, 330,* 699–704.

Welton, J. M., Fischer, M. H., DeGrace, S., & Zone-Smith, L. (2006). Nursing intensity billing. *Journal of Nursing Administration, 36,* 181–188.

Welton, J. M., Unruh, L., & Halloran, E. J. (2006). Nurse staffing, nursing intensity, staff mix, and direct nursing care costs across Massachusetts hospitals. *Journal of Nursing Administration, 36,* 416–425.

Welton, J. M., Zone-Smith, L., & Fischer, M. H. (2006). Adjustment of inpatient care reimbursement for nursing intensity. *Policy, Politics, & Nursing Practice, 7,* 270–280.

West, T. D., Balas, E. A., & West, D. A. (1996). Contrasting RCC, RVU, and ABC for managed care decisions. *Healthcare Financial Management,* 54–61.

Williams, R. M. (1996). The costs of visits to emergency departments. *New England Journal of Medicine, 334,* 642–646.

Wilson, L., Prescott, P. A., & Aleksandrowicz, L. (1988). Nursing: A major hospital cost component. *Health Services Research, 22,* 773–796.

Wong, R., Gordon, D. L., Cassard, S. D., Weisman, C. S., & Bergner, M. (1993). A cost analysis of a professional practice model for nursing. *Nursing Economics, 11,* 292–297, 323.

# 19 Outcomes Evaluation

LEAH L. SHEVER

Evaluation of outcomes in health care is drawing increasing attention from health care providers, consumers, regulatory bodies, and policymakers. The shift in focus to health care outcomes has been driven by the fact that while health care costs have continued to soar, reaching $2.4 trillion in 2007 (The National Coalition on Healthcare, 2009), the quality of health care in the United States is dismally low compared to that in other nations (Anderson & Frogner, 2008; Nolte & McKee, 2008). Although there are a number of factors that contribute to the broken health care system in the United States, such as absence of health care insurance, lack of access to care, inappropriate use of limited resources (e.g., lack of limits on the number of unnecessary tests, failure to focus on prevention, lack of limits on length of stay in an intensive care unit at the end of life)—one of the most disturbing factors, and one that also affects quality of care, involves the alarming number of errors and adverse events that are, in fact, largely preventable (Institute of Medicine, 2000). And, while defining quality in health care is commonly difficult, examining outcomes is an essential part of the process.

At its most basic level, health care quality can be defined as keeping patients safe and not inflicting further harm. Two Institute of Medicine (IOM) reports, *To Err Is Human: Building a Safer Health System* (2000) and *Crossing the Quality Chasm: A New Health System for the*

**387**

*21st Century* (2001), illustrate the opposite: the current U.S. health care system too often does a poor job of keeping patients safe. In a more recent report, the IOM asserts that nurses are the health care providers most likely not only to prevent adverse events or complications but also to identify them and to activate appropriate responses after a complication occurs (Institute of Medicine, 2004). It is, therefore, imperative that nurses monitor and evaluate health care outcomes beginning at the patient level and that they have an understanding of how aggregated patient outcomes are an indication of quality at the system or institution level.

## EVOLUTION OF OUTCOMES EVALUATION

### Agencies Impacting Health Care Outcomes and Quality

Outcomes in health care have always been important. Specific measures of outcomes, their definitions, how they are collected and reported, and their implications have evolved greatly over time. Although outcomes evaluation in nursing really started with one nurse, Florence Nightingale, during the Crimean War, many organizations have guided outcomes evaluation in the United States. A brief description of these organizations follows.

Hospitals in the United States must be accredited by an agency recognized by the U.S. government in order to receive reimbursement for patients whose health insurance is provided by Medicare or Medicaid. For most hospitals, this agency is the Joint Commission on Accreditation of Healthcare Organizations, or the "Joint Commission." This organization has been accrediting hospitals for more than 50 years. Hospitals must meet or exceed performance measures in order to be accredited and receive reimbursement from the federal government (Joint Commission, 2008). The performance measures set by the Joint Commission are a combination of process and outcome measures that evaluate hospitals' efforts to ensure patient safety.

Another influential agency that focuses on quality in U.S. health care is the Agency for Healthcare Research and Quality (AHRQ). AHRQ is a part of the U.S. Department of Health and Human Services (DHHS) and not only funds health services research but also is active in disseminating research results and evidence-based practices, which greatly influence health care outcomes. AHRQ has many resources for health care providers to help them positively impact patient outcomes, including evidence-based guidelines and outcome evaluation tools (Agency for Healthcare Research and Quality, 2002).

Specific to nursing, the American Nurses' Credentialing Center offers Magnet recognition for hospitals that draw and retain nurses. This work began in the early 1980s, when the American Academy of Nursing's (AAN) Task Force on Nursing Practice in Hospitals conducted a survey of approximately 160 hospitals in the United States and identified 41 hospitals with environments beneficial to nurses. In the early 1990s, the first U.S. hospital gained Magnet recognition, and today "Magnet" status is an international recognition available both for acute-care hospitals and long-term-care facilities (American Nurses Credentialing Center, 2008).

In addition to attracting and retaining nurses, these hospitals have demonstrated high quality in specific nursing-sensitive outcomes (Aiken, Havens, & Sloane, 2000a, 2000b; Scott, Sochalski, & Aiken, 1999). Magnet recognition, which identifies hospitals with exceptional nursing care and positive patient outcomes, is unlike other accreditations, which demonstrate satisfaction of minimum requirements. Starting in the fall of 2009, Magnet recognition will become even more dependent on health care outcomes, specifically those that are nursing-sensitive (American Nurses Credentialing Center, 2008).

In 1999, the nonprofit National Quality Forum (NQF) developed a strategy for measuring quality in health care, specifically related to valid and reliable performance indicators. Indicators endorsed by NQF are developed by consensus, and outcome measures are divided into three categories: patient-centered outcomes, nursing-centered intervention measures, and system-centered measures (National Quality Forum, 2004).

## Current Trends in Reporting Outcome Measures

Making specific hospital measures available to the public has also prompted significant change in how health care outcomes are utilized. Health care consumers are now able to access the Centers for Medicare and Medicaid Services' (CMS) Web site (http://www.hospitalcompare. hhs.gov/) to see not only how their local hospital performs in process measures (like the administration of aspirin to patients suspected of having acute myocardial infarction [AMI] or the timely delivery of antibiotics) but also how hospitals compare to one another. Currently, measures related to AMIs, heart failure, pneumonia, and surgical infections are publicly reported (U.S. Department of Health and Human Services, 2008). In theory, potential patients/health care consumers can examine the data related to specific health care problems and make a more informed decision on what hospital fits their care needs best.

CMS has now taken outcomes evaluation to the next level by no longer reimbursing hospitals for certain complications that patients incur while hospitalized, referred to as *hospital-acquired conditions* (HACs). Previously, if a patient covered by Medicare or Medicaid experienced an HAC that required additional care (e.g., surgical repair of a fracture from a fall), the hospital would be reimbursed by CMS for the costs associated with treating the fracture. Currently, hospitals will no longer receive reimbursement for treatment of the following HACs: a foreign object retained after surgery, air embolism, blood incompatibility, stage III and IV pressure ulcers, falls and injuries from falls (fractures, dislocations, intracranial injuries, crushing injuries, burns), catheter-associated urinary tract infection (UTI), vascular catheter-associate infection, and surgical-site infection-mediastinitis after coronary artery bypass graft (CABG) (Centers for Medicare and Medicaid, 2008).

The reasoning for nonreimbursement is simple: there is substantial evidence to support that these HACs can be prevented when proper processes are in place (from adequate nurse staffing and proper risk assessment to evidence-based interventions targeted to specific risk factors). As the implications of nonreimbursement are vast, hospitals are working to reduce the numbers of HACs in order to avoid potential future costs.

## DEFINITION AND INTRODUCTION OF TERMS

### Health Outcomes Research

Health outcomes research evaluates the end result of specific health care treatments or interventions (Agency for Healthcare Research and Quality, 2000). The difference between outcomes research and other medical research is that the definition of the treatment is broader in health outcomes research. Typical medical research examines the impact of a specific surgical procedure or the effect of a medication, whereas outcomes research broadens the definition of *treatment* to include such things as counseling, staffing, and care delivery models and how they impact outcomes (Kane, 2006). This type of research is also sometimes referred to as *intervention research* (Burns & Grove, 2001).

## Efficacy Versus Effectiveness Research

Often, when the general public hears "research" they think of randomized controlled trials (RCTs). RCTs are a type of *efficacy* research where the *potential* benefits of the treatment or intervention are studied under ideal, controlled conditions (Brown, 2002; Shwartz & Ash, 2003; Sidani & Epstein, 2003; Sidani, Epstein, & Moritz, 2003; Whittemore & Grey, 2002). In comparison, *effectiveness* research refers to studies of the impact of interventions or treatments on patient outcomes in a real-world situation where multiple other factors influence the outcome (Brown, 2002; Sidani & Epstein, 2003; Sidani, Epstein, & Moritz, 2003; Titler, Dochterman, & Reed, 2004; Whittemore & Grey, 2002).

For a number of reasons, efficacy research in nursing poses many problems. One issue is the feasibility of conducting such research. It is difficult from a practical point of view to randomize patients to nursing treatments. From an ethical standpoint, it is difficult to randomize patients to treatment if there is evidence to suggest that the treatment will provide an improved outcome or comfort to the patient. Furthermore, it is rarely the case that only one specific nursing treatment is provided for a patient with any type of health concern. Typically, nursing takes a multifaceted approach to treating individuals with health care concerns, recognizing that each patient is an individual and therefore has a unique set of needs and wishes. Nursing is also only one health care discipline attempting to effectively treat a patient. Pharmacy, medicine, physical therapy, and others all work with nursing in a variety of settings to achieve desired patient outcomes. To conduct nursing efficacy research in vacuum, thinking that only one specific nursing treatment is going to influence patient outcomes, appears to be a waste of time and resources given how nursing actually operates in collaboration with the patients, families, and other health care disciplines in a real-life setting. In short, the generalizability of nursing efficacy studies is very limited (Sidani, Epstein, & Moritz, 2003).

## Risk Adjustment

Risk adjustment refers to accounting, or controlling, for patient-specific factors that may impact outcomes (Iezzoni, 2003). If risk adjustment is not done, it is possible to reach a wrong conclusion about the treatment (Smith, Nitz, & Stuart, 2006). To illustrate the need for risk adjustment, consider two patients treated for a fracture of the tibia. Both require surgery to set the bone, followed by weeks in a cast while the bone heals. The first patient is 17-year old healthy male who broke his leg playing football. He experiences no complications during or following surgery and is able to have the cast removed in the expected time frame. The second patient is an 83-year old female who resides in a skilled-nursing facility, has a history of diabetes and dementia, and broke her leg when she tripped over a footstool. This patient has her leg set surgically and has a cast applied but develops pneumonia following surgery. She is hospitalized an additional 5 days and never regains the mobility she had prior to the fracture. If no risk adjustment were done, we would evaluate the treatment (i.e., surgery and cast) solely on the basis of the patients' outcomes—one regained full mobility and the other did not. An incorrect conclusion that the treatment is not effective may be drawn if the risk factors present in the second patient, such as her advanced age and comorbid conditions of diabetes, dementia, and pneumonia are not considered or adjusted for.

There are varying methods of risk adjustment, and selection of the most appropriate method depends on which outcomes are being evaluated, the time period, the study population, and the purpose of the evaluation (Iezzoni, 2003). The factors or variables most frequently used for risk adjustment include age, severity of illness, and comorbid conditions (Iezzoni, 2003; Smith, Nitz, & Stuart, 2006).

## CONSIDERATIONS FOR OUTCOMES EVALUATION

Whether conducting or evaluating an outcomes study or simply examining outcomes in a clinical setting, one must consider certain key components of outcomes measurement to ensure that the data are valid and reliable.

### Conceptual Model

The first step in evaluating health care outcomes is to consider the *conceptual model.* This can sound like an intimidating process, but it saves a lot of work if done at the beginning of the process. This first step is important whether one is conducting or evaluating an outcomes study or evaluating outcomes in a clinical setting. This first step is critical to ensure that relationships and/or processes that impact the outcome are considered (Kane, 2006). Spending time on the conceptual model helps delineate the processes that contribute to the outcome. It then becomes easier to explain or understand the research findings.

Consider central line-associated bloodstream infection rates on a nursing unit. A researcher may be interested in studying whether an antimicrobial dressing decreases the rate of infections. In constructing their conceptual model, they consider other factors, or variables, that may also impact infection rates, such as hand hygiene and aseptic technique when the line is first placed. By developing a conceptual model that carefully considers the variables that impact central line–associated bloodstream infections, the researcher realizes that they must also measure those additional factors (e.g., hand hygiene, aseptic placement) that impact infection rates if they want to have a full understanding of the impact of the antimicrobial dressing. The study findings will be more robust as a result of the careful consideration of factors that influence central line–associated bloodstream infections.

There are many conceptual models available to help guide outcomes evaluation, and many of these are based on or influenced by the work of Donabedian (2005). Donabedian created a model to describe how health care outcomes occur and how structure and process influence these outcomes. Examples of structure might include a hospital, a nursing unit, a patient's home, a clinic, or an operating room. Processes describe what is done within the structure. Processes can include such things as medical procedures, medication delivery, and nursing treatments (Donabedian, 2005).

## Data Sources and Measurement Issues

After the conceptual model has been carefully developed and key relationships defined, the next step is to identify the *data source* for each identified variable. The ideal data source is valid and reliable and lends itself well to precise or detailed measurement (Burns & Grove, 2001). In RCTs, the researcher has tight control over the variables to ensure that they are valid and reliable; this degree of control is not possible in effectiveness research.

In research that uses clinical data or data not collected for the purposes of research, it is much more difficult to identify valid and reliable data sources because the data sources were not designed to be

394 Part IV Evaluating the Impact of Evidence-Based Practice

measurement tools but were instead designed for clinical purposes related to patient care. Although this problem doesn't mean that the data cannot be useful, it is certainly a limitation and must be taken into consideration when evaluating the data.

## Episode of Care or Time Period

The *episode of care,* or time period, is the designated time that interventions and outcomes will be monitored or measured. It is important to designate an episode of care that is in keeping with the conceptual model. The time frame for data collection needs to capture the phenomenon of interest; that is, it must contain the time when the intervention is going to achieve a measurable effect (Strickland, 1997). As an example, consider a congestive heart failure patient who received targeted education on daily weight monitoring and proper diet, in the expectation that education will reduce the likelihood of the patient's readmission to the hospital. If the episode of care for data collection is hospital admission up to 30 days after discharge, the impact of the education intervention will probably not be captured, since it takes longer than 30 days to see a change in a person's health as a result of diet and close monitoring of weight.

Typically, the episode of care for acute-care settings is the patient's stay in the hospital. Often the focus is on interventions or treatments provided while the patient is in the hospital, and the associated outcomes are those that are observable while the patient is still in the hospital. For example, if the intervention of interest is whether or not hourly rounding by nurses on patient care units reduces fall rates, it would not be appropriate to continue to monitor patient falls after the patient has been discharged from the hospital. The designated episode of care would be the patient's stay on the care unit.

In an ambulatory setting, the episode of care could be a visit or a series of visits to a clinic until the problem is resolved. The time period, or episode of care, for data measurement and collection is an important concept that should be carefully considered along with the key concepts in the conceptual model.

## Level of Analysis

Health care is delivered in multiple environments at multiple levels that are integrated, at various points, with one another. Just as when one is defining the episode of care, one should consider carefully the level of analysis to be undertaken in view of the conceptual model being used. The person conducting outcomes evaluation needs to determine at what level the intervention, or treatment, of interest occurs. Using hourly rounding and falls again as an example, one could examine the findings at multiple levels. If the research question was whether patients who received the treatment of interest (i.e., hourly rounding) had a lower probability of falling, the level of analysis would be the patient, and data collection would occur at the individual patient level (e.g., whether the patient received hourly rounding and whether the patient fell). If the research question was whether nursing units that conducted hourly rounds had lower fall rates, the level of analysis would be the nursing unit. In this case, the intervention of interest (i.e., hourly rounding) would be calculated at the nursing-unit level (e.g., more than 90% of patients on the unit received hourly rounding) and the outcome of interest (i.e., fall rates) would also be measured at the nursing-unit level. If the question were changed to "Do hospitals that conduct hourly rounding have significantly lower fall rates?" then the level of analysis would be at the hospital level.

## OUTCOME MEASURES: NURSING, ORGANIZATIONAL, AND PATIENT-SPECIFIC

Because of the extremely large number of potential health care outcomes, we cannot discuss them all. Therefore, we will focus on outcomes most closely related to nursing care. Outcomes that have been associated with nursing care are often referred to as being *nursing-sensitive.*

### Nursing-Sensitive Outcome Measures

The National Quality Forum breaks its health care performance measures into three categories: patient-centered outcomes, nursing-centered intervention measures, and system-centered measures. These can be seen in Table 19.1. It is important to note that there are very few *nursing-centered intervention* measures. In other words, the only nursing intervention that NQF has designated as impacting patient outcomes is *smoking cessation counseling* (National Quality Forum, 2004). To grow the evidence in this area, a revolutionary study was funded in 2000 by the National Institute for Nursing Research (NINR) (Titler, 2000). This

Table 19.1

## NATIONAL VOLUNTARY CONSENSUS STANDARDS FOR NURSING-SENSITIVE CARE

| FRAMEWORK CATEGORY | MEASURE | DESCRIPTION |
|---|---|---|
| Patient-centered outcome measures | 1. Death among surgical inpatients with treatable serious complications (failure to rescue) | Percentage of major surgical inpatients who experience a hospital-acquired complication (i.e., sepsis, pneumonia, gastrointestinal bleeding, shock/cardiac arrest, deep vein thrombosis/pulmonary embolism) and die |
| | 2. Pressure ulcer prevalence | Percentage of inpatients who have a hospital-acquired pressure ulcer (Stage 2 or greater) |
| | 3. Falls prevalence | Number of inpatient falls per inpatient days |
| | 4. Falls with injury | Number of inpatient falls with injuries per inpatient days |
| | 5. Restraint prevalence (vest and limb only) | Percentage of inpatients who have a vest or limb restraint |
| | 6. Urinary catheter-associated urinary tract infection (UTI) for intensive care unit (ICU) patients | Rate of UTI associated with use of urinary catheters for ICU patients |
| | 7. Central line catheter-associated bloodstream infection rate for ICU and high-risk nursery (HRN) patients | Rate of bloodstream infections associated with use of central line catheters for ICU and HRN patients |
| | 8. Ventilator-associated pneumonia for ICU and HRN patients | Rate of pneumonia associated with use of ventilators for ICU patients and HRN patients |

| | |
|---|---|
| Nursing-centered intervention measures | 9. Smoking-cessation counseling for acute myocardial infarction (AMI) | Percentage of AMI inpatients with history of smoking within the past year who received smoking-cessation advice or counseling during hospitalization |
| | 10. Smoking-cessation counseling for heart failure (HF) | Percentage of HF inpatients with history of smoking within the past year who received smoking-cessation advice or counseling during hospitalization |
| | 11. Smoking-cessation counseling for pneumonia | Percentage of pneumonia inpatients with a history of smoking within the past year who received smoking-cessation advice or counseling during hospitalization |
| System-centered measures | 12. Skill mix (Registered Nurse [RN], Licensed Vocational/Practice Nurse [LVN/LPN], unlicensed assistive personnel [UAP], and contract) | ■ Percentage of RN care hours to total nursing-care hours<br>■ Percentage of LVN/LPN care hours to total nursing-care hours<br>■ Percentage of UAP care hours to total nursing-care hours<br>■ Percentage of contract hours (RN, LVN/LPN, and UAP) to total nursing-care hours |
| | 13. Nursing-care hours per patient day (RN, LVN/LPN, and UAP) | ■ Number of RN care hours per patient day<br>■ Number of nursing-care hours (RN, LVN/LPN, UAP) per patient day |
| | 14. Practice Environment Scale-Nursing Work Index (PES-NWI) (composite and five subscales) | Composite score and mean presence scores for each of the following subscales derived from the PES-NWI<br>■ Nurse participation in hospital affairs<br>■ Nursing foundations for quality of care<br>■ Nurse manager ability, leadership, and support of nurses<br>■ Staffing and resource adequacy<br>■ Collegial nurse-physician relations |
| | 15. Voluntary turnover | Number of voluntary uncontrolled separations during the month for RNs and advanced practice nurses, LVN/LPNs, and nurse assistants/aides |

397

study was one of the first to use nursing interventions captured in electronic medical records for research purposes. This study showed that specific nursing interventions impact hospital cost (Shever et al., 2008; Titler et al., 2005, 2007, 2008), failure to rescue from a medical complication (Shever, 2007), medication errors (Picone et al., 2008), and discharge disposition (Titler et al., 2006).

Before NQF, the American Nurses' Association (ANA) produced the Nursing Care Report Card for Acute Care, which identified, defined, and measured nursing-sensitive quality indicators (American Nurses Association, 1995). This work evolved into the National Database of Nursing Quality Indicators (NDNQI), a database to which more than 1,200 hospitals currently contribute data. The data are collected at the nursing-unit level rather than at the broader hospital-level (Montalvo, 2007). The NDNQI process and outcome indicators are these:

- Patient falls with injury
- Pressure ulcers:
  - Community acquired
  - Hospital acquired
  - Unit acquired
- Staff mix
- Nursing hours per patient day
- RN surveys:
  - Job satisfaction
  - Practice environment scale
- RN education and certification
- Pediatric pain assessment cycle
- Pediatric IV infiltration rate
- Psychiatric patient assault rate
- Restraints prevalence
- Nurse turnover
- Nosocomial infections:
  - Ventilator-associated pneumonia (VAP)
  - Central-line-associated bloodstream infection (CLABSI)
  - Catheter-associated urinary tract infections (CAUTI)

## Organizational Outcome Measures

The outcome indicators outlined in the preceding section can be measured or analyzed at multiple levels that include the nursing unit, the hospital, the hospital system, and so on. There are, however, multiple indicators that should not be measured and compared at levels below that of the hospital level because of their rarity. Two of those measures, mortality and failure to rescue, are discussed here.

## Mortality

Mortality (death) is typically reported as a rate. This outcome is frequently examined when one is comparing quality across hospitals. Mortality is a great example of an outcome that requires careful risk adjustment. It is typically dichotomous; death either occurred or did not occur. What often varies is the episode of care. In other words, the outcome may be death during hospitalization, death during a specific medical treatment, death so many days after discharge from a hospital, and so on.

## Failure to Rescue

Failure to rescue from a medical complication, usually referred to as *failure to rescue* in the literature, is defined as death following a complication during hospitalization. This variable was developed in 1992 at a time when hospitals were often ranked according to their complication and mortality rates, which may put hospitals that treat more critically ill patients at a disadvantage (Silber, Williams, Krakauer, & Schwartz, 1992). This outcome was developed by the researchers as a way to measure health care providers' recognition of a complication and how quickly they respond to the complication.

Failure to rescue is typically reported as a rate. The denominator is a count of the number of patients who experienced one or more complications during hospitalization. The numerator is a count of deaths that occurred in patients included in the denominator (Silber et al., 1992). For example, if 1,200 patients in a hospital experienced a complication during one year and 200 of those 1,200 patients died, the failure to rescue rate would be 16.7% (200/1200). Examples of complications include a deep vein thrombosis (DVT), pneumonia, and gastrointestinal bleed.

Failure to rescue is an example of a health care outcome where it is very important to pay attention to how the variable is defined or calculated. In the previous paragraphs, failure to rescue was defined as death *occurring after a complication during hospitalization,* which may seem straightforward. However, there has been variability in how failure to rescue has been operationally defined and calculated. While the operational definition of death may be clear, definitions of *complications* have varied greatly across failure to rescue studies.

A number of studies have used a broader definition of *complications*. Many studies have included any death after surgery as a failure to rescue even if there were no documented complications (Aiken, Clarke, Cheung, Sloane, & Silber, 2003; Aiken, Clarke, Sloane, Sochalski, & Silber, 2002; Silber et al., 2000; Silber et al., 2002; Silber, Rosenbaum, Schwartz, Ross, & Williams, 1995; Silber et al., 1992). The rationale behind this definition is that a physician deemed the patient healthy enough to survive surgery; therefore, when the patient died following surgery, the patient must have experienced a complication, even if it was not documented.

In contrast, other researchers and organizations have defined failure to rescue as death that occurs after a patient experiences one of *five complications:* pneumonia, shock or cardiac arrest, upper gastrointestinal (GI) bleed, sepsis, and deep vein thrombosis (DVT) (Agency for Healthcare Research and Quality, 2007; National Quality Forum, 2006; Needleman, Buerhaus, Mattke, Stewart, & Zelevinsky, 2002). Needleman states that this definition of failure to rescue was "developed as a part of a project to identify nursing sensitive measures" (Needleman & Buerhaus, 2007). The original definition essentially included all deaths after surgery, whereas this newer definition greatly limits the number of complications eligible for inclusion and therefore also limits the number of deaths included.

## Patient Outcomes

### Nursing Outcomes Classification

While the majority of outcomes discussed earlier have been negative in nature (e.g., hospital-acquired conditions, falls, and infection rates), outcome evaluation can also involve neutral outcomes. The Nursing Outcomes Classification (NOC) is a patient-level outcomes classification system that captures positive and negative changes to a patient's condition, as well as cases where there is no change. Although the title Nursing Outcomes Classification may imply that the classification is sensitive to nursing care, it is actually patient focused and is sensitive to more than that one aspect of care (Moorhead, Johnson, Maas, & Swanson, 2007).

There are many advantages to using NOC rather than other outcomes measures. First, NOC employs a standardized language that can be used across a variety of settings and therefore across the continuum of care. It enables health care providers to track patient outcomes across settings and time. Second, it is easily linked to nursing diagnoses and nursing interventions. Another benefit of NOC is that it is organized in such a manner that it can be built into electronic documentation systems (Moorhead, Johnson, Maas, & Swanson, 2007).

## Patient Satisfaction

The first patient satisfaction tool to address nursing care was developed in 1975. The name of this tool is the Patient Satisfaction Scale (PSS), and it addresses three aspects of nursing care: (1) technical-professional area, (2) interpersonal educational relationship, and (3) interpersonal trusting relationship. It was developed for primary-care settings (Risser, 1975).

Hinshaw and Atwood (1981) took Risser's tool for primary-care settings and adapted it for acute-care settings. Their tool was called the Patient Satisfaction Instrument, and it covered the same three aspects of nursing care that were the focus of the PSS (Hinshaw & Atwood, 1981). A number of studies and tools to measure patient satisfaction have been developed since this time.

Some of the key principles when evaluating patient satisfaction tools are to examine their reliability and validity, the specific concepts the tool is measuring, and the setting and sample on which the tool was tested. Most studies include these items in the study description. Keep in mind that the reliability and validity are applicable only to the setting in which the tool was tested. A tool that is found to be highly valid and reliable in the acute-care setting may not be valid and reliable in a home-care setting (Burns & Grove, 2001; Lin, 1996).

One of the drawbacks of using patient satisfaction as an outcome is the difficulty in determining what care delivery process is affecting the patient's response. For example, patients are often asked to rate their overall hospital stay. When a patient states that he or she was "not satisfied," it is often impossible to know whether the person was dissatisfied with the nursing care received or the lack of cleanliness of the patient's room. Although it is important for patients and families to be satisfied with the overall hospital experience, it is not possible to make process changes from this type of aggregated information.

## SUMMARY

A large part of outcomes evaluation is ensuring quality in health care. Quality in health care continues to be a priority for providers, consumers, regulatory agencies, and the U.S. government. Quality, as well as outcomes measurement and evaluation, will continue to be an important issue in the United States as costs remain astoundingly high. Nurses must be able to demonstrate how the care they provide impacts patient outcomes in order to ensure that nurses' work is valued and appropriate resources are dedicated to ensure delivery of high-quality care. Outcomes evaluation helps guide practice change to help achieve desired outcomes.

## SUGGESTED ACTIVITIES

1    Go to the CMS Hospital Compare Web site (http://www.hospital compare.hhs.gov/Hospital/Search/Welcome.asp), and compare two hospitals in your area. On the basis of the information presented, how would you decide which hospital is the best one in which to receive care?

- Develop a conceptual model that explains part or all of one of the reported outcomes. Consider the episode of care as defined on the CMS Web site and what processes could be measured and obtained that contribute to the outcome.

2    Go to the Joint Commission Web site (http://www.jointcommis sion.org/), and examine the patient safety goals related to your care setting (e.g., hospital, critical-access hospital, home health). Select one or two goals, and then identify outcomes related to those specific goals that can be measured and monitored.

## REFERENCES

Agency for Healthcare Research and Quality. (2000). *Outcomes research: Fact sheet.* AHRQ Publication No. 00-P011. Rockville, MD: Agency for Healthcare Research and Quality. Retrieved May 19, 2008, from http://www.ahrq.gov/clinic/outfact.htm

Agency for Healthcare Research and Quality. (2002). *What is AHRQ?* Retrieved May 19, 2008, from http://www.ahrq.gov/about/whatis.htm

Agency for Healthcare Research and Quality. (2007). *AHRQ Patient Safety Network Glossary: Failure to rescue.* Retrieved October 9, 2007, from http://psnet.ahrq.gov/glossary.aspx#F

Aiken, L. H., Clarke, S. P., Cheung, R. B., Sloane, D. M., & Silber, J. H. (2003). Educational levels of hospital nurses and surgical patient mortality. *Journal of the American Medical Association, 290*(12), 1617–1623.

Aiken, L. H., Clarke, S. P., Sloane, D. M., Sochalski, J., & Silber, J. H. (2002). Hospital nurse staffing and patient mortality, nurse burnout, and job dissatisfaction. *Journal of the American Medical Association, 288*(16), 1987–1993.

Aiken, L. H., Havens, D. S., & Sloane, D. M. (2000a). The Magnet Nursing Services Recognition Program. *American Journal of Nursing, 100*(3), 26–35; quiz 35–26.

Aiken, L. H., Havens, D. S., & Sloane, D. M. (2000b). Magnet nursing services recognition programme. *Nursing Standard, 14*(25), 41–47.

American Nurses Association. (1995). *Nursing care report card for acute care.* Silver Spring, MD: Author.

American Nurses Credentialing Center. (2008). *History of the Magnet Program.* Retrieved May 19, 2009, from http://www.nursecredentialing.org/magnet/history.html

Anderson, G. F., & Frogner, B. K. (2008). Health spending in OECD countries: Obtaining value per dollar. *Health Affairs, 27*(6), 1718–1727.

Brown, S. J. (2002). Nursing intervention studies: A descriptive analysis of issues important to clinicians. *Research in Nursing and Health, 25*(4), 317–327.

Burns, N., & Grove, S. (2001). *The practice of nursing research: Conduct, critique and utilization* (4th ed.). Philadelphia: W. B. Saunders.

Centers for Medicare and Medicaid. (2008). *Hospital acquired conditions.* Retrieved May 18, 2008, from http://www.cms.hhs.gov/HospitalAcqCond/06_Hospital-Acquired%20Conditions.asp#TopOfPage

Donabedian, A. (2005). Evaluating the quality of medical care. 1966. *Milbank Quarterly, 83*(4), 691–729.

Hinshaw, A. S., & Atwood, J. R. (1981). A Patient Satisfaction Instrument: Precision by replication. *Nursing Research, 31*(3), 170–175, 191.

Iezzoni, L. I. (2003). Getting started and defining terms. In L. I. Iezzoni (Ed.), *Risk adjustment for measuring health care outcomes* (3rd ed., pp. 17–32). Chicago: Health Administration Press.

Institute of Medicine. (2000). *To err is human: Building a safer health system* Washington, DC: National Academy of Sciences.

Institute of Medicine. (2001). *Crossing the quality chasm: A new health system for the 21st century.* Washington, DC: National Academy of Sciences.

Institute of Medicine. (2004). *Keeping patients safe: Transforming the work environment of nurses.* Washington, DC: National Academies Press.

Joint Commission. (2008). Hospital Accreditation Program. Retrieved May 19, 2008, from http://www.jointcommission.org/AccreditationPrograms/Hospitals/

Kane, R. L. (2006). Introduction. In R. L. Kane (Ed.), *Understanding health care outcomes research* (2nd ed.). Boston: Jones & Bartlett.

Lin, C. C. (1996). Patient satisfaction with nursing care as an outcome variable: Dilemmas for nursing evaluation researchers. *Journal of Professional Nursing, 12*(4), 207–216.

Montalvo, I. (2007). The national database for nursing quality indicator (NDNQI). *The Online Journal of Issues in Nursing.* Retrieved May 17, 2008, from www.nursingworld.org/MainMenuCategories/ANAMarketplace/ANAPeriodicals/OJIN/TableofContents/Volume122007/No3Sept07/NursingQualityIndicators.aspx

Moorhead, S., Johnson, M., Maas, M., & Swanson, E. (Eds.). (2007). *Nursing Outcomes Classification (NOC)* (4th ed.). St. Louis: Mosby.

National Coalition on Health Care. (2009). Facts on the cost of health insurance and health care. Retrieved May 3, 2009, from http://www.nchc.org/facts/cost.shtml

National Quality Forum. (2004). *National Voluntary Consensus Standards for Nursing-Sensitive Care: An initial performance measure set.* Washington, DC: National Quality Forum.

National Quality Forum. (2006). Nursing Care Performance Measures. Retrieved April 29, 2007, from http://www.qualityforum.org/nursing/#measures

Needleman, J., Buerhaus, P., Mattke, S., Stewart, M., & Zelevinsky, K. (2002). Nurse-staffing levels and the quality of care in hospitals. *New England Journal of Medicine, 346*(22), 1715–1722.

Needleman, J., & Buerhaus, P. I. (2007). Failure-to-rescue: Comparing definitions to measure quality of care. *Medical Care, 45*(10), 913–915.

Nolte, E., & McKee, C. M. (2008). Measuring the health of nations: Updating an earlier analysis. *Health Affairs, 27*(1), 58–71.

Picone, D. M., Titler, M., Dochterman, J., Shever, L., Kim, T., Abramowitz, P., et al. (2008). Predictors of medication errors among elderly hospitalized patients. *American Journal of Medical Quality, 23*(2), 115–127.

Risser, N. L. (1975). Development of an instrument to measure patient satisfaction with nurses and nursing care in primary care settings. *Nursing Research, 24*(1), 45–52.

Scott, J. G., Sochalski, J., & Aiken, L. (1999). Review of magnet hospital research: Findings and implications for professional nursing practice. *Journal of Nursing Administration, 29*(1), 9–19.

Shever, L. (2007). *Predictors of failure to rescue and failure to rescue from an adverse incident with closer examination of nursing surveillance.* Unpublished doctoral dissertation, University of Iowa, Iowa City.

Shever, L. L., Titler, M., Kerr, P., Qin, R., Kim, T., & Picone, D. M. (2008). Effects of nursing surveillance on hospital cost for older adults at risk for falling. *Journal of Nursing Scholarship, 40*(2), 161–169.

Shwartz, M., & Ash, A. S. (2003). Estimating the effect of an intervention from observational data. In L. Iezzoni (Ed.), *Risk adjustment for measuring health care outcomes* (3rd ed., pp. 275–295). Chicago: Health Administration Press.

Sidani, S., & Epstein, D. R. (2003). Enhancing the evaluation of nursing care effectiveness. *Canadian Journal of Nursing research, 35*(3), 26–38.

Sidani, S., Epstein, D. R., & Moritz, P. (2003). An alternative paradigm for clinical nursing research: An exemplar. *Research in Nursing and Health, 26*(3), 224–255.

Silber, J. H., Kennedy, S. K., Even-Shoshan, O., Chen, W., Koziol, L. F., Showan, A. M., et al. (2000). Anesthesiologist direction and patient outcomes. *Anesthesiology, 93*(1), 152–163.

Silber, J. H., Kennedy, S. K., Even-Shoshan, O., Chen, W., Mosher, R. E., Showan, A. M., et al. (2002). Anesthesiologist board certification and patient outcomes. *Anesthesiology, 96*(5), 1044–1052.

Silber, J. H., Rosenbaum, P. R., Schwartz, J. S., Ross, R. N., & Williams, S. V. (1995). Evaluation of the complication rate as a measure of quality of care in coronary artery bypass graft surgery. *Journal of the American Medical Association, 274*(4), 317–323.

Silber, J. H., Williams, S. V., Krakauer, H., & Schwartz, J. S. (1992). Hospital and patient characteristics associated with death after surgery. A study of adverse occurrence and failure to rescue. *Medical Care, 30*(7), 615–629.

Smith, M. A., Nitz, N. M., & Stuart, S. K. (2006). Severity and comorbity. In R. L. Kane (Ed.), *Understanding health care outcomes research* (2nd ed.). Boston: Jones & Bartlett.

Strickland, O. L. (1997). Challenges in measuring patient outcomes. *Nursing Clinics of North America, 32*(3), 495–512.

Titler, M. (2000). *Nursing interventions and outcomes effectiveness in 3 older populations.* R01 No. NR05331–02. Rockville, MD: National Institute of Nursing Research.

Titler, M., Dochterman, J., Kim, T., Kanak, M., Shever, L., Picone, D. M., et al. (2007). Cost of care for seniors hospitalized for hip fractures and related procedures. *Nursing Outlook, 55*, 5–14.

Titler, M., Dochterman, J., Picone, D. M., Everett, L., Xie, X., Kanak, M., et al. (2005). Cost of hospital care for elderly at risk of falling. *Nursing Economics, 23*(6), 290–306.

Titler, M., Dochterman, J., & Reed, D. (2004). *Guideline for conducting effectiveness research in nursing and other health services.* Iowa City: University of Iowa, College of Nursing, Center for Nursing Classification & Clinical Effectiveness.

Titler, M., Dochterman, J., Xie, X. J., Kanak, M., Fei, Q., Picone, D. M., et al. (2006). Nursing interventions and other factors associated with discharge disposition in older patients after hip fractures. *Nursing Research, 55*(4), 231–242.

Titler, M., Jensen, G., Dochterman, J., Xie, X., Kanak, M., Reed, D., et al. (2008). Cost of hospital care for older adults with heart failure: Medical, pharmaceutical and nursing costs. *Health Services Research, 43*(2), 635–655.

U.S. Department of Health & Human Services. (2008). *Hospital compare.* Retrieved May 19, 2008, from http://www.hospitalcompare.hhs.gov/Hospital/Search/Welcome.asp

Whittemore, R., & Grey, M. (2002). The systematic development of nursing interventions. *Journal of Nursing Scholarship, 34*(2), 115–120.

# 20 Ethical Aspects of a Study

## MARQUIS D. FOREMAN AND JULIE JOHNSON ZERWIC

The process of obtaining approval to conduct a research study varies among clinical settings. Some organizations favor a committee structure consisting of two review bodies: a *nursing research committee* (Kirchhoff & McGuire, 1985) to examine scientific merit and resource consumption issues, and a *human subjects review committee* (also known as the *institutional review board* [IRB] or the hospital research committee) to examine issues related to the protection of subjects from the risks of participating in research.

## REVIEW COMMITTEES

If a committee structure exists, whether a nursing research committee or an IRB, the investigator must also consider the following:

- *Frequency of the committee meetings.* Some organizations schedule meetings on an as-needed basis if the volume of clinical studies is small. If both a nursing research committee and an IRB exist, the investigator will need to determine whether a proposal for review can be submitted to both simultaneously or whether one must approve the proposal before it can be submitted to the other for review. This must be factored into the timeline for the study, possibly adding several months to the process.

- *Composition of the review committees.* It cannot be assumed that all review committees include a member who is familiar with nursing research. Therefore, it is important to write the proposal for readers who may not have expertise in that particular content area and may not be familiar with nursing research.
- *The presence of site-specific idiosyncrasies.* For example, some institutions require that an employee or physician be listed as the Principal Investigator (PI) in a submission. Both of these may require that the researcher set up collaborations in advance. An IRB may require initial training in research ethics before a protocol can be submitted. The Collaborative Institutional Training Initiative (CITI) provides online training for participating institutions. Although these issues may seem trivial, such things can delay the process of approval while the committees seek out additional information, and they can become obstacles to the study. By dealing directly and proactively with these issues, the investigator establishes credibility and demonstrates professionalism.

## Nursing Research Committees

Nursing research committees were initiated for the review of (a) the scientific merit of a proposal for which an investigator is seeking support from nursing services, and (b) the nature and magnitude of the resources required of nursing services to implement the proposed research.

The nature and magnitude of resource consumption can range from minimal (e.g., a request merely to access subjects for the study) to significant (e.g., an expectation that nursing staff will both implement various elements of an intervention and collect data regarding the feasibility and efficacy of the intervention).

## Institutional Review Boards

IRBs, also called human subject review committees, exist to provide fair and impartial reviews of research proposals to protect human subjects from any unnecessary risks associated with participation in research. The federal government requires that any institution receiving federal funding set up IRBs. Institutions that do not receive federal funding, that are small, or that produce a limited volume of research may have no formal review structure; however, they may have negotiate an agreement with a larger institution to provide the required oversight.

In major organizations, or in organizations where a large volume of research is conducted, there may be more than one IRB (e.g., a biomedical committee, a social-behavioral committee, and a biobehavioral committee). In the absence of federal funding and a formal review structure, the review may be done informally by an administrator of the institution. In this instance, the investigator should obtain a review from an external human subjects committee to document that the researcher has adhered to federal guidelines concerning the protection of human subjects from risks. Several independent IRBs can be found on the Internet. Having approval from some type of IRB may be a requirement for publication of the results.

## Professional Groups

Some professional groups or national health organizations may be willing to conduct research reviews in the absence of an IRB or when an investigator is conducting research independent of a sponsoring body. In any case, the guarantee of protection of human subjects from undue risks is a joint responsibility of the investigator and the data collection site. Failure to comply with federal regulations regarding the protection of human subjects from research risks can result in withdrawal of current federal funding and loss of eligibility for future federal funding (NIH, 1991).

### Guidelines for Review

IRBs usually have a set of guidelines or principles that govern their procedures and reviews. Institutions that receive federal funding must follow federal code 45 CFR 46. This code of federal regulations can be obtained at http://www.hhs.gov/ohrp/humansubjects/guidance/45cfr46.htm.

Some small IRBs may use the principles set forth in the Belmont report, which can be accessed at http://ohsr.od.nih.gov/guidelines/belmont.html. International review committees tend to use principles from the World Medical Association in the Declaration of Helsinki, found at http://www.wma.net/e/policy/b3.htm.

Federal code stipulates the composition of the IRB (U.S. Department of Health and Human Services, 2005). An IRB must consist of a minimum of five members with varying backgrounds to ensure a complete and adequate review of the research activities commonly conducted by the institution. Furthermore, by regulation, an IRB may not consist entirely of members of one profession, gender, or racial group. Collectively, the IRB must be sufficiently qualified through the experience and expertise of its membership, the diversity of their personal backgrounds (e.g., sex, race and cultural heritage), and members' knowledge of and sensitivity to prevailing community attitudes (Office for Protection from Research Risks, 1993, pp. 1–3). If the particular IRB routinely reviews research involving vulnerable subjects, then the composition of the board must include individuals knowledgeable about and experienced with such vulnerable populations. Also, the IRB must include at least one member whose primary concerns are in nonscientific areas and one who is not otherwise affiliated with the institution or a family member of one who is. One of the members should be able to discuss issues emanating from the perspective of the community and its values. Last, an IRB may invite additional individuals with special areas of expertise to participate in the review and discussion of research proposals to enable the IRB to fulfill its purpose. These individuals, however, are not able to vote on the disposition of the proposed research.

## Jurisdiction of an IRB

The jurisdiction of an IRB is determined by answering two fundamental questions: "Is the activity research?" and "Does the activity involve human subjects?" For health care professionals, the first question may not be so easily answered because the distinction between research and therapy is not always readily apparent. Federal policy defines research as "a systematic investigation, including research development, testing, and evaluation designed to develop or contribute to generalized knowledge." (U.S. Department of Health and Human Services, 2005, 45 cfr 46.102[d]). Furthermore, research itself is not inherently therapeutic in that the therapeutic benefits of experimental interventions are unknown or may prove to be ineffective (Office for Protection from Research Risks, 1993, pp. 1–3). If the focus of the proposed activity is currently accepted and standardized methods of care or if the research addresses institutional or patient-specific case issues, then the activity is generally not considered research and consequently does not require IRB reporting and review. However, if there is any uncertainty as to whether the activity is research, the activity should be treated as research and reported to the IRB. An activity is research if the answers to the following two questions are "yes": if the answer to *either* question is "no," then the activity is not research. The two questions are: Does the activity employ a systematic approach involving predetermined methods for studying a specific topic, answering a specific question, testing a specific hypothesis, or developing a theory? and is the activity intended to contribute to generalizable knowledge by extending the results (e.g., publication of presentation) beyond a single individual or an internal unit? (45 CFR 46.102(d)).

There is one caveat. It is a common, although not universal, standard within the health care community that even though an activity may not be "research," if the activity is to be disseminated (i.e., reported in a publication or presentation), the general practice is to consider the activity research and to report it to the IRB. An activity that causes great confusion as to whether or not it constitutes research is continuous quality improvement. Quality improvement is considered an essential component of responsible professional health care (Cretin et al., 2000) and a means for improving the processes, efficiencies, safety, and quality of care while preventing substandard care (Bellin & Dubler, 2001; Casaret, Karlawish, & Sugarman, 2000; Johnson, Vermeulen, & Smith, 2006). However, quality improvement activities frequently consist of methods traditionally associated with randomized clinical trials, blurring the distinction between quality improvement activities and research (Johnson et al., 2006). As a result, it is not always easy to determine whether the activity is research, warranting review by the IRB, or quality improvement and therefore exempt from review. This issue prompts some observers to suggest that all activities should be reviewed by the IRB to ensure that the activity, be it research or quality improvement, does not compromise patient autonomy or safety (Bellin & Dubler, 2001; Miller & Emanuel, 2008). Those who advocate the review of all activities contend that if this were the practice, once the activity receives IRB approval, it is sanctioned, thereby assuring the public and health care community that the activity complies with commonly accepted ethical practices and involves a consequent minimal level of risks for all participating parties, that is, the human subjects, investigators, and institution. However, the majority of the heath care community believe that review of all activities would stall the research enterprise and have instead proposed criteria (e.g., Casaret et al., 2000; Johnson et al., 2006) by which to determine whether an activity warrants review by the IRB. According to Johnson et al. (2006), if any of the following apply to the activity, it should be considered research and submitted to the IRB for review:

- Results are to be disseminated.
- Results contribute to generalized knowledge.
- Conditions are systematically assigned to patients.

- Conditions are other than a standard of care.
- Risks of participation exceed those of usual care.
- Information collected goes beyond routine patient care.
- Personal health information will be sent outside institution.
- Risks to privacy and confidentiality exist.

Only if all of these points do not apply should the activity be considered quality improvement.

Once the activity has been deemed research, the investigator should ask whether the research activity involves human subjects, and, if so, whether the activity falls within the jurisdiction of the IRB. This question must be answered "yes" if the activity consists of any systematic collection of data about human beings, including data obtained from surveys and observations, as well as from any human tissues, including embryonic or cadaveric tissues. A human subject is a living individual about whom an investigator obtains data through intervention or interaction or identifiable private information (45 CFR 46.102(f)). For example, an investigator whose research activities involves accessing health records of only patients who have died is not conducting research with human subjects.

## Levels of Review

Once it has been established that the activity falls within the jurisdiction of the IRB, the level of IRB reporting and review must be identified. There are three levels of review, determined on the basis of the degree of risk inherent in the proposed research. Risk is defined by federal policy as "the probability of harm or injury (physical, psychological, social, or economic) occurring as a result of participation in research. Both the probability and magnitude of risk can vary from minimal to significant" (Office for Protection from Research Risks, 1993, pp. 1–3). The three levels of review are exempt, expedited, and full. It is important to determine which level of review is required because, typically, the extent of information required, the forms to be completed, and the time necessary for the review are determined by the type of review. Any questions about the level of review or the submission process generally can be discussed with the chair of the IRB. When a proposed research activity does not clearly fall into a distinct level of review, submission of materials for the next higher level of review is prudent and expeditious. The IRB can determine the risk level and may assign the activity a lower risk than the level at which it was initially submitted.

### Exempt From Review

Research activities that are *exempt* from review by the IRB are those that pose no risks to subjects, have no means by which a subject can be identified, and use human subjects who are capable of freely consenting to participate (Office for Protection from Research Risks, 1993). Even though a research activity falls into the exempt category, it still must be submitted to the IRB for affirmation. Examples of activities that are exempt from review are listed in Exhibit 20.1.

Copies of surveys, interview guides, or questionnaires and the exact introductory remarks and consent forms to be used must be submitted. If advertisements for subjects are used, copies of the text for the planned advertisement must also be submitted. Although these materials are not formally reviewed, a member of the IRB will assess the materials to verify that the activity meets the stipulations for an exemption. This verification generally requires a few days (but may take a few weeks), after which the investigator receives a document from the IRB indicating the exact criteria used to judge whether the activity does or does not meet the requirements for an exemption. If the initial assessment determines that the activity does not fulfill the requirements for an exemption, the investigator may be asked to submit an additional justification or the appropriate materials for an expedited review.

### Expedited Review

There are three types of activities that may receive an expedited review:

1  Activities that pose no more than minimal risk to subjects for participation in the activity. Minimal risk is defined as "a risk where the probability and magnitude of harm or discomfort in the proposed research are not greater, in and of themselves, than those ordinarily encountered in daily life or during the performance of routine physical or psychological examinations or tests" (U.S. Department of Health and Human Services, 2005, 45 cfr 46.102[i]). If the risks are greater than minimal and if precautions, safeguards, or alternatives cannot be incorporated into the research activity to minimize the risks to such a level, then a full review is required.

2  Activities in which subjects are capable of providing consent to participate. If subjects are unable to freely choose whether to participate in the activity (e.g., cognitively impaired individuals or comatose patients), are particularly vulnerable subjects (e.g.,

Exhibit 20.1

## RESEARCH ACTIVITIES EXEMPT FROM 45 CFR 46

Research in which the involvement of human subjects will be in one or more of the following categories is exempt from coverage under this Assurance:

- Research conducted in established or commonly accepted educational settings, involving normal educational practices such as (1) research on regular and special educational instructional strategies, or (2) research on the effectiveness of or the comparison among instructional techniques, curricula, or classroom management methods.
- Research involving the use of educational tests (cognitive, diagnostic, aptitude, achievement), survey procedures, interview procedures or observation of public behavior, unless (1) information obtained is recorded in such a manner that human subjects can be identified directly or though identifiers linked to the subjects, and (2) any disclosure of the human subjects' responses outside the research could reasonably place the subjects at risk of criminal or civil liability or be damaging to the subjects' financial standing, employability, or reputation.
- Research involving the use of educational tests (cognitive, diagnostic, aptitude, achievement), survey procedures, interview procedures, or observation of public behavior that is not exempt above, if (1) the human subjects are elected or appointed officials or candidates for public office, or (2) federal statute(s) require(s) without exception that the confidentiality of the personally indefinable information will be maintained throughout the research and thereafter.
- Research, involving the collection or study of existing data, documents, records, pathological specimens, or diagnostic specimens, if these sources are publicly available or if the information is recorded by the investigator in such a manner that subjects cannot be identified, directly or through identifiers linked to the subjects.
- Research and demonstration projects that are conducted by or subject to the approval of department or agency heads and that are designed to study, evaluate, or otherwise examine (1) public benefit or service programs, (2) procedures for obtaining benefits or services under those programs, (3) possible changes in or alternatives to those programs or procedures, or (4) possible changes in methods or levels of payment or services under those programs.
- Taste and food evaluation and consumer acceptance studies (1) if wholesome foods without additives are consumed, or (2) if a food is consumed that contains a food ingredient at or below the level and for a use found to be safe or agricultural chemical or environmental contaminant at or below the level found to be safe by the Food and Drug Administration or approved by the Environmental Protection Agency or the Food Safety and Inspection Services of the U.S Dept. of Agriculture.

Adapted from *Protection of Human Subjects,* by U.S. Department of Health and Human Services, 2005, Title 45, Code of Federal Regulations, part 46.101 revised June 23, 2005. Washington, DC: Office of Protection from Research Risks. Retrieved April 8, 2008, from http://www.hhs.gov/ohrp/humansubjects/guidance/45cfr46.htm

children, and minors), prisoners, pregnant women, mentally disabled persons, or economically or educationally disadvantaged persons, a full review by the IRB is required.

**3** Activities requiring minor changes in previously approved research during the period for which approval is authorized (1 year or less) (U.S. Department of Health and Human Services, 2005, 45 cfr 46.110[b]).

Activities that are considered within the exempt category but that provide a means by which individual subjects can be identified must be reviewed at the expedited level because of the potential risk resulting from loss of anonymity and confidentiality. Materials required for an expedited review generally consist of an abbreviated research protocol that presents the objectives, methods, subject selection criteria, theoretical or potential risks and benefits, precautions and safeguards, and a sample informed consent. An expedited review typically requires a couple of weeks. The proposal may be reviewed by a member of the IRB.

As with all levels of review, the investigator receives a document from the IRB, indicating the exact criteria used to determine that the activity fulfills the requirements for an expedited review. If the initial assessment determines that the activity does not fulfill the requirements, the investigator may be asked for additional justification or to submit the appropriate materials for a full review. Federal policy requires that all members of the IRB be advised of all proposals that have been approved under the expedited review process U.S. Department of Health and Human Services, 2005, 45 cfr 46.110[c]).

**Full Review**

A full review of any proposed research activity involving human subjects must occur in all other situations, such as those in which participation in the activity poses greater than minimal risk; those for which a subject, for whatever reason, cannot freely consent and those involving vulnerable populations as subjects. Materials required for a full review are identical to those required for an expedited review; it is the review process that differs. A full review typically requires at least 1 month from the submission of materials to the notification of the disposition of the proposal. The proposal is reviewed by at least three members of the IRB. (A member cannot participate in the discussion and determination of disposition of a project in which the member is an investigator. In such cases, the investigator member must be absent from the discussion, and this absence must be reflected in the minutes of the meeting.)

The review of the proposed research activity, which is to focus on the aspects listed in Exhibit 20.2 and Exhibit 20.3, must occur at a convened meeting at which a majority of the members of the IRB are present. The impartial review conducted by the IRB typically focuses on the mechanisms within the proposed research by which the subjects are safeguarded or protected from any undue risks of participation, and the process and content of the informed consent, that is, the ethics of the research. However, scrutiny of the research methodology also falls within the purview of the IRB because research that is so poorly designed as to be invalid exposes the subjects, the investigator, and the institution to unnecessary risks. So, although a proposal may be deemed to be ethically sound, if it is methodologically unsound, the IRB must disapprove the application. For proposed research to be approved, it must receive the approval of a majority of those members present at the meeting (U.S. Department of Health and Human Services, 2005, 45 cfr 46.108[b]).

A research proposal must receive approval from the IRB before the collection of data can be initiated. Once permission has been granted by

Exhibit 20.2

**CRITERIA FOR APPROVAL OF RESEARCH PROPOSALS**

All of the following requirements must be satisfied to be approved:

1. Risks to subjects are minimized.
2. Risks to subjects are reasonable relative to anticipated benefits.
3. Selection of subjects is equitable.
4. Informed consent is sought as required.
5. Informed consent is documented.
6. There is adequate provision for the monitoring of data collected to ensure the safety of subjects.
7. There are adequate provisions to protect the privacy of subjects to maintain confidentiality.
8. If any subject is vulnerable to coercion, additional safeguards are included to protect their rights and welfare.

Adapted from *Protection of Human Subjects,* by U.S. Department of Health and Human Services, 2005, Title 45, Code of Federal Regulations, part 46.111 revised June 23, 2005. Washington, DC: Office of Protection from Research Risks. Retrieved April 8, 2008, from http://www.hhs.gov/ohrp/humansubjects/guidance/45cfr46.htm

Exhibit 20.3

## BASIC INSTITUTIONAL REVIEW BOARD REVIEW

In the review of research proposals, the members of the IRB must:

- Identify the risks associated with participation in the research.
- Determine that the risks will be minimized to the extent possible.
- Identify the probable benefits to be derived form the research.
- Determine that the risks are reasonable in relation to the benefits to the subjects and the importance of the knowledge to be gained.
- Ensure that potential subjects will be adequately informed as to the risks or discomforts and anticipated benefits.
- Determine the intervals for periodic review.
- Determine the adequacy of the provisions to protect privacy and maintain confidentiality of the data.
- In the case of vulnerable population, determine that appropriate additional safeguards are in place to protect their rights and welfare.

the IRB, the researcher is obligated to conduct the study as proposed. If it becomes necessary to alter the study in any way, the researcher must report those alterations to the IRB for review and approval before implementing the changes. The IRB also must be notified if any unforeseen problems arise during the conduct of the study. Although investigators are required to provide a progress report on at least an annual basis (see Exhibit 20.4), any changes in procedure, risks, or unforeseen problems should be reported to the IRB immediately. For example, if an investigator wants to enroll more subjects than originally requested, this step needs to be approved in advance. Similarly, any changes in the methods of recruitment or changes in questionnaires must receive IRB approval. The individual study participants from whom data that are collected should not be identifiable. This can be achieved by protecting health information. (See Table 20.1).

The process of providing informed consent is not a distinct moment in time at which the subject simply signs a form; it is an ongoing educational process between the investigator and subject, and it reflects the basic principle of respect for persons. Consequently, informed, voluntary participation of the subject should be verified at every interaction between the investigator or a representative of the research team and the subject. Because of the nature and complexity of some studies (e.g., longitudinal, multiphase studies), informed consent may be required for the various phases of the study.

Exhibit 20.4

### ELEMENTS OF A PERIODIC REVIEW

Periodic reviews of research should include:

- Any amendment to the currently approved research (e.g., the addition of research personnel, or a change in funding, research protocol, consent documents, HIPAA authorization, or any other change to the research)
- Preliminary results, especially those that might suggest one intervention is better or worse than the other with respect to risks, benefits, alternatives, or willingness to participate
- Subject enrollment and demographics
- Information about any subject complaints, refusals or withdrawals from participation, and safety
- Reportable events (e.g., study-related adverse events) and protocol violations
- Review by other IRBs
- Suspension of research activity
- Presentations and publications
- Conflicts of interest

*Note:* Periodic reviews are mandatory for all ongoing studies, the intervals between the re-evaluations are to be appropriate to the degree of risk but are to take place not less than once a year (IRB guidebook).

Although some IRBs require the use of a standardized format for consent procedures, modifications are usually permitted as long as the process provides for full disclosure, adequate comprehension, and voluntary choice—elements easy to enumerate but not so easy to achieve (see Exhibit 20.5) (U.S. Department of Health and Human Services, 2005).

Usually any element may be omitted that is not relevant to the study; however, a statement that the subject understands what will occur as a result of his or her participation in the study and affirming that the subject freely agrees to participate must be included at the end of the form, followed by a place for the subject's and witness' signatures and date (see Exhibit 20.6). When a parent or guardian signs for a subject, the subject's name should be clearly identified, as should the signatory's relationship to the subject. If the research is complex or poses a significant risk, the IRB may encourage the investigator to develop a "patient information sheet" that presents the information from the formal consent form in simple, unambiguous language that is devoid of all "legalese." In other instances, audiotaped verbal consents may be acceptable, for example, with interviews. With questionnaire or survey research, it is commonly

Table 20.1

## PROTECTED HEALTH INFORMATION

1. Names
2. Any geographic subdivision smaller than a state (including street names, city, county, precinct, ZIP code)
3. Any element of dates directly related to an individual (e.g., birth date, admission date, date of death)
4. Telephone numbers
5. Facsimile numbers
6. Electronic mail addresses
7. Social security numbers
8. Medical record numbers
9. Health plan beneficiary numbers
10. Account numbers
11. Certificate/license numbers
12. Vehicle identifiers
13. Devise identifiers
14. Web universal resource locators (URLs)
15. Internet protocol (IP) address numbers
16. Biometric identifiers (e.g., fingerprints and voiceprints)
17. Full-face photographic images
18. Any other unique identifying number, characteristic, or code

Adapted from *Protecting Personal Health Information in Research: Understanding the HIPAA Privacy Rule,* by U.S. Department of Health and Human Services. Revised July 13, 2004. Retrieved April 8, 2008, from http://privacyruleandresearch.nih.gov

assumed that the return of a completed questionnaire implies consent. However, in any of these situations, the investigator is obligated to fully disclose the nature and extent of the subject's participation in such a way that the subject can understand and freely decide whether to participate. Guidelines for developing a consent form as well as sample consents can usually be obtained from the IRB.

In providing the information for consent, the investigator may want to consider using such devices as audiovisual aids, tests of the information provided, or consent advisers to verify that each potential subject understands the nature of the research (Office for Protection from Research Risks, 1993). Each oral presentation of the information for consent must be witnessed by a third person, who must sign both the consent form and, if used, a copy of the written summary of the presentation (also known as the patient information sheet). Copies of each are given to the subject, and the investigator should retain the originals for at least 5 years.

Exhibit 20.5

### GENERAL REQUIREMENTS FOR INFORMED CONSENT

In seeking informed consent, the following information is to be provided to each subject:

1. A statement that the activity is research, including an explanation of the purpose, expected duration, and procedures, especially if procedures are experimental
2. A description of all reasonably foreseeable risks or discomforts associated with the research
3. A description of all reasonably expected benefits to the subjects from participating in the research
4. Disclosure of appropriate alternative procedures
5. A description of how confidentiality of records is to be maintained.
6. If research is greater than minimal risk, a description of compensation for participation and what is to occur in the occurrence of injury from participation
7. An explanation with contact information for persons who can provide additional information about (a) the research, (b) the rights of subjects, and (c) research-related injury
8. A statement that participation is voluntary and that refusal has no consequent penalties or loss of benefits to which the subject is otherwise entitled
9. Additional elements when appropriate:
   a. Acknowledgment if procedure may involve currently unforeseeable risks to subject, embryo, or fetus if subject becomes pregnant.
   b. Circumstances under which the subject's participation may be terminated by the investigator without regard to the subject's consent
   c. Additional costs resulting form the subject's participation in the research
   d. Consequences of withdrawal and procedures for orderly termination of participation by the subject
   e. The approximate number of subjects involved in the research
   f. Provision of new information that may influence the subject's willingness to continue to participate

Adapted from *Protection of Human Subjects,* by U.S. Department of Health and Human Services, 2005, Title 45, Code of Federal Regulations, part 46.116 revised June 23, 2005. Washington, DC: Office of Protection from Research Risks. Retrieved April 8, 2008, from http://www.hhs.gov/ohrp/humansubjects/guidance/45cfr46.htm

Few circumstances allow for the waiver of consent. Situations in which waivers may be approved include the following: (a) the research involves no more than minimal risk to subjects; (b) the waiver or alteration will not adversely affect the rights and welfare of subjects; (c) the research could not practically be carried out without the waiver or

Exhibit 20.6

## A SAMPLE CONSENT FORM

You are being asked to be a subject in research under the direction of Dr._____, a professor in the College of Nursing at the University of _____. Many older patients get confused while in the hospital. This confusion can affect their recovery from illness. Although you are not now confused, confusion may occur while you are in the hospital. You are being told about this research and may be able to take part because of your current illness and hospitalization. Before you agree to be in this research, please read this form. Your participation is completely voluntary. Your decision will not affect your relations with the university, your physicians, or the hospital staff or your care. If you decide to participate, you are free to quit at any time.

The purpose of the research is to study the effects of confusion on the health of older patients who are in the hospital. Approximately 720 patients may take part in this research. We are interested in looking at the effects of confusion on bathing and eating; memory and thinking; the use of health care services; and the severity, length, and return of any confusion.

If you agree to take part, I, or another member of the research team, will visit you daily while you are in the hospital to ask you questions about your thinking and your ability to perform daily activities. The first interview will last about 20 minutes. All other daily visits will last about 10 minutes. These visits will be scheduled at a time that is convenient for you and your care. Each day, we would like to review your hospital record to obtain information about your care, medications, and any tests and their results. We would also like your permission to talk with a relative, friend, or caregiver about your recent illness. When you leave the hospital, we would like to get a copy of your hospital bill.

The risks of being in this research include possible inconvenience of interviews and possible breach of privacy and confidentiality.

There is no direct benefit to you. This research will not help in your current care or treatment. We hope that what we learn from this research will help to improve the care to patients like you in the future.

If you decide to take part, we will be careful to keep all information about you strictly confidential. Only members of the research team will have access to this information. All information about you will be kept under lock and key in the research office of Dr. _____. When results are published or discussed, no information will reveal your identity.

There is no payment for your participation.

You may ask questions now. If you have questions later, you may contact Dr. ____ _____ at XXX.XXX.XXXX or by e-mail at _____

If you have questions about your rights as a research subject, you can call the Office for Protection of Research Subjects at the University of Illinois at Chicago at XXX.XXX.XXXX.

*(Continued)*

Exhibit 20.6

**A SAMPLE CONSENT FORM (CONTINUED)**

Your participation in this research is entirely voluntary. Your decision will not affect your care. You can refuse to answer any question or stop answering altogether. You can quit the research at any time without any consequences of any kind. You will be given a copy of this form for your information and to keep for your records.

I have read (or someone else has read to me) the above information. I have been given a chance to ask questions, and my questions have been answered to my satisfaction. I have been given a copy of this form.

Signature of the Subject


Signature of Researcher Date

alteration; and (d) whenever appropriate, the subjects will be provided with additional pertinent information after they have participated (U.S. Department of Health and Human Services, 2005, 45 cfr 46.116[d]). An example of a situation in which a waiver of consent is granted is a study that uses only data that have been previously collected for nonresearch purposes, such as the medical record. The investigator must demonstrate that it would not be practicable to go back and obtain consent from the individuals whose records are to be used. It may be the case that a large number of individuals cannot not be reached because their contact information has changed, because the patients are no longer affiliated with the medical center, or because they are deceased.

For individuals experiencing health emergencies, there is a provision by the Federal Drug Administration (FDA) and the Department of Health and Human Services (DHHS) that allows emergency research to proceed without voluntary prospective informed consent by the patient (21 CFR 50.24). However, these health emergencies must render the patient incapable of providing informed consent. Examples of such health emergencies include patients who are experiencing life-threatening illnesses or trauma and those requiring resuscitation in which research is clearly necessary to identify safe and effective therapies (Sugarman,

2007). These health emergencies may occur out-of-hospital or in the emergency department or intensive-care unit. According to 21 CFR 50.24, "Exception from informed consent requirements for emergency research" (FDA, 2007), the potential subject must be in a life-threatening situation and current treatments must be either unproven or unsatisfactory. Obtaining informed consent is not feasible, because the subject in unable to consent as a result of the health emergency, a surrogate is not readily available, and there is a limited window of opportunity to intervene. Participation may provide direct benefit to the subject, and the project must have been prospectively reviewed and approved with waiver of consent by an IRB. Additional protections of the rights and welfare of the subjects also must be ensured; for example, either the patient or their surrogate must provide informed consent as soon as is practicable (21 CFR 50.224).

However, research in which participation does not hold the potential for "therapeutic benefit" continues to require informed consent of either the patient or a legal surrogate (Chen, Meschia, Brott, Brown, & Worral, for the SWISS investigators, 2008).

At the end of the study as approved by the IRB, the researcher may need to complete a form telling the IRB how many subjects were taken in, any adverse events that occurred, when the data collection ended, and when the study will conclude with IRB supervision. The de-identification of the data may be considered the last step in reporting required by the IRB.

## SUMMARY

Obtaining ethical review and approval of a study is an essential preliminary step for conducting research. It can consume large amounts of time and provide numerous opportunities for success or failure. The recommendations offered are intended to facilitate development of a partnership in pursuing knowledge that results in a positive research experience for all, as well as the successful completion of the research.

## SUGGESTED ACTIVITIES

Persons who sustain a mild brain injury (MTBI) have been reported to experience difficulties with memory. It has been reported in the literature that using a handheld personal digital assistant (PDA) might help persons with MTBI with their memory. On the basis of your review of the literature, you decided to recruit participants for a study. Participants will be randomly assigned to times when they are scheduled to call a research voicemail. A two-week predetermined call schedule will be assigned to each participant; half of the participants will use a PDA as a reminder, and half will not.

Before conducting the study, you are required to obtain IRB approval.

1    Acquire and complete the IRB forms at your institution.
2    Write an informed consent for potential participants to complete.
3    Write a script that will be used when recruiting a participant.

## REFERENCES

Bellin, E., & Dubler, N. N. (2001). The quality improvement—research divide and the need for external oversight. *American Journal of Public Health, 91*(9), 1512–1517.

Casarett, D., Karlawish, J. H. T., & Sugarman, J. (2000). Determining when quality improvement initiatives should be considered research. Proposed criteria and potential implications. *Journal of the American Medical Association, 283*(17), 2275–2280.

Chen, D. T., Meschia, J. F., Brott, T. G., Brown, R. D., & Worrall, B. B., for the SWISS investigators. (2008). Stroke genetic research with adults with impaired decision-making capacity. A survey of IRB and investigator practices. *Stroke, 39,* 2732–2735.

Cleary, M., & Freeman, A. (2005). Facilitating research within clinical settings: The development of a beginner's guide. *International Journal of Mental Health Nursing, 14,* 202–208.

Cretin, S., Keeler, E. B., Lynn, J., Batalden, P. B., Berwick, D. M., & Bisognano, M. (2000). Should patients in quality-improvement activities have the same protections as participants in research studies? [letter] *Journal of the American Medical Association, 284*(14), 1786.

Hodgman, E.C. (1978). Student research in service agencies. *Nursing Outlook, 26,* 558.

Johnson, M. S., Gonzales, M. N., & Bizila, S. (2005). Responsible conduct of radiology research. Part V. The health insurance portability and accountability act and research. *Radiology, 237*(3), 757–764.

Johnson, N., Vermeulen, L., & Smith, K. M. (2006). A survey of academic medical centers to distinguish quality improvement and research activities. *Quality Management and Health Care, 15*(4), 215–220.

Kirchhoff, K. T., & McGuire, D. B. (1985). The nursing review process in a clinical setting. *Journal of Professional Nursing, 1,* 311.

Larson, E., Bratts, T., Zwanziger, J., & Stone, P. (2004). A survey of IRB process in 68 U.S. hospitals. *Journal of Nursing Scholarship, 36*(3), 260–264.

Miller, F. G., & Emanuel, E. J. (2008). Quality-improvement research and informed consent. *New England Journal of Medicine, 358*(8), 765–767.

Ness, R. B. for the Joint Policy Committee, Societies of Epidemiology. (2007). Influence of the HIPAA privacy rule on health research. *Journal of the American Medical Association, 298*(18), 2164–2170.

Office for Human Subjects Protection. (1993). *Institutional review board: Guidebook.* Retrieved April 8, 2008, from http://www.hhs.gov/ohrp/irb/irb_guidebook.htm

Office for Protection from Research Risks. (1993). *National Institutes of Health: Protecting human research subjects: Institutional review board guidebook.* Washington, DC: U.S. Government Printing Office. Retrieved April 8, 2008, from http://www.hhs.gov/ohrp/irb/irb_guidebook.htm

Sugarman, J. (2007). Examining the provisions for research without consent in the emergency setting. *Hastings Center Report, 37(1),* 12–13.

U.S. Department of Health and Human Services. (2004). *Protecting personal health information in research: Understanding the HIPAA privacy rule.* Revised July 13, 2004. Retrieved April 8, 2008, from http://privacyruleandresearch.nih.gov

U.S. Department of Health and Human Services. (2005). Protection of human subjects: Title 45, Code of Federal Regulations, part 46, revised June 23, 2005. Washington, DC: Office of Protection from Research Risks. Retrieved April 8, 2008, from http://www.hhs.gov/ohrp/humansubjects/guidance/45cfr46.htm

U.S. Food and Drug Administration. (2007). Exception from informed consent requirements for emergency research. 21 CFR 50.24. Retrieved April 8, 2008, from http://www.accessdata.fda.gov/scripts/cdrh/cfdocs/CFRSearch.cfm?FR = 0.24

Williams, M. A. (1989). Research and the acute care setting (Editorial). *Research in Nursing & Health, 12*(1), iii.

# WEB RESOURCES

## General Resources

Department of Veterans Affairs, Protection of Human Subjects: http://www.access.gpo/gov/nara/cfr/waisdx_98/38cfr16_98.html

FDA guidelines: http://www.cfsan.fda.gov/~lrd/cfr50.html

IRB Guidebook: http://www.hhs.gov/ohrp/irb/irb_guidebook.htm

Office for Human Subjects Protection: http://www.hhs.gov/ohrp/

Protection of Human Subjects: http://www.hhs.gov/ohrp/humansubjects/guidance/45cfr46.htm

U.S. Food and Drug Administration: http://www.accessdata.fda.gov/scripts/cdrh/cfdocs/CFRSearch.cfm?FR = 0.24

## For information about the registration of clinical trials

"Is this clinical trial fully registered?": http://www.icmje.org/clin_trialup.htm

NIH Office of Extramural Research, "Guidance on new law (Public Law 110–85): http://grants.nih.gov/grants/guide/notice-files/NOT-OD-08-014.html

"Registration at ClinicalTrials.gov as required by Public Law 110–85, Title VII: http://prsinfo.clinicaltrials.gov/s801-fact-sheet.pdf

## For online ethics training

Collaborative Institutional Training Initiative: http://www.citiprogram.org

# 21 Communicating Research Through Oral Presentations

SUZANNE P. SMITH AND MAGDALENA A. MATEO

Communicating information about a completed study or a study in progress is a vital aspect of evidence-based practice. Advance practice nurses (APNs) have numerous ways for sharing information on studies, such as oral presentations made in a clinical unit or at an event sponsored by an organization, at conferences through paper or poster sessions, via the Internet, and through the media. The heightened interest of the media in topics related to health is shown by the increased presence of reporters at scientific conferences. The availability of technology such as podcasting, broadcasting, and blogging has led to the expedited dissemination of information, allowing it to reach a large and varied audience.

## PREPARING THE PRESENTATION

After a study has been implemented, the researcher must identify opportunities for presentations at research or clinical conferences. Sponsors of a conference solicit presenters by announcing a call for papers or abstracts. Review the conference focus to determine whether your study fits the focus of the conference. If your topic is congruent with the conference objectives and the specialty group that is most likely to attend the conference, carefully review the detailed requirements for submitting an abstract (e.g., online submission).

Abstracts of completed research are reviewed for oral or poster presentations, whereas ongoing research is considered only for a poster session. The abstract, usually ranging from 200 to 500 words in length depending on the organization, is used by reviewers to determine the worthiness of a study, making it vital that the researcher follow submission guidelines. Most guidelines for research abstracts require a summary of the major aspects of the study (Starver & Shellenbarger, 2004), including:

1   Title—key variables, participants, setting
2   Purpose of the study
3   Brief description of sample—number of subjects, distinct characteristics such as diagnosis, age range, and gender
4   Methods—design of the study, setting, procedure for collecting data, instruments (including reliability and validity)
5   Findings—data and significant statistical (level of significance) or clinical differences
6   Conclusions—summary of the results in relation to the purpose of the study and meaning of the data

In addition to major aspects of a study, an organization may require a brief author biography and bibliography. The American Association of Neuroscience Nursing publishes the required information at http://www.aann.org. Criteria often used to evaluate abstracts are originality, scientific merit, clinical relevance, soundness of findings, overall quality, and relevance to conference theme and objectives. Organizations sponsoring research conferences publish information in their call of abstracts, which can be accessed through their Web site. For example, one can access information from the Eastern Nursing Research Society, whose Web site is at http://www.enrs-go.org. It is important to keep these criteria in mind when writing the abstract in order to increase the likelihood that your research will be accepted for presentation.

Presentation of research-related activities may be included in scientific conferences. The format of an abstract meant for clinical presentations includes:

1   Why? Relevance, importance of topic
2   Where? Setting, clients (specific needs)

**3**  How? Overview of initiative, preparation, issues, challenges and strategies in achieving goals of a program
**4**  What? Observed outcomes
**5**  What now? Structured evaluation findings; implications for practice; lessons learned (Happell, 2007)

Acceptance of an abstract for paper or poster presentation triggers the need to start preparing for a successful event. The letter of acceptance usually includes presentation guidelines. Although different organizations' guidelines vary, most paper presentations are scheduled for a total of 20 minutes, with 15 minutes for content delivery and 5 minutes for questions. Poster presentations may occur over several days, with the presenter expected to be at the poster at designated times to interact with conference participants.

Things to keep in mind when developing a paper presentation include the target audience (researchers, clinicians, lay people); the setting (size of the room and seating arrangement); and the time allotted. Adapt the language to match the audience's level of sophistication and expertise; for example, use research language if the audience is composed primarily of researchers.

## Identifying the Content

Develop a detailed outline to serve as a roadmap when you write your script to practice the presentation. Include the segments that were included in the abstract you submitted. An important aspect of your preparation is determining the audiovisual aids you will use; for example, will you use slides and distribute handouts?

## Developing Slides

The purpose of slides is to enhance the presentation of your content. As you develop your presentation, determine the types and number of slides that you will use—word or pictorial or a combination. There are numerous computer software programs (e.g., Harvard Graphics, PowerPoint, and Presentation) that can be used for making slides. PowerPoint is the most commonly used software at conferences. Several Web sites are available to develop you slides for effective presentations (http://www.iasted.org/conferences/formatting/Presentations-Tips. ppt#256,1, Making PowerPoint Slides; http://www.skagitwatershed.org/~donclark/leader/leadpres.html).

Developing digital slides on a computer allows for easy previewing and re-ordering if necessary. You can also preview color combinations before producing the slide. Using contrasting colors is vital for readability; for example, words set in light pink against a light blue background are difficult to read. There are several other considerations when developing slides: (1) use a consistent simple template; (2) pick a font such as Arial or Sanserif, and use a font size of 40 to 44 for main headings and between 28 and 32 for text; (3) use the 5-7-7 rule: 5 words in title, 7 words per line, and 7 lines per slide, and left-justify the text; (4) when using graphs, orient the audience to essential aspects of the graph (Hardicre, Coad, & Devitt, 2007; Shepherd, 2006; Vollman, 2005).

Using a computer for a slide presentation saves money because it eliminates the need to physically produce a large number of slides. If your slide presentation is saved to a disk to be used on another computer, make sure your slide program is compatible with the host computer system. You may need to save more than one version of the file to be safe. Always bring a flash drive with a copy of your slide presentation to the presentation. In addition, always bring a print copy of your slide files; this ensures that you can give your presentation effectively in the event of a technological or electric power malfunction. If at all possible, preview your slides using the equipment available during the presentation, and practice delivering your presentation.

## Using Strategies for Public Speaking

Despite the anxiety most people feel when speaking publicly, the experience can be rewarding and exciting. Public speaking, like any skill, requires learning and practice (Engelhart, 2004). There are several Web sites that give a good overview of presentation skills. In addition to a discussion of the skills essential to developing presentation aids and delivering oral and poster presentation, tutorials are available at the following sites:

- http://www.skagitwatershed.org/~donclark/leader/leadpres.html,
- http://www.kumc.edu/SAH/OTEd/jradel/effective.html,
- http://www.aresearchguide.com/3tips.html,
- http://presentationsoft.about.com/od/powerpointtips/qt/planningppt.htm.

Nurses have much to say that will positively impact health care delivery. Public speaking by nurses will surely increase in the coming years. This may occur secondary to the vast amount of research that is currently under way in clinical and administrative practice. Another factor that will contribute to nurses' mandate to present research publicly is the move to community health, wellness, and prevention models of care. While nurses have always played important roles in teaching self-care to patients, the demand for such instruction is increasing in a pay-for-performance environment. It is necessary that nurses engage in research and seek appropriate opportunities to present their findings publicly.

There are many strategies that you can use to help make this experience exciting and worthwhile (Barton, Reichow, & Wolery, 2007; McConnell, 2002):

- Know your audience. Speak their language and present your material in a way that is meaningful to them.
- Organize your thoughts.
- Use audiovisual aids.
- Use charts and graphs. Research findings can often best be displayed with the use of tables, charts, graphs, and figures. These tools help you better organize your findings for the audience.
- Speak to the audience, and maintain eye contact.
- Rehearse your presentation and time it so that you can fit the schedule.
- Dress appropriately. If you are doing a presentation during working hours or on site at your organization, work clothes may be appropriate. If you are presenting off site, business clothing is the appropriate attire.
- Elicit audience participation by asking questions or presenting a concept, idea, or finding and then asking, "What does this mean to you" or "What do you think about this study result?"
- Vary your tone of voice.
- Provide time for questions, and always repeat the question. The nature of research stimulates inquiry, so people will likely have questions; plan to leave time for the audience to ask questions.
- Use tact in responding to criticism to your research, and keep an open mind.
- Recognize people who have made significant contributions to the research.
- Thank the audience, and let them know where you may be reached by phone or provide an address or business cards.

## CONDUCTING THE PAPER PRESENTATION

Review your notes on the day of your presentation. Arrive early at the room where you are scheduled to present so that you can meet the moderator and any fellow speakers and review the podium and audiovisual setup. As you start your presentation, take time to introduce yourself to the audience; often, an interesting or humorous anecdote related to the conference location or focus or to your content serves to relax both you and the audience. Presentations scheduled after lunch, late in the afternoon or evening, or at the end of a conference can be challenging because the audience may have particularly low levels of energy at those times. Include humor so that the presentation is lively, or develop strategies that frequently encourage audience participation (Goldman & Schmalz, 2007; McConnell, 2002).

Although most presentations are delivered to a live audience at the same location as the speaker, there are times the audience may be in another location, such as when a satellite teleconference or video presentation format is used. Conducting face-to-face oral presentations gives you the opportunity to see your audience, interact with them, and receive verbal and nonverbal feedback about the presentation. On the other hand, you reach only a small number of people. Regardless of the medium used, the strategies for preparing the presentation are the same.

## CONDUCTING THE POSTER PRESENTATION

Like the paper presentation, the poster used to present your work should include the major categories covered in the abstract. Since the primary purpose of a poster is to visually communicate research in a simple way, it is necessary that it present the information in a concise and clear manner (Hardicre, Devitt, & Coad, 2007). A poster should be easily understood within 5 minutes. Readability is enhanced when the text is concise, the flow of the segments is logical (left to right in the Western world), and the font is readable from a distance of at least 4 to 6 feet. Several authors have suggested methods for preparing for poster presentations (http://people.eku.edu/ritchisong/posterpres.html; http://www.pitt.edu/~etbell/nsurg/PosterGuide.html; http://www.ucmo.edu/x8700.xml). Steps in preparing a poster presentation usually include:

1   Information gathering
    ■ Conference date and location

- Length of time for poster session and requirement for being present at poster
- Type of display—table or board is usually 4 feet x 8 feet. When a table is provided, use a stand-alone table-top display. A stand-alone display can be constructed by using a foam board or a portable commercial stand and Velcro fasteners to mount segments of the poster. A cork board requires that you use an aid such as pins to mount the poster

2   Types of information to be included
- Title, author names, and affiliation
- Problem and a brief background
- Method—design, sample, setting, data collection process
- Data analysis
- Results and implications
- Acknowledgment—sources of funds

3   Marketability of the poster
- Layout of poster—consider the sequence of ideas, and use headings, arrows or broken lines to guide the reader
- Use of color—pictures, title of sections
- Self-explanatory graphs or tables

4   Poster assembly
- Resources—audiovisual department or self-assembly
- Use poster boards in separate pieces for portability
- Use a computer to print texts of sections

5   Other considerations
- Use of handouts (e.g., abstract that includes authors, affiliation, address, and telephone number)
- Use of display items such as data collection tools marked "for display only"

6   Poster session
- Set up the poster and take it down at designated times
- Be at the poster and interact with participants—introduce yourself and ask attendees their research interests
- Note participant requests for information by asking individuals to write their request on the back of their business card or on a clipboard at the poster
- Look at other posters and seek permission from authors to take a picture of posters you find attractive

7   Evaluation
- Immediately following the presentation, jot down things you would do differently—format, colors, written content, type

and number of handouts. Consider the following criteria when evaluating posters that you viewed

- Overall appearance—attractiveness, accuracy of information, color combination, readability, inclusion of only necessary information, uncluttered appearance
- Content—current, logical, grammatically correct, inclusion of components of the research
- Presentation—author's knowledge of the study, professional appearance of the presenter, availability of presenter to participants

Poster presentations have distinct advantages over oral presentations or publications for researchers wishing to disseminate their work. By conducting a poster presentation, they can communicate with conference participants in an informal way. The informal exchange of ideas between the author and the participant promotes immediate feedback to the author, which may be useful when the author is preparing future presentations or manuscripts or for clarifying unclear or confusing aspects of the study and for networking. Editors of nursing journals often solicit manuscripts after viewing posters and talking to the presenter.

Posters are excellent vehicles for disseminating research findings to the community, as well as to the profession. They can easily be used at community health fairs and at local professional meetings and seminars and can be developed for display in shopping malls, physicians' offices, and community and social service agencies. When the plan is to use a poster for different types of audience, it is helpful if the entire poster is not developed as a whole piece. Develop separate segments for each section (e.g., the research methods and the conclusions) so that these sections can be adapted to the audience.

## Disseminating Research Findings Through the Media

The media—newspapers, newsletters, television, radio, and the Internet—are powerful vehicles for disseminating nursing research. Before considering the media as an outlet for disseminating information, check with your employer about existing policies. There may be a staff member who is charged with assisting those who wish to communicate research findings to the media. Some organizations submit press releases, written overviews of events that are occurring. If your organization does this, find out how you could submit your research findings.

Professional organizations often invite reporters from local television stations to conferences so that research of interest to the public can be identified. Because of this possibility, many organizations will ask you to sign a document indicating your willingness to share the study with the media.

Another outlet for research findings is the lay literature. Articles published in consumer magazines related to nursing research often focus on topics such as acquiring a healthy life style, getting enough exercise, and avoiding various diseases. Once you have selected appropriate consumer magazines for your topic, examine physical copies of the journal to see how others have formatted information similar to yours. Then peruse the magazine's Web site to obtain the e-mail addresses of editors and assistant and associate editors to whom you might submit a query. A query e-mail should be sent to ascertain whether the editor is interested in your topic. Be brief and to the point, highlighting the benefits of your topic to the readership. Under no circumstance should you attach documents to your e-mail unless the editor requests additional material. To find out more about how to query a magazine editor, go to http://www.associatedcontent.com/article/125070/how_to_query_a_magazine.html.

Web sites that are useful in preparing researchers to disseminate their study findings include "A Communications Toolkit for Health Researchers" (www.ruralhealthresearch.org/pdf/toolkit.pdf) and the Canadian Health Services Research Foundation's tools for disseminating research (http://www.chsrf.ca/keys/use_disseminating_e.php).

## Television and Radio

Television, radio, and newspaper reporters often search the Internet for evidence-based research reports on their topic of interest. If you have disseminated research in any way, always do an Internet search on your topic to see if you find mention of yourself and your work. If you do, be prepared for the possibility of being contacted by a reporter. Develop key talking points related to your topic to manage the interview and make sure your message is heard. Also always know, and be ready to talk about, the implications of your topic for the public. The University of Arizona's "Media Interview Guide" (cals.arizona.edu/pressrelease/interviewguide.pdf) and the "Media Manual Samples" provided by the County of Santa Clara (www.sccgov.org/SCC/docs/Public%20Health%20Department%20(DEP)/attachments/Tool9MediaManualSamples.doc) provide an excellent overview and strategies for effectively dealing with media representatives.

Television is a powerful medium for disseminating research. Studies show that people today spend an inordinate number of hours watching television. And, most homes have at least two television sets. One study of older women ages 50 and older with HIV (n = 514) reported that their most frequent sources of information were television (85%), friends (54%), and newspapers (51%). Only 38% identified health professionals as their source of information (Henderson et al., 2004).

Nurses must seek out this medium by contacting local television stations and meeting with producers. Before contacting the local station, ensure that your institution is supportive of your effort. Have a clear idea of the type of local show that might broadcast your findings, know the type of people who watch particular shows, determine the fit between your topic and the show, and maintain the confidentiality of study participants. If an interview is granted, inquire whether the interview will be live or taped and whether you are the only person to be interviewed or there will be other participants. If there are other participants, find out the background of each participant. Start preparing by doing an outline and a script and practicing with a colleague or by videotaping your presentation and reviewing the tape. Suggestions for preparing for an oral presentation and public speaking strategies presented in this chapter are useful.

It is important to prepare carefully for an interview with the media. This includes becoming familiar with the mechanics that will be used (i.e., face-to-face or telephone interview, videotaping or audiotaping for television or radio). Several strategies for conducting a successful interview are presented at www.cals.arizona.edu/pressrelease/interviewguide. They include these pointers:

1   Be clear on the ground rules related to topics you will and will not address and the opportunities to review and correct misstatements.
2   Identify possible questions that support and do not support your study and formulate a 10- to 30-second response.
3   Respond directly to a question, use citations, and do not predict the unknowable when presented with hypothetical situations for which answer is being sought.
4   Determine the key points of your interview, and emphasize these points each time you have the opportunity.

**5** Look at the interviewer during the taping or when you are not being addressed and above the camera when you are speaking.
**6** Use terms that lay people will understand.
**7** Limit your movements during the interview.
**8** Immediately correct the interviewer when something that is said is incorrect.
**9** Communicate enthusiasm and smile.
**10** Wear a solid-color outfit.
**11** Write a thank-you note to the host and the producer.

A local news channel is likely to be open to allowing a short segment presentation when the topic is one that is of great interest to its viewers. Also, consider a national channel. If your research findings have major implications for the health of society, this may not be so implausible an idea. By reading newspapers and magazines that the public reads, you will acquire an idea of topics that are relevant and interesting to the public, as well as how information is presented.

The radio is also a powerful medium for research dissemination. Most people invest daily time in radio listening, so the audience potential is vast. Many local channels host special-interest shows and talk shows and invite people to participate. It would be wise to invest time in searching out these likely opportunities.

There are advantages and disadvantages to the use of the media in disseminating research findings. Distinct advantages are that the media have the potential to reach a large audience and to influence the public's perception of nurses' contributions to their health. On the other hand, television and radio are likely to allot only a short time for your presentation, thereby increasing the possibility that your message will be misinterpreted. Thus, researchers are challenged to provide a comprehensive presentation of the research methodology and findings and their implications in an understandable and concise manner. To help compensate for the simplicity and brevity of the presentation, provide your name and a phone number or address where you can be reached so that the community may have further access to you to learn more about your studies. This is also a helpful way to solicit participants for future studies.

## The Internet

Technology continues to play a major role in providing new opportunities and vehicles by which we can disseminate our research. The Internet is a fast and easy way not only to obtain information but to effectively disseminate research findings. Connecting to the Internet allows users to transfer vast amounts of knowledge through new and sophisticated means. This means of knowledge transfer is rapidly and radically transforming how we disseminate nursing knowledge and influence the health of the nation. As example, YouTube.com is a video-sharing Web site where users can upload, view, and share video clips. A quick search of YouTube with the key words "nursing research" provides many ideas for disseminating your research findings to the world. More and more frequently, journal Web sites are technology enabled, allowing authors of articles to post supplemental content, such as a video clip of the author discussing recent research. Blogs, Twitters, and listservs are more informal ways of sharing your ideas, getting feedback from others, and identifying potential colleagues with whom to collaborate.

## Digital Video Discs (DVDs)

Producing a DVD may be one of the easiest ways to disseminate ideas. DVDs of a research presentation can be made and given to colleagues, patient-care units in the hospital, television stations, community agencies, and professional organizations. In addition, all or just segments of the DVD can be broadcast through selected Internet venues.

There are advantages and disadvantages to using DVDs. The advantages are that DVDs enable the researcher to reach a large number of people and, if creatively done, are an exciting and interesting way to present content. Disadvantages include the cost, the difficulty, and the length of time needed for production. The right physical setting is required—lighting, reduced noise level, staged settings. When planning the DVD, mention the target audience, the desired outcomes, and the content. Identify the most effective ways to communicate your message—often this means the use of visual aids that support the script or photography.

Using a DVDR to record can be intimidating to presenters, especially when done without a live audience. It is, therefore, a good idea to write a script to ensure that the message is succinct and delivered within the allotted time. During the recording, it is helpful to consider the camera as the audience and to pretend that you are in your living room speaking to guests. A researcher can market a DVD by giving a copy to professional organizations who may find it useful for its members.

## SUMMARY

Whatever method is chosen, effective communication with the target audience is crucial. It is essential that researchers conform to the guidelines set by the journal or organization that is sponsoring a publication or an event and that they employ numerous strategies to evaluate their presentation and public-speaking skills in order to enhance their oral presentation abilities.

## SUGGESTED ACTIVITIES

1   After reviewing your research findings and the University of Arizona's "Media Interview Guide" (cals.arizona.edu/pressrelease/interviewguide.pdf), answer these questions:
   - What is new or unique about your findings?
   - Why are your findings important? To whom? In what way?
   - Who or what benefits as a result of your findings?
2   Within the context of your oral presentation content and your desire to maintain audience attention:
   - Develop an analogy that illustrates complex content (as example, childbirth process as analogy for the thesis/dissertation process).
   - Identify a few key points in your talk that might be illustrated with humor (an anecdote, a cartoon, a poem).
   - Identify content points or time in your presentation where you might ask hypothetical questions to engage your audience (e.g., If you had a patient with X, what would you do? Why would you think it was a problem?).

## REFERENCES

Barton, E. E., Reichow, B., & Wolery, M. (2007). Guidelines for graphing data with Microsoft PowerPoint. *Journal of Early Intervention, 29,* 320–336.

Black, S. (2005). In the public interest. *Nursing Standard, 19*(29), 16–18.

Engelhart, N. (2004). Giving effective presentations. *Canadian Operating Room Nursing Journal, 22*(1), 22–24.

Goldman, K. D., & Schmalz, K. J. (2007). Speech righting: Presentation preparation principles for potent performances. *Health promotion Practice, 8,* 114–118.

Happell, B. (2007). Hitting the target! A no tears approach to writing an abstract for a conference presentation. *International Journal of Mental Health Nursing, 16,* 447–452.

Hardicre, J., Coad, C., & Devitt, P. (2007). Ten steps to successful conference presentations. *British Journal of Nursing, 16,* 402–404.

Hardicre, J., Devitt, P., & Coad, C. (2007). Ten steps to successful poster presentation. *British Journal of Nursing, 16,* 398–401.

Henderson, S. J., Bernstein, L. B., St. George, D. M., Doyle, J. P., Paranjape, A. S., & Corbie-Smith, G. (2004). Older women and HIV: How much do they know and where are they getting their information. *Journal of the American Geriatric Society, 52*(9), 1549–1553.

Longman, P. (2004). Tips on media management. *Nursing Standard, 18* (33), 16–17.

McConnell, E. A. (2002). Making outstandingly good presentations. *Dimensions of Critical Care Nursing, 21*(1), 28–31.

Shepherd, M. (2006). How to give an effective presentation using PowerPoint. *European Diabetes Nursing, 3*(3), 154–158.

Starver, K. D. & Shellenbarger, T. (2004). Professional presentations made simple. *Clinical Nurse Specialist, 18*(1), 16–20.

Vollman, K. M. (2005). Enhancing presentation skills for the advanced practice nurse. *AACN Clinical Issues, 16,* 67–77.

## 22  Reporting Results Through Publication

SUZANNE P. SMITH AND MAGDALENA A. MATEO

As the value and quality of clinical research in nursing have increased, more and more nurses are making concerted efforts to disseminate their findings though multiple channels. Since disseminating research findings is an integral part of the research process, the plan for communicating findings must be developed at the time a study is proposed.

Some funding agencies and organizations require a review of results before these can be made public. Since these reviews may delay the dissemination process, it is important that researchers be familiar with the requirements of funding agencies and their organization of employment before initiating plans for presentations or publications.

Although the traditional approach to publishing research findings and study outcomes is to present these in professional journals, other publication options include cyberspace, electronic journals, newsletters of organizations and professional societies, and newspapers. This chapter examines strategies for successfully disseminating research findings through publications. Emphasis is placed on process and on strategies to develop high-quality, professional presentations of your work. Although strategies pertinent to different types of publications are described, the cited principles apply to most types of publications.

## PRINT JOURNALS

While the Citations in Nursing and Allied Health Web site (http://www.eb scohost.com/thisTopic.php?marketID=1&topicID=53) "provides indexing for 2,928 journals from the fields of nursing and allied health," only a small percentage are exclusively research journals. Publishing research reports in these research journals has the advantage of allowing nurse researchers to report the conduct of their investigation using the standard, structured research report format: background, review of the literature, methods, findings, and implications (Tornquist, 1999). The primary focus of review for the research journal is scientific merit—be the study consists of quantitative or qualitative research. Publishing in a research journal is ideal for disseminating your research if you wish to showcase your methods (Oermann, Galvin, Floyd, & Roop, 2006). Research journals use the IMRAD format, which includes introduction, methods, result, and discussion. The introduction includes a brief background of the topic and the study purpose(s). The methods section comprises the design, setting, sample description, intervention, and outcome measures. Results include the primary findings. Finally, the discussion section is the place where conclusions and implications for practice and research are presented. A structured abstract format is suggested because it helps readers to select articles that are appropriate to their topic (Nakayama, Hirat, Yamazaki, & Naito, 2005).

If you wish to highlight, instead, your research outcomes and their applicability to a certain nursing audience, you may want to write for a nonresearch journal (Tornquist, 1999; Webb, 2007). This may require a more labor-intensive effort, because you cannot follow the traditional research report format. The nonresearch journal requires that you use less formal language, take a process approach to your topic (what was the problem you faced, how did you go about solving it, and what did you discover?), and provide creative, interesting headings.

Editors are critically aware of the need to have a data-driven practice base and are eagerly seeking research-based information that holds the potential for transforming nursing practice. Thus, whatever type of journal you choose to publish your research findings, you will find editors receptive.

## CYBERSPACE PUBLICATION

Cyberspace is the electronic medium of computer networks in which online communication takes place. By publishing in cyberspace by using the Internet and its best-known part, the World Wide Web, researchers can "publish" and retrieve vast amounts of information. Every day, more and more businesses and people establish Web sites to promote themselves, supply information, and sell their products. Because of its great use and unlimited potential, the Internet is an easy, quick, and inexpensive way to disseminate research findings. By visiting the site of a nursing journal publisher (http://www.nursingcenter.com) or simply by searching any search engine (e.g., Google.com) for keywords such as "nursing listserv," "nursing twitter," or "nursing blog," you will find hundreds of possible vehicles (lists, bulletin boards, user groups, podcasts, and wikis) that can be used to disseminate ideas related to your research.

## Web-Based Tools

YouTube.com, founded in 2005, is an increasingly popular place for nurses to watch and share original videos through Web sites, mobile devices, blogs, and e-mail. A simple YouTube search using the keywords "nursing research" produces a plethora of narrated videos about all aspects of nursing research conducted by faculty, students, and practitioners. Searching the term "writing for publication" yields a similar result. So, if you learn best through visual representations, YouTube may be for you.

A Wiki, a mass communication mechanism that allows anyone to edit all posted content, is rapidly being used in health care to share common work and ideas, including research. You can go to http://en.wikipedia.org/wiki/Nursing_research/ or http://en.wikipedia.org/wiki/Nursing and then click various links to learn about the potential of these sites to assist you as you proceed through the nursing research process (from idea generation to dissemination). Not finding what you need related to your research? It's easy to start your own Wiki and get all the assistance you desire from around the world. To see how a cardiovascular service line administrator set up a Wiki in her health system to connect key nurses, physicians, managers, and support staff regarding specific issues, see Clancy (2007).

One note of caution when using any interactive Internet site: what you post to any open-access Web site can easily be taken and used by someone without your knowledge. Likewise, what you post has the potential to exist forever. So make sure that what you post today will not be an embarrassment years later when seen by a potential employer or school admissions officer.

Numerous health care organizations have their own Web sites, which are copyrighted and where nurse researchers may post their studies. Another possibility is to develop your own dedicated Web site. Almost every Internet service provider (e.g., Google, Yahoo, AOL) provides free Web site space with building instructions, as does FreeWebs (http://members.freewebs.com/). Almost every journal publisher has its print journal content available on its Web site in an electronic format. This process gives an author who is published in the print version exposure to readers who prefer to search the Internet for information rather than use a library indexing reference. Electronically search the Internet addresses given previously to find print journals that also have an electronic version.

## Linking Print and Online Versions of Manuscripts

Almost all publishers are using Web-based systems to acquire, review, edit, and produce their journals' content. While there are a few long-standing online-only nursing journals (the *Online Journal of Issues in Nursing, the Online Journal of Nursing Informatics, and Worldviews on Evidence-Based Nursing*), most publishers maintain a print product, with content duplicated and enhanced on a Web site. The online version of an author's article can include additional material related to the research but not appropriate for the print product. A few examples are a lengthy appendix, a podcast, hyperlinks from the print article's reference list to the actual reference, a PowerPoint presentation, and photos. The *American Journal of Nursing*'s Web site (ajnonline.com) illustrates this concept nicely.

Publication in an electronic peer-reviewed journal has the advantage of almost immediate publication—material is submitted electronically to an editor, forwarded by the editor to reviewers electronically, and revised and published electronically. Publication in a print journal with an online Web site usually involves posting a pre-print copy of the article on the Web site of the author's revised paper after peer review. The Web site clearly indicates that this is not the final version. When the production staff has produced the version that will appear in the print journal, that final version replaces the pre-print version online.

Because of technology, there is little delay between the generation of knowledge and its dissemination to those who can use it. Resources (time, money, energy) are conserved as authors, peer reviewers, editors, and publication staff use nonpaper means to generate and publish ideas. In addition, content can be updated easily by adding new information and hypertext links to other sites related to your topic. Readers can enter into a dialogue with you and the editor through electronic mail, blogs, listservs, and tweets, which can be appended to the electronic article.

## CRITICAL SUCCESS FACTORS FOR PUBLISHING

Journal publication is the most frequent method for research dissemination because many nurses can be reached by one effort—writing a high-quality, focused manuscript. To increase the chance of having your manuscript accepted for publication (Happell, 2005; Smith, 2009), the following guidelines are recommended.

### Select the Appropriate Audience

The first step in any writing project is selecting the appropriate audience. To whom do you wish to convey your findings? Who would benefit most from your research findings? When writing your paper, be specific in the introduction as to your intended audience. If you focus on a particular audience, you can present your research findings to meet that audience's needs. For example, if your research findings suggest a cost-effective way to deliver nursing care, both practitioners and administrators would be interested in the topic. However, practitioners would be interested in the clinical implications, whereas administrators would be interested in the management aspects.

### Select the Appropriate Journal

The most innovative, well-written manuscript will be rejected if it is submitted to the wrong journal (Smith, 2009). Having identified your audience, you can now select the journals that are edited for that group. Once you have selected your potential journals, obtain the guidelines for authors that most journals publish in each issue. These guidelines frequently include a short mission statement highlighting the major focus of the journal, the intended readership profile, and the types of topics that are appropriate for submission. In addition to seeking this information, examine several recent issues to assess the preferred format approach of the journal.

### Query the Editor

As you plan your writing project, it is a good idea first to query editors of potential journals that might be appropriate for your topic. While queries can be made by mail, telephone, or e-mail, almost all editors prefer electronic queries. They are fast and can be answered at the editor's convenience. Do not attach files to your queries; place your query in the e-mail message area. Information for Authors guidelines often include which approach the editor prefers. Exhibit 22.1 shows an acceptable format for an e-mail query. Please note while an e-mail query has a more casual format than a formal mailed letter, it is still professional. Exhibit 22.2 illustrates a query to a consumer journal on the same topic as that in Exhibit 22.1. Note the change in language and tone.

Querying the editor can save you time and effort. Although it is acceptable to query several editors at the same time, it is not acceptable to send a manuscript to more than one journal at the same time.

Editors are professionals and experts in writing for publication. Editors know the types of manuscripts they would like to obtain for publication. When querying an editor, explain in detail your research and plans for the manuscript's content (Smith, 2009). The editor may discuss your thoughts and approach for organizing the manuscript content. The editor may persuade you to use a different focus to increase the chance that

Exhibit 22.1

## SAMPLE E-MAIL QUERY LETTER FOR NURSING JOURNAL

Dear (name of editor):
I wish to submit a manuscript to (name of publication). Our research examined processes of change used in smoking cessation by 190 smokers and former smokers selected through random digit dialing. A mailed cross-sectional survey had an 84% response rate. Multivariate analysis of variance of 10 processes of change across five stages of smoking cessation (precontemplation, contemplation, relapse, recent quitting, and long-term quitting) was significant, $F(40,590) = 5.02$, $p = 0.0001$. Post hoc analysis revealed statistically significant differences on 7 of the 10 processes of change ($p < .05$). The readers of your journal can apply our study findings in their practice to help clients stop smoking.
(Optional to add content outline here if first paragraph is not self-explanatory as to approach.)
(Optional brief paragraph here indicating your qualifications to write on your topic if that is not obvious in your ending signature information.)
The manuscript will be ready for submission within 6 weeks of receiving your positive reply. I look forward to hearing from you.
(Contact Person)
(Work or home address and telephone number; work information preferred.)

Exhibit 22.2

---

**SAMPLE E-MAIL QUERY LETTER FOR CONSUMER MAGAZINE**

---

Dear (name of editor):

Smoking is an addiction with severe consequences—cancer, emphysema, circulatory problems, to name a few. Despite the widely known negative effects of smoking, people have great difficulty quitting, spending millions to beat their addiction.

As a nurse expert with years of helping people stop smoking, I would like to write a manuscript for (magazine name). The manuscript will present 10 significant strategies, shown in a recent nursing research study to assist people advance successfully through the five stages of smoking cessation.

This practical manuscript to assist your readers to stop smoking can be submitted now according to your requirements. I look forward to hearing from you.

(Your name)

(Address and telephone number)

---

your manuscript will be accepted for publication. And, the editor may inform you that the particular journal is not interested in your manuscript because it is similar to already published or soon-to-be published papers. Receiving this type of information allows you to tailor your manuscript to the journal whose editor has expressed the most interest in your topic.

## Include Implications for Practice

Often a good manuscript is rejected for publication because the author does not discuss the implications of the research findings for the journal's readership. Readers expect the author, as the topic expert, to discuss the utility of findings to practice. The length of the implications section will vary depending on the journal's purpose. The implications section in a research journal is often shorter than that in a clinical journal, which focuses on application.

When discussing implications for the study, present your findings in relation to similar studies. Highlight how your findings support as well as differ from those of others of any similar studies that have been reported. Finally, suggest directions for future research that is needed to further apply your research to practice.

## Conform to the Submission Requirements

All journals have requirements for how you format and submit your manuscript. While these requirements are not often printed in the journal, they can usually be found on the journal's Web site. Journal editors have a bias toward manuscripts that are correctly formatted. An incorrectly formatted manuscript can be a "red flag." Often, editors assume that if the author of a paper were serious about its publication in the journal, the author would have made an effort to send it properly formatted. A lingering thought in the editor's mind will be, "If the author did not pay attention to simple formatting requirements, what attention has been paid to ensure the integrity of the research and the manuscript?"

## Adhere to Copyright Laws

Once a manuscript is accepted for publication, authors are required by the publisher to sign an agreement that transfers copyright of the author's material to the publisher (Rhoads & White, 2008). Once signed, the agreement makes the manuscript the copyrighted work of the publisher. The author must have the publisher's written permission to use a significant part of the article in another medium, whether oral, written, or electronic. When in doubt about using copyrighted work, call and/or write the copyright holder (Dobbins, Souder, & Smith, 2005; Rhoads & White, 2008).

## Use Recent References

References used in your manuscript should be current and relevant to your topic. The definition of current varies from editor to editor, but, generally, a 3-year range is acceptable. Obvious exceptions to this rule of thumb might be "classic" works related to your topic. Use of older references is also acceptable when you are replicating a study. Using current references conveys to the editor and your readers that your research has been placed in the context of contemporary concerns and that you are making a new contribution to the health care literature.

## Maintain Organization

A manuscript with a logical flow of ideas is easy to read and understand. Developing an organized, orderly paper, however, requires work, particularly when you are presenting a complex research protocol that was not necessarily linear. Facilitate order and clarity by outlining your content and using headings and subheadings. Always have a colleague read a draft of your paper solely to evaluate the logical progression of its content.

## Use Tables and Graphs

Tables, graphs, and illustrations add significantly to the overall sophistication of your manuscript. They also serve to clarify concepts and present research findings and outcomes in an easily understood way. The use of tables and graphs also helps you organize your information. Before writing the paper, decide which concepts lend themselves to display in a graphic form. When discussing table or graph information in the text, do not restate every piece of information that is in the graph. Highlight one or two key points and refer the reader to the table or graph. Refer to Chapter 13 for further information on using tables to present results.

Develop tables that are self-explanatory by keeping in mind the following guidelines:

- Keep the title clear and concise
- Label each row and column and provide units of measure for the data
- Include notes (general, specific, and probability note) below the table. General notes provide information applicable to the table (e.g., abbreviations, symbols). Specific notes refer to an entry, column, or row. Notes on probability indicate results of tests of significance. (American Psychological Association, 2001; Rice University, 2008)

You can use graphs to synthesize data and show the relationship between two or more variables. Effective graphs are accurate, simple, clear, neat, professional, and attractive. There are several points to consider when developing graphs (American Psychological Association, 2001; Rice University, 2008), including these: (1) use a frame to establish a boundary between the data and other information, (2) use prominent symbols to plot data, and (3) employ a scale appropriate to the data.

## Determine Authorship Entitlement

Authorship implies significant involvement in writing a paper and in the work that led up to that writing. It implies "substantial intellectual contribution" (Nativio, 1993, p. 358). The reality is that authorship is often given to (or insisted on by) people with minimal involvement in the writing project—perhaps a supervisor, a data collector, or a statistician. Guidelines for authorship make it clear that "Authorship credit should be based on (1) substantial contributions to conception and design, or acquisition of data, or analysis and interpretation of data; (2) drafting the article or revising it critically for important intellectual content; and (3) final approval of the version to be published. Authors should meet conditions 1, 2, and 3. Acquisition of funding, collection of data, or general supervision of the research group, alone, does not justify authorship" (International Committee of Medical Journal Editors, 2008). For large, multisite research projects, it is becoming common to list the research group as the author, with individuals mentioned in a footnote. When this is the case, all members of the group still must meet the stringent requirements for authorship.

There is no rule for order of authorship. The order of authorship should be the joint decision of the co-authors, after analysis of each author's contribution to the work. This analysis is best done at the start of a project so that expectations are clear and conflicts are later avoided. In general, order of authorship should run from person who made the greatest contribution to the person who made the smallest. This order might be determined by the amount of time put into the project or the importance of the contribution (Erlen, Siminoff, Sereika, & Sutton, 1997).

## Acknowledge Appropriately

If not everyone who contributed to a research project is entitled to authorship, then certainly all those who help in some way should be acknowledged. But, there is almost as much controversy about who is entitled to acknowledgment as there is about authorship entitlement. Although some editors feel that authors who blindly acknowledge family, friends, and colleagues are frivolous, others feel that generous acknowledgments reflect the humanity of authors (Mundy, 2002). As a rule of thumb, acknowledgments are reserved for those who have made a substantial contribution to the project being reported in a paper, including those who provided editorial and writing assistance (Flanagin & Rennie, 1995). People who might be acknowledged include data collectors, a project director, an editorial assistant, or a faculty adviser. Be aware that not everyone wishes to be acknowledged publicly. For this reason, obtain written permission from those named in an acknowledgment to assure that they approve your use of their name in material that will be published and widely disseminated before you include their names in the manuscript. Some journals require a signed statement from those acknowledged.

## Conform to Ethical Practices

Adhering to ethical practices when publishing is vital; unethical practices can ruin your chances for future publication. Two easily avoided unethical practices are submitting the same manuscript to different journals at the same time and committing plagiarism.

It is unethical to submit a manuscript to more than one journal at the same time. Every journal's guidelines for authors include a statement to the effect that the author warrants that he or she is submitting original, unpublished material that is under consideration by no other publisher. So, while it is acceptable to query as many editors as desired about interest in your manuscript, you can submit it to only one journal at a time. If your manuscript is rejected, you may then send it to another journal.

Plagiarism is the act of claiming someone's ideas and work, published or unpublished, as your own. The four common types of plagiarism are (1) verbatim lifting of passages, (2) rewording ideas from an original source in an author's own style, (3) paraphrasing an original work without attribution, (4) noting the original source of only some of what is borrowed (American Medical Association, 2007). Be acutely aware of material in your paper that reflects the ideas of others and appropriately reference the original source. If you borrow a significant amount of material (copyright law does not define significant) through paraphrasing or direct quotation, write the copyright holder, which is usually the publishing company, and obtain written permission. Likewise, use of any published item, no matter how large or small, that is complete unto itself, such as a table, figure, chart, graph, art work, poem, or picture, requires that you have permission from the copyright holder to reproduce. For further discussion of the intricacies of copyright in order to avoid plagiarism or copyright law violation, see publications such as Rhoads and White (2008) and American Medical Association (2008), or visit the federal government copyright office's Web site (http://www.lcweb.loc.gov/copyright/).

## MANUSCRIPT REVIEW PROCESS

Peer review is the process that editors use to help ensure the professional integrity of nursing knowledge. This process has three main purposes—detection of errors, fair and impartial treatment of authors' ideas, and identification and publication of innovative and new ideas to advance the profession (Clarke, 2006; Miracle, 2008; Spear, 2004; Swartz, 2008). To accomplish these purposes, editors assume the responsibility of selecting reviewers who have demonstrated advanced knowledge or practice in a particular nursing role (administrator, researcher, educator) or patient care specialty. Manuscripts then are reviewed by at least two reviewers, often three. Reviewers screen the manuscripts for quality, accuracy, timeliness, relevance, and appropriateness before the editor considers the paper for publication.

Peer review has been criticized as not always being an effective means to ensure the validity of the content published or the fairness of the manuscript selection process (Miracle, 2008). Despite its potential weaknesses, peer review is the most appropriate means for selecting manuscripts for publication. It gives readers assurance that the journal's content meets acceptable standards of scholarship, conferring validity and credibility on an author's work (Dougherty, 2006; Froman, 2006).

When journals are not peer reviewed, the editor reviews manuscripts and decides which manuscripts will be published, using criteria similar to those used by peer-reviewed journals. Although the articles in such journals may be excellent, the lack of peer review lessens their credibility. Journals that are peer reviewed state that fact somewhere within each issue. If such a statement is not found, contact the journal's editorial office and seek clarification.

Promotion and tenure criteria require that faculty in institutions of higher education and in some major academic health science centers receive credit only for publications in peer-reviewed journals. While the quality of material published in a nonpeer-reviewed journal may not be any different from that in a peer-reviewed journal, your choice of journal should be made in light of the requirements of your current job and your planned career track.

## DEALING WITH REJECTION OF A MANUSCRIPT

If your manuscript is not accepted for publication by your first-choice journal, do not give up. Many published authors have had their works rejected for publication. The art of writing requires practice and study. Receiving feedback about your manuscript's strengths and weaknesses from reviewers and editors helps you focus on developing the skills you need to publish your work.

If your manuscript is rejected, there are two options (neither of which is never writing again!). First, you can call and speak to the editor personally. Ask what you can do to revise the work to have it published. Editors are very quick to acknowledge such requests and most will work with you to recommend suggestions for revision and resubmission. A good editor will be honest about the quality of your manuscript and may recommend other journals that may be more appropriate for your work.

The second option is to revise and submit the manuscript to another journal. Remember to focus your revised content to the new journal's readership and editorial purpose. Many excellent manuscripts are needlessly rejected because the author did not target the content to a journal's readership or conform to its style.

There are advantages and disadvantages to publishing research findings in a print journal, with the advantages outweighing the disadvantages. Some of the advantages include:

- Enhanced self-esteem
- National recognition of work
- Achievement of professional goals
- Identification as an expert in topic area
- Ability to appropriately disseminate research
- Contribution to the nursing profession

Some disadvantages are:

- Inability to interact with the audience
- Inability to personally answer questions
- Inability to provide clarification of content without additional effort on the part of the reader
- Limited space in which to present your work
- Lack of honorarium or royalty
- Lack of retention of copyright, limiting your use of the manuscript content in the future

## SUMMARY

Nursing research contributes positively to the health care delivery system. As more nurses are prepared at the graduate and doctoral levels, more and more nursing research is being conducted in clinical, administrative, and education settings. Nurses who conduct research have a professional obligation to share their findings. This is how a profession grows and matures. In the past, nurses have been shy about presenting their findings (Winslow, 1996), but this is changing. Nurses are making outstanding contributions to the future health state of the world.

## SUGGESTED ACTIVITIES

The Owl at Purdue (http://owl.english.purdue.edu/owl//) is an excellent site at which to hone your writing and research skills.

1   Go to http://owl.english.purdue.edu/owl/resource/629/02/ and complete an "Audience Analysis."

2   Go to http://owl.english.purdue.edu/owl/resource/567/01/ and identify your blocks to writing and try two of the suggested intervention strategies.

3   Go to http://owl.english.purdue.edu/owl/resource/553/02/ and evaluate the value of the next three sources of information that you plan to use in your research.

## REFERENCES

American Medical Association. (2007). *AMA manual of style* (10th ed.) New York: Oxford University Press.

American Psychological Association. (2001). *Publication manual of the American Psychological Association* (5th ed.). Washington, DC: Author.

Clancy, T. R. (2007). Organizing: New ways to harness complexity. *Journal of Nursing Administration, 37,* 534–536.

Clarke, S. P. (2006). Reviewing peer review: The three reviewers you meet at submission time. *Canadian Journal of Nursing Research, 38*(4), 5–9.

Dobbins, W. N., Souder, E., & Smith, R. M. (2005). Living with fair use and TEACH: A quest for compliance. *Computers Informatics Nursing, 23*(3), 120–124.

Dougherty, M. C. (2006). The value of peer review. *Nursing Research, 55*(2), 73–74.

Erlen, J. A., Siminoff, L. A., Sereika, S. M., & Sutton, L. B. (1997). Multiple authorship: Issues and recommendations. *Journal of Professional Nursing, 13*(4), 262–270.

Flanagin, A., & Rennie, D. (1995). Acknowledging ghosts. *Journal of the American Medical Association, 273*(1), 73.

Froman, R. D. (2006). The importance of peer review. *Research in Nursing and Health, 29*(4), 253–255.

Happell, B. (2005). Disseminating nursing knowledge: A guide to writing for publication. *International Journal of Psychiatric nursing Research, 10*(3), 1147–1155.

International Committee of Medical Journal Editors. (2008). *Authorship and contributorship.* Retrieved January 10, 2009, from http://www.icmje.org

Miracle, V. A. (2008). The peer review process. *Dimensions in Critical Care Nursing, 27*(2), 67–69.

Mundy, D. (2002). A question of missing acknowledgement. *Science Editor, 25*(2), 58–59.

Nakayama, T., Hirat, N., Yamazaki, S., & Naito, M. (2005). Adoption of structured abstracts by general medical journals and format for a structured abstract. *Journal of the Medical Library Association, 93*, 237–242.

Nativio, D. G. (1993). Authorship. *IMAGE: Journal of Nursing Scholarship, 25*, 358.

Oermann, M. H., Galvin, E. A., Floyd, J. A., & Roop, J. C. (2006). Presenting research to clinicians: Strategies for writing about research findings. *Nursing Research, 13*, 66–74.

Rhoads, J., & White, C. (2008) Copyright law and distance nursing education. *Nurse Educator, 33*(1), 39–44.

Rice University. (2008). *Displaying data in written documents.* Retrieved January 10, 2009, from http://www.owlnet.rice.edu/~cainproj/courses/comp482/Data_Written_Docs.doc

Smith, S. P. (2009). The manager as published author: Tips on writing for publication. In M. Harris (Ed.), *Handbook of home health care administration* (5th ed.). Sudbury, MA: Jones & Bartlett.

Spear, H. J. (2004). On ethical peer review and publication: The importance of professional conduct and communication. *Nurse Author Editor. 14*(4), 1–3.

Swartz, M. (2008). The importance of peer review. *Journal of Pediatric Health Care, 22*, 333–334.

Tornquist, E. M. (1999). *From proposal to publication: An informal guide to writing about nursing research.* Menlo Park, CA: Addison Wesley.

Webb, C. (2007). Publishing from a research thesis. *Nurse Author & Editor, 17*(3). Retrieved December 30, 2008, from http://www.nurseauthoreditor.com/article.asp?id = 86

Winslow, E. H. (1996). Failure to publish research: A form of scientific misconduct? *Heart and Lung: The Journal of Acute and Critical Care, 25*, 169–171.

# Appendix A: Preparing Families for Withdrawal

In the ICU, families may choose to be with their loved one following withdrawal of equipment, which leads to the patient's death. Families therefore witness their loved one's progress toward death. This form aims to collect information from you, to help us formulate a message for families to prepare them for this experience ahead of time. As a nurse, please describe your various objective findings and observations based on your experience by completing the following sections.

**A. Physical sensations/observations** (what you see, hear, smell, and feel [or touch] in a withdrawn dying patient). Complete as many sections as possible.

1. Respiratory:

_____

_____

_____

2. Skin:

_____

_____

_____

3. Neurological:

_____

_____

_____

4. Musculoskeletal:

_____

_____

_____

5. Sense organs (eyes, ears, nose, tongue, & their functions):

_____

_____

_____

6. Gastrointestinal:

_____

_____

_____

7. Genitourinary:

_____

_____

_____

8. Others:

_____

_____

_____

_____

_____

_____

**B. Temporal Characteristics** (duration and sequence of events from withdrawal of equipment to death of the patient).

_____

_____

_____

_____

_____

_____
_____
_____

**C. Environmental Features** (the kind of environment the withdrawn patient is in, such as the characteristics of the ICU cubicle or unit; transfer of the patient to a different unit after withdrawal of equipment; the people in the cubicle or unit; the activities taking place).

_____
_____
_____
_____
_____
_____
_____

**D. Cause of Sensations, Experiences** (what do you tell families are the physiological causes of the physical observations that you have identified?).

_____
_____
_____
_____
_____
_____
_____

**E.** Other information that you think is important to be included in the **"Family Intervention"** that prepares families for the death of their loved one.

_____
_____
_____
_____
_____
_____
_____

Thanks for your time!!

## POLICY AND PROCEDURE MANUAL

### Nursing: Medical-Surgical Services
### N-MSS-7JCE-10.002

**SUBJECT/TITLE:**  Guidelines for Gastrointestinal Assessment After Abdominal Surgery—7 JCE.

**PURPOSE:**  To outline routine nursing practice for abdominal assessment following abdominal surgery.

To promote early identification of return of gastrointestinal (GI) motility To promote early identification of potential complications following abdominal surgery.

**POLICY:**  Following abdominal surgery, abdominal assessment is completed at least every 8 hours until the patient experiences first flatus and first bowel movement, and then BID and PRN until discharge.

## PROCEDURE

**A**  Explain the procedure to the patient.

**B**  Interview the patient for the following subjective symptoms indicative of postoperative ileus or return of GI motility, including assessment of presence or absence of:

   **1**  Abdominal pain/discomfort

   **2**  Flatus, within last 8 hours[R1, R6, R12, L3]

   **3**  Bowel movement/stool, within last 12–24 hours[R1, R6, R12, L3]

   **4**  Nausea and/or vomiting

**461**

  **5** Feeling bloated
  **6** Return of appetite/feeling hungry[R5, L4]
  **7** Abdominal cramps
  **8** Referred pain (e.g., shoulder pain)
**C** Position the patient supine and to promote comfort (e.g., supine with HOB slightly elevated).
**D** Inspection of the patient's abdomen including assessment of presence or absence of:
  **1** Distention
  **2** Drainage from the wound
**E** If the patient's abdomen is distended, palpation of the patient's abdomen is preformed in a systematic fashion and with care to avoid discomfort. Palpation includes assessment of presence or absence of:
  **1** Abdominal firmness
  **2** Abdominal tenderness

## PRECAUTIONS, OBSERVATIONS, GENERAL CONSIDERATIONS

**A** Follow universal precautions.
**B** Auscultation of the abdomen during the early recovery phase after surgery does not serve to monitor recovery of postoperative motility.[R7] Early postoperative bowel sounds may not represent return of normal GI motility.[R3, R10, L2] Return of GI motility begins in the small intestine and proceeds to the stomach and finally the colon.[R8, R11, L1] Auscultation of early returning bowel sounds likely represents discoordinated early contraction in the small intestine, not coordinated propulsive contractions of the colon.[R2, R7, R9] Progression from IV fluids to oral intake is dependent on return of coordinated GI motility in the stomach.[R4, R8, R10]
**C** The primary markers for return of GI motility after abdominal surgery are return of flatus and bowel movement.[R1, R6, R12, L3] An additional indication of ileus recovery is the patient's ability to tolerate oral solids without nausea or vomiting.[R5]
**D** Palpation of the abdomen may contribute to discomfort, especially near the surgical site.
**E** Postoperative assessment must not be limited to abdominal assessment. Additional postoperative assessment includes, but is

not limited to: vital signs, level of consciousness, urinary output, intake and output, etc.

F   The RN will notify the physician on-call of concerns or deterioration in patient clinical condition.

## RESEARCH REFERENCES

R1  Bauer, JJ., Gelernt, IM., Salky, BA., Kreel, I. (1985). Is Routine Postoperative Nasogastric Decompression Really Necessary? *Annals of Surgery,* 201(2), 233–236.

R2  Benson, MJ., Roberts, JP., Wingate, DL., Rogers, J., Deeks, JJ., Castillo, FD., & Williams, NS. (13994). Small bowel motility following major intra-abdominal surgery: The effects of opiates and rectal cisapride. *Gastroenterology,* 106(4), 924–936.

R3  Boghaert, A., Haesaert, G., Mourisse, P., & Verlinden, M. (1987). Placebo-controlled trial of cisapride in postoperative ileus. *Acta Anaesthiologica Belgica,* 38(3), 195–199.

R4  Cali, RL., Meade, PG., Swanson, MS., & Freeman, C. (2000). Effect of morphine and incision length on bowel function after colectomy. Diseases of the Colon and Rectum, 43(2), 163–168.

R5  Condon, RE., Cowles, VE., Ferraz, AAB., Carilli, S., Carlson, ME., Ludwig, K., Tekin, E., Ulualp, K., Ezberci, F., Shoji, Y., Isherwood, P., Frantzides, CT., & Schulte, WJ. (1995). Human colonic smooth muscle electrical activity during and after recovery from postoperative ileus. American Journal of Physiology, 269(3 pt. 1), G408–G417.

R6  Ducerf, C., Duchamp, C., & Poyet, M. (1992). Postoperative electromyographic profile in human jejunum. Annals of Surgery, 215(3), 237–243.

R7  Huge, A., Kreis, ME., Zittel, TT., Becker, HD., Starlinger, MJ., & Jehle, EC. (2000). Postoperative colonic motility and tone in patients after colorectal surgery. Diseases of the Colon and Rectum, 43(7), 932–939.

R8  Hotokezaka, M., Mentis, E.P., & Schirmer, B.D. (1996). Gastric myoelectric activity changes following open abdominal surgery in humans. Digestive Diseases and Sciences, 41(5), 864–869.

R9  Morris, IR., Darby, CF., Hammond, P., & Tayloe, I. (1983). Changes in small bowel myoelectrical activity following laparotomy. British Journal of Surgery, 70(9), 547–548.

R10 Nachlas, MM., Younis, MT., Roda, CP., & Wityk, JJ. (1972). Gastrointestinal motility studies as a guide to postoperative management. Annals of Surgery, 175(4), 510–521.

R11 Schippers, E., Holscher, AH., Bollschweiler, E., & Siewert, J.R. (1991). Return of interdigestive motor complex after abdominal surgery: End of postoperative ileus? Digestive Diseases and Sciences, 36(5), 621–626.

R12 Tollesson, PO., Cassuto, J., Faxen, A., & Bjork, L. (1991). A radiology method for the study of postoperative colonic motility in humans. Scandinavian Journal of Gastroenterology, 26(8), 887–896.

## LITERATURE REFERENCES

L1  Livingston, EH., & Passaro, EP. (1990). Postoperative Ileus. Digestive Diseases and Sciences, 35(1), 121–132.

L2  Rothnie, NG., Harper, RAK., & Catchpole, BN. (1963) Early postoperative gastro-intestinal activity. The Lancet, July 13, 64–67.

L3  Thoren, T., Sundberg, A., Wattwil, M., Garvill, J.E., & Jurgensen, U. (1989). Effect of epidural bupivicaine and epidural morphine on bowel function and pain after hysterectomy. Acta Anaesthesiologica Scandinavica, 33(2), 181–185.

L4  Madsen, D., Sebolt, T., Cullen, L., Folkedahl, B., Mueller, T., Richardson, C., & Titler, M. (2005). Listening to Bowel Sounds: An Evidence-Based Practice Project. *American Journal of Nursing*, 105(12), 40–50.

# Index

Absolute size (of samples), 164
Abstract section (of research article),
9, 21, 73, 74. *See also* Database of
Abstracts of Reviews of Effects
calls for (at conferences), 427–429
citation (display) with, 38
described, 74
links from websites to, 109
in poster presentations, 432, 433
structured format (in print journals),
442
Academic detailing (educational
outreach), 345
Accelerating Translation of Research Into
Practice project, 89
Accidental (nonprobability) sample, 159
ACE Star Model of Knowledge
Transformation (Stevens), 6–7, 8,
49, 269
ACP Journal Club, 8
Adams, Susan, 329–353
Adolescent Self-Report (CASS), 222
Advanced search mode, 29, 35
"Advancing Quality Care through
Translation Research" conference,
351–352
Adverse events, 54–55, 57, 58, 91, 387
Agency for Healthcare Research and
Quality (AHRQ), 6, 7–9, 34, 52, 270
EBP research reports on website, 34
Evidence-Based Practice Centers, 61
Health Care Innovations Exchange, 61
Knowledge Transfer Framework, 339
Knowledge Transfer Framework
developed by, 339
quality focus of, 388–389
role of, 388
on systematic reviews, 259, 263–264
Translation Research Model funded
by, 337

AGREE collaboration. See Appraisal of
Guidelines Research and Evaluation
(AGREE) collaboration
AHRQ. See Agency for Healthcare
Research and Quality
Ambiguous temporal precedence,
124–125
American Academy of Nursing (AAN),
389
American Association of Critical-Care
Nurses (AACN), 157
American Association of Neuroscience
Nursing, 429
American College of Cardiology (ACC),
89, 278
American Diabetes Association, 8
American Heart Association (AHA),
89, 278
American Nurses' Association (ANA), 43,
66, 395, 398
American Nurses' Credentialing Center,
389
American Nurses Recognition
Credentialing Center, 67
Analysis of covariance (ANCOVA), 121
AOL search engine, 444
Applicability concerns, 11, 105–106, 107,
149, 150
Appraisal of Guidelines Research and
Evaluation (AGREE) collaboration,
8, 275–277, 282
Appraisal of performance, 214
Appraising clinical practice
guidelines (CPGs)
AGREE, 275–277
*Brief Summary* feature (NGC), 277
*Critically Appraised Topics* (CAT),
277
evidence grading systems, 277–279
"three Rs" (Haynes), 280

**465**